ABDOMINAL ULTRASOUND

ABDOMINAL ULTRASOUND

Mike Stocksley

MSc CertEd MDCR DMU

Senior Lecturer
Faculty of Health
South Bank University
London, UK

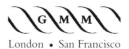

London • San Francisco

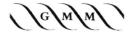

Greenwich Medical Media
4th Floor, 137 Euston Road,
London
NW1 2AA

870 Market Street, Ste 720
San Francisco
CA 94109, USA

ISBN 1900151669

First Published 2001

www.greenwich-medical.co.uk

Distributed worldwide by Plymbridge Distributors Ltd and in the USA by Jamco Distribution

Typeset by Phoenix Photosetting, Chatham, Kent
Printed by MPG Books, Bodmin, UK

CONTENTS

Preface vii
Foreword ix
Acknowledgements xi

1   Essential Preliminaries 1
2   Basics of Doppler Ultrasound 19
3   The Liver 29
4   The Biliary System 61
5   The Pancreas 91
6   The Spleen 107
7   Lymph Nodes 119
8   Abdominal Aorta and Inferior Vena Cava 125
9   Kidneys and Ureters 141
10 The Bladder and Lower Ureters 181
11 Prostate 195
12 The Adrenal Glands 203
13 Bowel 213
14 Muscle 227
15 Fluid 237
16 Miscellaneous Information 245

Appendices
1   Common Abdominal Conditions 256
2   Common Blood Tests 260
3   Abdominal Aortic Aneurysm – Monitoring Intervals . . 261
4   Renal Failure 262
5   Reporting 263
6   General further reading 271

Index 273

PREFACE

The rapid expansion of abdominal ultrasound examinations within the field of medical imaging worldwide has led to a need for an increasing number of health care professionals to be trained in its use.

This book, whilst no substitute for practical experience, is aimed at those healthcare professionals starting or who have already started their training in this field and who are beginning to enjoy the challenge of abdominal scanning. It is hoped that those already scanning in a team with support from experienced colleagues or those practising single handed in less than ideal conditions might also find it useful. Most of all, I hope the book is used and not left on a shelf.

The intention is to provide sufficient ultrasound and clinical information to enable the sonographer to identify normal appearances and variations, to show what to look for in a problematic and methodical way, to help form an opinion of the patient's condition from both the ultrasound appearances and overall clinical picture and to recognise the limitations of the ultrasound examination when they exist.

As the success of any ultrasound scan is dependent on the skill of the operator, it is hoped that this book will encourage and enable the sonographer to go some way in achieving a high standard of scanning in abdominal ultrasound which in turn will provide a quality service that the patient deserves.

Mike Stocksley
May 2001

FOREWORD

This book is a labour of love by Mike Stocksley who, after years of clinical ultrasound, has devoted his time to teaching students on the postgraduate ultrasound course. He, like myself, started in the days of static ultrasound scanning.

Mr Stocksley has written a book which is extremely practical, easy to read and beautifully illustrated. It is a testament to his understanding of the complexities of teaching that he has included an excellent chapter on the practical side of ultrasound.

I have had the pleasure of lecturing to his students over the last eight years. We have changed the course emphasis to become problem orientated rather than just technical and this book has expanded on that.

In each chapter, he has outlined the anatomy, physiology, variations in normal anatomy, followed by the ultrasound examination and relevant pathology. I particularly liked the boxes which draw the reader's attention to practical advice on either how to improve the scan or to an explanation of what has been seen.

This book emphasises the fact that medical and non-medically qualified practitioners should be considering an ultrasound investigation, not as a technical exercise to produce pretty images, but as an examination, which asks questions in order to solve specific problems. His objective has been achieved.

It has been written as a source of reference, a book to be read in conjunction with a teaching programme and can be used as a teaching aid in its own right.

In summary, this book will more than likely become a standard text for sonographers, medical students and a bench book in ultrasound departments.

Lesley MacDonald
Consultant Radiologist
St Thomas' Hospital
Guy's and St Thomas' Hospital

ACKNOWLEDGEMENTS

I would like to thank Greenwich Medical Media for their patience and encouragement; Dr B. Al-Murrani, Dr R. de Bruyn, T.S. Evans, P. Keane, A. Lund, Dr L. MacDonald, F. Pocock and M. Shah for providing some of the ultrasound images; J. Hughes, E Gannon, S. Brown and Emma, M. Gradwell and Child A for the positioning images and all who have supported me while the book was in the making.

1

ESSENTIAL PRELIMINARIES

Technical aspects
Setting up the equipment to scan
Patient preparation
Basic scanning techniques

As with any kind of ultrasound scan, there are many elements that contribute to a successful scan apart from a knowledge of the relevant anatomy and where it lies, surface markings and sectional anatomy. These are:

- up-to-date equipment offering the latest technology

- a knowledge of the capabilities and facilities of the scanning equipment used and how to manipulate the equipment in order to obtain optimal images of the anatomy and pathology, (if present)

- quality assurance tests to ensure optimum performance and accuracy of equipment

- an appropriate transducer for the investigation

- sufficient coupling medium to allow good transmission of sound into the patient

- a well-prepared patient

- good patient cooperation

- a knowledge of the clinical background of the patient before beginning the scan

- an understanding of the relevance of the body's own acoustic windows and how to use them to the best advantage

- an understanding of how to obtain the most information possible based on ultrasound scanning technique and a knowledge of how the patient's posture produces changes in anatomy

- the use of techniques to avoid scanning through intestinal gas

- the ability to give a clear indication of what has been observed (the report).

In brief, all the above can be found in three interdependent areas: equipment, operator and patient.

Technical aspects

The choice of equipment

Equipment chosen for an abdominal ultrasound unit must reflect the present and projected workload and practice. Important considerations are the ability to upgrade the software and the availability of hardware such as different transducers, needle guides and remote monitors required for changing practice and protocols.

As the highest quality image is required, it is a false economy to buy relatively inexpensive equipment as the main ultrasound scanner for the department. Up-to-date technology, although costly to finance initially, can now offer the latest facilities, allowing improved results and a potentially better diagnostic pick-up rate. Amongst these facilities are:

- tissue harmonic imaging – which can provide significant increases in detail on difficult-to-scan patients: the overweight, elderly or those with a thick body wall

- broadband digital beamforming technology – which can improve contrast and axial and spatial resolution said to reveal subtle tissue features

- real-time compound imaging – which can be used to reduce speckle and small shadows cast by normal or benign structures and can improve the visualization of linear structures.

The equipment must also be user friendly and, among many other facilities, allow easy switching between several transducers, have clear output displays, power output control, a large memory cine facility, good Doppler sensitivity, programmable presets and an appropriate number of clearly marked focusing zones which, along with gain and pre- and postprocessing controls, should be simple to use and easily at hand.

Ergonomics and operator health and safety must also be considered. The equipment must be suited to the operator and feel comfortable during long periods of use. Operator neck, shoulder and wrist strain can be considerable if the scanning position is awkward with the patient too high or the operator too low although this is often a couch or operator's stool height problem. Swivel monitors and keyboards can often add flexibility and afford a more comfortable scanning position for the operator.

The choice of probe

A correct choice is essential to obtain the optimum sections in an area that is anatomically difficult to scan. You may not have the choice with existing equipment. If choosing from new, consider the following.

- Frequencies required will be from about 7.5 MHz in a baby to 3.5–5 MHz in an adult. A variety of frequencies is not always available.

- When imaging the liver, ultrasound will have to penetrate to a depth of approximately 5 cm in a baby and 15–20+ cm in an adult.

- Some surfaces are quite superficial so a transducer with a good near-field resolution will be required in order to produce the most accurate examination.

- The footprint of the transducer (the part in contact with the skin) needs to be small enough to make contact with small, rather inaccessible areas such as the intercostal spaces and to allow a degree of angulation without loss of contact.

Large linear array transducers are generally not suitable for abdominal scanning owing to their large footprint although they can be useful when scanning superficial gallbladders. They are better suited to the larger, flatter areas such as superficial vascular, joint, limb muscle, small part, anterior abdominal wall, superficial organ scanning in small patients and in obstetric scanning. These transducers usually have a good near-field resolution capability and a wide field of view.

Curved linear transducers are often supplied with new equipment. They have become smaller and more user friendly in recent years. Their advantages are that they have electronic phased-array technology which gives good near-field resolution and quite a wide field of view in the near-field. They are sometimes awkward to use intercostally and when dipping or angling up or down when scanning longitudinally, they can lose much contact with the skin surface (Fig. 1.1).

Sector transducers have a small footprint and are ideal for scanning in intercostal and subxiphisternal spaces. They are good for angling without losing contact with the skin surface. The near-field is comparatively small and superficial information can be missed. They sometimes suffer from slightly inferior near-field resolution and the mechanical sector transducers eventually suffer from wear and tear which results in inferior image quality.

Therefore, as usual, there is a compromise between sector and curved linear; you will often have to use what is available. Check which probes are supplied with the equipment when purchased; you may be supplied with ones which are not appropriate for your workload. Paediatric scanning, for example, requires small footprint probes. Multifrequency or dynamic frequency probes, when available, are useful and cost-effective alternatives to fixed-frequency probes, reducing the need to purchase several probes. Biopsy attachments are essential if this work forms part of the departmental workload.

The choice of image recording equipment

Images are taken for teaching, illustrating, reminding, monitoring, record keeping, discussion, quality assurance and possibly medicolegal situations. However, they should not be used to make a diagnosis. Depending on the use to which images taken during ultrasound scans of the abdomen will be put, there are several ways of producing images, both hard copy and paperless. Below is a list of available imaging equipment and associated features.

THERMAL PRINTERS

- Black and white and colour available

- Low initial cost and running costs for black and white, more for colour although usually colour is used less frequently

- Simple to install

- Immediate images

- Low maintenance

- Quality of image good and improving

VIDEOPRINTERS

- Pictures available quickly

- 1–12 images on an A4 sheet

- Long archival life

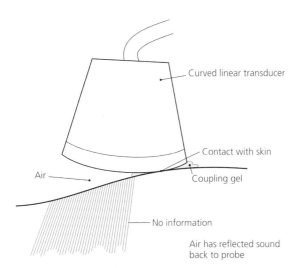

Fig. 1.1 Loss of contact with skin surface.

- Colour and black and white images can be mixed on each sheet
- Film or photographic paper can be used
- Relatively inexpensive

MULTIFORMAT IMAGERS

- Uses single-sided emulsion film or photographic paper (up to six images on one film)
- Initially expensive to buy
- Bulky
- Excellent detail. Not often used now owing to cost of film and development
- Requires darkroom to load and unload and processor to develop

LASER IMAGER

- Choice of laser imager with wet processor or dry laser equipment
- Equipment is large and remote
- Suited to connection to other diagnostic imaging equipment
- Used in busy imaging departments
- Variety of image sizes on 35 × 43 cm film
- Film expensive compared to thermal paper
- Good-quality images
- Expensive to maintain when service contracts are considered

PICTURE ARCHIVING AND COMMUNICATION SYSTEMS (PACS)

- Digital and paperless
- No films needed
- Excellent detail
- Quick and convenient
- Can be viewed remote from the site of scan
- Huge storage capacity
- High capital cost initially but low running costs

- Sometimes difficult to match different systems together

For ease of connecting the ultrasound scanner to your choice of imager, especially the more sophisticated types, ensure that your scanner and imager are DICOM (Digital Imaging and Communications in Medicine) compatible. This is an industry standard for transference of medical images from computer to computer and ensures compatibility between equipment.

Safety in ultrasound

Laboratory tests have shown that ultrasound can cause harmful effects. These are classed as thermal and mechanical effects.

Thermal effects are noticed as a rise in temperature, usually highest at bone/tissue interfaces but more frequently encountered in abdominal scanning near the probe/skin interface. It is therefore prudent not to hold the probe over the same area for too long. B-mode imaging using modern equipment uses acoustic outputs incapable of producing harmful temperature rises (i.e. of more than 1.5°C). Pulsed Doppler produces a greater heating effect but this is more of a concern when scanning the developing embryo, rather than the abdomen.

Mechanical effects arise when stress in tissues is caused by the amplitude of the ultrasound pulse and this has, under laboratory conditions, caused rupture of small blood vessels in the lungs. Mechanical effects are greatest in gas-filled organs (lungs, bowel).

Two indices are used to monitor these effects.

- The thermal index (TI) which is an estimate of the tissue temperature rise in °C that could happen as a worst case. Three thermal indices have been defined: two bone indices, which are less relevant for abdominal scanning, and one soft tissue index.
- The mechanical index (MI) is an indication of the amplitude of the ultrasonic pulses being used at any time and consequently an indication of the potential for cavitation.

In future, new ultrasound equipment will have to indicate thermal and mechanical indices as the output display standard (ODS). This is a calculation for any scanner-generated beam and should help to remind the operator to reduce the power and/or the scanning time. The operator has an increasing role to play in reducing the potential for ultrasound bioeffects to occur. The American Institute for Ultrasound in Medicine (AIUM) has proposed that all users employ the ALARA principle (as low as reasonably achievable) with regard to insonation of the patient.[1]

Reducing the insonation time to the patient can be carried out by several direct and indirect means.

- By reducing the power output to the lowest level possible and increasing the amplification to the returning echoes (gain).

- By not resting the probe on the abdomen or using it to spread newly applied contact gel while the probe is active.

- By taking the least possible time to scan while being thorough (as a result of good training).

- By not repeating scans or performing unnecessary scans.

Visual safety checks can be carried out on a daily basis by the operator. Check for:

- broken or cracked probe casings

- split or bare wires

- clogged cooling fan filters.

A quality assurance programme should be instigated if not already in progress. Written and photographic records can be made of the equipment's performance with the aid of tests carried out on one of the widely available tissue-mimicking phantoms (Fig. 1.2).

Tests that can be carried out by sonographers include:

- sensitivity

- axial resolution

- lateral resolution

- dead zone

- caliper measurement accuracy.

These tests can be carried out on a regular basis. If a linear or curvilinear probe has been dropped accidentally or knocked, a crystal drop-out test can quickly be carried out. Apply some gel over the footprint of the probe and run an open paper-clip or small screwdriver gently over the surface at right angles to the length of the probe. Crystal drop-out will show as a small dark shadow where the non-functioning crystal is positioned.

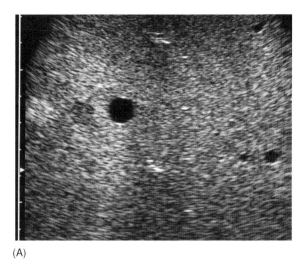

(A)

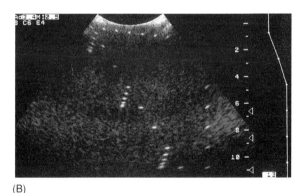

(B)

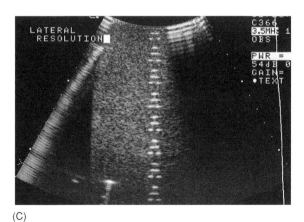

(C)

Fig. 1.2 Tissue-mimicking phantom tests. (A) Scan of tissue-mimicking test object. (B) Test for axial resolution. (C) Test for lateral resolution.

Other safety tests must be carried out by service engineers or by medical physics personnel. If there is any doubt as to the safety of any equipment, leave well alone and label the machine as unsafe, warning others not to use it.

Coupling gel

Coupling gel is the universal medium used to exclude the tiny amount of air between the probe and the skin. The air acts as a barrier to sound entering the body and it reflects about 99.5% of the sound back to the probe. Little has been written about the history of coupling media but for many years, vegetable or mineral oil was used as a cheap and readily available source. These oils were extremely messy to use; they stained clothing and transferred easily from patient to hand to machine. It was not long before the oil-covered machines (usually large static B-scanners) would start attracting dust, giving the equipment a suede appearance, much to the disgust of those about to service the equipment.

It was also found that this oil attacked the rubber cabling and would, if used these days, invalidate any manufacturer's warranty. Thus the rise in the number of available gels. Differences are not only in colour and cost but also in viscosity, something that must be considered when choosing what gel to purchase for abdominal scanning. Some gel is of low viscosity and is better suited to obstetrics and gynaecology examinations. This covers extremely well but tends to be too runny for abdominal scanning. Some is of high viscosity and is more appropriate for examinations where the transducers have a limited range of movement, such as cardiac and Doppler studies. Gel with a medium viscosity is a good compromise between the two and avoids both dredging of thick gel and frequent reapplication of the thinner product.

Ultrasound should ideally travel through the gel as near to the velocity of sound through skin as possible (1518 m/s) so that refraction of the sound beam at the gel/skin interface does not occur. Also, manufacturers use silicone, epoxy materials or plastic on the face of their transducers with the idea of matching this material to the acoustic impedance of skin. If there is a large difference between the acoustic impedance of the transducer face and the gel, sound beam refraction can occur, altering the focusing characteristics and beam profile, causing phase changes in the acoustic wave and resulting in degradation of image quality.

Therefore the optimal acoustic impedance of the gel should be between that of the transducer and that of the skin.

With silicone transducer faces, the optimal acoustic impedance of the gel should be somewhere between 1489 m/s and 1561 m/s.[2]

Other considerations for a coupling medium

Dermatologically, it should not contain irritants or sensitizers such as dyes, fragrances and propylene glycol. These are often found in cosmetics but have no place in an ultrasound coupling medium. Propylene glycol is a documented contact allergen and can cause contact dermatitis. Modern gels contain more beneficial constituents such as glycerine and aloe vera, although to maintain the benefits, the aloe must contain at least 20% of aloe vera gel.

A research paper published in 1988 discussed the risks of cross-infection when scanning by testing transducers, coupling gel and stand-off blocks.[3] The results may have prompted the inclusion of antimicrobial additives as by 1992 it was noted that some gels contained propylene glycol to inhibit the growth of *Staphylococcus aureus* and *Escherichia coli*, this having to be >10% in order to be effective. However, propylene glycol can sensitize the skin and can, in high amounts, contribute to the swelling of plastics and elastomers in the transducer.[2] Some gels contain cosmetic-grade antimicrobial substances. A test of the preservative system in the ultrasound gel is the USPXX11 Antimicrobial Preservation Effectiveness Test in which the gel is subjected to inoculation by *Staphylococcus aureus*, *Escherichia coli*, *Pseudomonas aeruginosa*, *Candida albicans* and *Aspergillus niger* and plate counts taken on four consecutive weeks.[2]

Gels should never contain mineral oil, silicone oil, alcohol, surfactants or fragrances as they can damage cables and the bonding of the transducer and can affect the acoustic lens.

Practically, the coupling gel should always be warmed to body temperature by use of a proprietary gel warmer or adapted baby's bottle warmer as cold gel spread on the upper abdomen is uncomfortable for the patient. Gel should always be wiped off the transducer between patients to avoid a build-up of dried gel which can degrade the image and shows the patient that they are being cared for and not being offered second-hand gel from a previous patient. This is bad practice.

Great care should also be taken with the transducer to minimize the spread of infection by means of thorough transducer cleaning between patients. For those patients with open wounds or drains, scanning with the use of sterile gel (available in sachets or in disposable syringes) should be mandatory, as should the use of a sterile transducer cover.

A stand-off gel block is sometimes used to reduce the amount of near-field reverberation. In effect, this moves the footprint of the transducer away from the skin surface and causes the near-field reverberation artefacts to occur within the gel block instead of superficially within the patient. Acoustic coupling medium is spread between the transducer and the top of the gel block and also between the bottom of the gel block and the skin surface to ensure exclusion of air between transducer and skin (Fig. 1.3).

The need for stand-off blocks has been reduced by the vastly improved near-field resolution seen in modern equipment, although if considering buying new sector transducers or scanning equipment with sector transducers, it would be of benefit to assess the near-field for minimal reverberation artefact before purchasing.

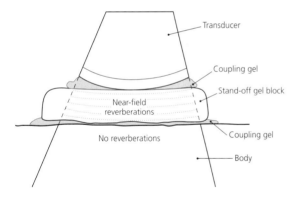

Fig. 1.3 Use of stand-off gel block to exclude near-field reverberation when scanning superficial structures.

On another practical note, when buying coupling media, try samples of available gel from different manufacturers before ordering to see which type of gel suits your workload. Find out the time taken to deliver from the time the order is placed, the cost per litre and discounts for bulk ordering, but ensure that you have sufficient storage space and estimate how much you will use before the gel is past its sell-by date.

Setting up the equipment to scan

With abdominal scanning, as with any other ultrasound scanning, the setting up of the controls that manipulate the image is important. Assuming that the contrast and brightness of the TV monitor and imaging systems have been checked, properly adjusted and set to their optimum positions, the time gain compensation (TGC) must be set. The normal liver is an ideal test object for setting up the TGC as it is an organ of homogeneous texture throughout a relatively large area. Sufficient coupling medium must be used for the entire scanning process otherwise very little information will be available on the screen, despite altering the power output or gain controls.

A longitudinal section of the right lobe of the liver is often used. While scanning this section, the idea is to produce an image giving a normal, even spread of grey tissue reproduction from the front to the back of the liver. This is done by adjusting the power output control to the lowest possible level, nominally 30–40%, and adjusting the TGC to demonstrate all returning echoes from the anterior to the posterior parts of the liver so that the spread of grey is even (Figs 1.4, 1.5). If the deepest part is too dark with the TGC at its highest level, the power output may be increased slightly. If separate sliding individual gain controls are available, they can be set to even up the image. There should be no banding seen on the screen. The focusing zone should include from front to back of the liver.

Compression should be set for the required contrast resolution. This is a basic set-up programme and may

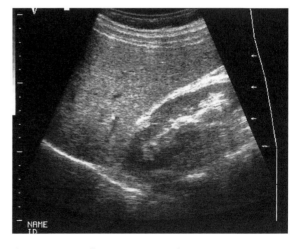

Fig. 1.4 Normally set-up image with correct gain settings.

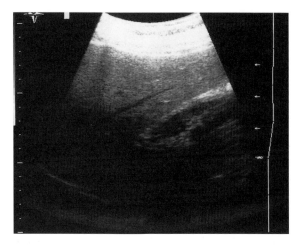

Fig. 1.5 Poor gain settings.

differ according to equipment and preference. The controls should be altered frequently according to the patient type and the anatomical structures being scanned.

Orientation

As with any conventional scanning, the patient's right side and head end is demonstrated on the left-hand side of the screen during transverse and longitudinal scans respectively (Fig. 1.6). The probe's position relative to the patient can be found by placing it longitudinally on the patient's midline and placing a finger at the head end of the probe between it and the skin. If a shadow appears on the right of the screen, turn the probe 180°.

General rules for obtaining the best image

- Use the highest frequency to obtain sufficient penetration to scan the region of interest when the power output is set at a low-medium level (see 'Setting up the equipment to scan'). This is prudent use of power levels and should give the best resolution.

- Always aim to position the ultrasound beam at right angles to the interface or structure under examination.

- Increase the line density by reducing the frame rate, reducing the sector angle or reducing the depth of field.

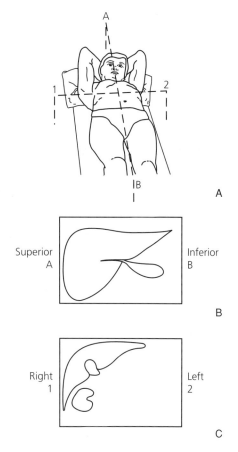

Fig. 1.6 Conventional orientation with head end and right side on left of screen, foot end and left side on right side of screen.

- Use harmonic tissue imaging, if available, for scanning the obese subject.

- Use the most appropriate focal zone for the structure under examination.

Measuring

When measuring relatively small structures, the image should be magnified greatly in order to improve caliper accuracy. On a small scale, the smallest movement from one point to another may register as much as half a centimetre.

Patient preparation

Upper abdominal preparation

Compared to some patient preparation used in radiological examinations, the preparation for upper abdominal ultrasound is relatively simple. Basically, the reason for preparing the patient is to obtain as clear and unequivocal a scan as possible with minimal patient disruption.

Avoiding disruption to the patient was not so important in the relatively early days of abdominal ultrasound scanning. Twenty years ago, aperients were suggested in order to cleanse the bowel, supposedly to improve the chances of completing a satisfactory study. It was suggested at the time that the cost to those centres that did not use aperients on their ultrasound patients was an increased failure rate. Some centres gave their patients aperients only when the first scan had been unsuccessful. An example of the regime in those days is:

- aperients 24 hours prior to examination
- fasting 12 hours prior to examination
- fluid restricted two hours prior to examination
- a possible low-residue diet during the day prior to the examination.

This was supposed to lead to a reduction in bowel contents and intestinal gas, which was admirable but probably gave the patients a headache. Purging and fasting when possible were the rule.

The rule of starving the patient prior to an abdominal ultrasound examination still holds true. However, the attitude to bowel gas is slightly less dogmatic. The following outlines the reasoning behind patient preparation. Different departments will issue their own preparation instructions to their patients, but they are all more or less variations on a theme.

A 6–8 hour fast will distend a normally functioning gallbladder. Whether or not the question asked on the request form concerns the gallbladder directly, a distended gallbladder acts as a landmark for the sonographer and helps avoid confusion with any pathology in the vicinity. If no fasting occurs and the patient has eaten, the gallbladder wall will thicken and the gallbladder reduce in size, appearing as a possible non-functioning gallbladder. If the patient has been fasting and the gallbladder appears small, this may suggest that

it is unable to distend in response to fasting. It could similarly be mistaken for a diseased or small gallbladder with cholecystitis. Thus it is essential to check that the patient has followed the preparation protocol closely.

Fasting ensures the gallbladder is as easily observed as possible, reducing the chances of missing pathology and thus avoiding confusion. Fasting also ensures that the stomach is empty and avoids the chances of the sonographer confusing stomach contents with pathology connected to the spleen, left kidney or pancreas, especially if there are no strong peristaltic surges visible during the scan. Several authors make this point. Late eating prior to a scan can confuse the appearances in the left upper quadrant. This may be the stomach with contents or genuine pathology. A fizzy drink may be given to differentiate between the stomach and a possible mass. If the gas bubbles are seen in the mass, the mass is the stomach. Fasting also helps reduce the content of the duodenum that may obscure the common duct and pancreas.

In addition, the portal vessels dilate to a degree after a meal, thus making any observations about their size less valid. Fasting is therefore desirable. To avoid headaches, water may be taken in moderation. In cases where the posterior gallbladder wall is situated close to the duodenum, acoustic shadowing can mimic gallbladder pathology. Giving water to drink usually helps outline the duodenum and demonstrate the gallbladder more clearly. Allowing any fluids to be taken will seemingly permit patients to consume milk (this contains fat and will contract the gallbladder), fizzy drinks (these will produce large quantities of gas) and soup (usually containing variable amounts of fat) among others. Strong cooking smells have also been known to contract the biliary system so the 'fair, fat, fertile, forty and flatulent female' cooking her partner's bacon and eggs before her morning appointment might well be advised to give him a bowl of muesli for once.

It has been said, on the other hand, that some fasting is recommended but not essential as it does little to improve visualization, can increase gas as a result of aerophagy and does not decrease intestinal gas. It has also been suggested that a light meal might, in fact, be advantageous as fasting tends to cause people to swallow more air than those who have eaten. In some situations, scanning an unprepared patient is unavoidable, especially if an urgent evaluation is required. Infants and neonates can be given a glucose drink to placate them during a scan but if the liver and biliary system are to be examined, milk (either maternal or substitute) must not be given.

Intestinal gas can be a reason for an examination failing, so ways to reduce or eliminate it must be considered at the preparation stage.

The following causes of intestinal gas have been suggested.

- Anxiety and excessive talking can cause an increase in gas in the upper abdomen. The anxiety can stem from the thought of visiting a hospital, what the scan involves, worry about the results of the scan, etc. One explanation for this phenomenon is that anxious patients may unconsciously relax their upper oesophageal sphincter and the negative intrathoracic pressures generated during respiration suck air into the oesophagus.

- Smoking and nervous inhalation. Smoking increases gastric motility and also prevents optimum visualization of the gallbladder and bile ducts as nicotine gives rise to the release of cholecystokinin, leading to a contraction of the gallbladder and bile ducts.

- Inactivity.

- Gulping water.

Suggested methods of ridding patients of intestinal gas include the following.

- Chewing gum can prevent excessive talking and air intake and helps to relax the patient.

- Reduce anxiety before the examination by a full explanation of the procedure to the patient. An explanation on the appointment form of what will happen to the patient during the scan is suggested. This is widely done at present. Patients will hopefully not present for the scan ignorant of what will happen to them.

- No smoking six hours before the examination (although some may argue that smoking may help alleviate anxiety!).

- Mobilize the patient if possible.

- Drink water before the examination; sipping water through a straw has been suggested rather than gulping it down quickly in an effort to please the staff.

- Allow the patient to drink 500–750 ml water when in the ultrasound room, sitting upright at first to fill the stomach then lying on the right side to chase water through the duodenum. Tomato juice, having a closer acoustic impedance to soft tissue than water, has been used in the past. It is unknown how the patients enjoyed drinking 750 ml tomato juice.

- In addition, with the patient supine, having ensured that there is no abdominal aortic aneurysm present, ask the patient to push their abdomen forward while pushing the transducer firmly over the mid-part of the upper abdomen. This should be done without the patient taking a deep breath in first, otherwise this air intake defeats the object of dispersing gas.

- Lie the patient prone to allow their own weight to disperse gas.

Preparation for children and infants

Where the liver and biliary system are to be investigated, it is suggested that:

- babies are scanned before a feed, this being available immediately after the scan (fractious babies may be soothed by a teat and water, although gas may arise from this)

- children 2–5 years should be nil by mouth for four hours except for water or weak squash

- children over 12 years of age should be prepared as for an adult although the bladder preparation should be to drink less.

Diabetics should be starved if the liver and biliary system are to be examined but discretion should be used. The diabetic patient, if starved, should be placed first on the list in the morning and should be advised to bring food and insulin, if used, to take after the scan. Non-fizzy glucose drinks may be taken prior to the examination if required.

Other more drastic measures to avoid the accumulation of intestinal gas include:

- nasogastric intubation to remove air and fluid

- glucagon injection to relax peristalsis and retain gastric fluid and the giving of dimethyl siloxane to prevent air bubbles forming

- prescan oxygen therapy 100% humidified at 10 l/min for 10–12 hours before the scan in addition to starving the patient six hours before. This is said to reduce the concentration of non-diffusible gases.[4]

> **Box 1.1   Advice**
>
> Suggested preparation for the upper abdomen including liver, gallbladder and ducts, pancreas, spleen, kidneys, aorta and inferior vena cava.
>
> - Fast for 6–8 hours prior to examination.
> - Drinks may be taken as long as they are not fizzy or milky.
> - No smoking before examination for same period.
> - If possible, keep active rather than sit around to try to reduce the presence of bowel gas.

Pelvic preparation

The urinary bladder requires filling if it forms part of a urological ultrasound assessment when the bladder and lower ureters are being investigated. Apart from aiding visualization of the uterus and ovaries when scanning transabdominally, it also helps to visualize the iliac arteries as the urine acts as an acoustic window. The prostate gland can also be seen more easily when scanning transabdominally.

Problems can arise when the bladder is overfilled, especially in the elderly and incontinent. In those who are not, an overfilled bladder can produce a small to moderate renal pelvicdilatation which may be reported falsely as such. The amount of fluid to be taken must be related to the patient's age and condition. The fluid must be taken sufficiently before the time of the examination to allow it to be absorbed by the small bowel. A suggested preparation for an average 30-year-old adult male would be 0.5–1 litre of clear still fluid one hour before arrival for the scan.

In addition to what is usually considered 'patient preparation', I would like to suggest a few other areas involved in the preparation stage before commencement of the scan.

ON RECEIVING THE REQUEST FORM

- Is the request urgent or non-urgent?
- Is the request relevant and useful?
- Has the patient had the examination before?

- Where is the patient – at home or in the hospital? Where is the preparation instruction sheet to be sent?
- Is the patient diabetic?
- Does the patient have any transport problems or special needs?

ON ARRIVAL IN THE ULTRASOUND DEPARTMENT

- Is the gel warm?
- Is the patient correctly identified?
- Is the patient ready for the scan; does the patient need to get changed?
- Is the room tidy and the paper or sheet on the couch replaced or tidied?

IN THE ULTRASOUND ROOM

- Introduce yourself.
- Explain what is going to happen and reassure the patient, especially if they are young.
- Ask if the preparation instructions have been followed.
- Have all the information to hand: clinical notes, when possible, results of laboratory tests, previous diagnostic imaging examination reports and their results in order to obtain as much information about the patient as a whole before starting to scan.
- Have the light in the room sufficiently bright at first to be able to observe the patient for skin colour, previous operation scars and oedema, amongst other things. Talk to the patient and listen to them.
- Assess their shape and size, making a mental note of the relative position of the organs and how to approach the scan before commencing (see body types below).

Body types

Knowing where the organs lie and their surface markings is an essential part of the preparation. Knowing where organs are situated in different body types is essential both for their accurate imaging and for their appropriate use as acoustic windows when imaging adjacent anatomy. Knowing where the organs lie is of paramount importance when a measurement of the longest axis of certain organs, such as the kidneys, is required.

People can be broad in relation to their height or vice versa. Two contrasting types are recognized: the one with the short, broad trunk (hypersthenic) and the other with a long, narrow trunk (asthenic). Two further divisions are termed hyposthenic and sthenic. The variation of types, their frequency in the population and the position of the relative organs is demonstrated in Figure 1.7.

If nothing else, it should be noted that the gas-filled bowel and stomach are considerably higher and closer to the liver in the hypersthenic and sthenic types and the gallbladder considerably higher in these types than in the asthenic and hyposthenic types. The liver tends to cover less of the area under the diaphragm in the hypersthenic and sthenic types and so these types tend not to have as good an acoustic window for scanning the pancreas and have more bowel gas in the vicinity of the upper abdominal organs. The saying that these types are 'gassy' may be unfair to them as they may not have any more flatulence than the thin types; however, it is the proximity of that gas to the organs of interest that is important to a sonographer.

Basic scanning techniques

Acoustic windows

An acoustic window is a region of tissue or fluid through which ultrasound can be easily transmitted. It contains no barriers to ultrasound such as gas or bone and allows visual access to other anatomy deeper in the body.

Acoustic windows tend to be relatively large and lie between the probe and the organ under examination. They are called windows as they specifically help to demonstrate structures positioned behind them.

Acoustic windows used in scanning the abdomen are:

- liver – helps in viewing the right kidney, pancreas, gallbladder and common duct, upper abdominal aorta and inferior vena cava

- spleen – helps in viewing the left kidney, tail of pancreas and upper abdominal aorta

- fluid-filled stomach and duodenum – helps to see the pancreas (Fig. 1.8)

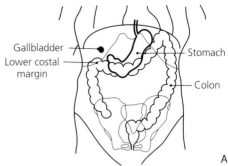

Hypersthenic 5% of population

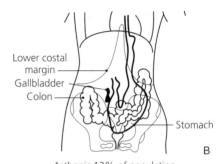

Asthenic 12% of population

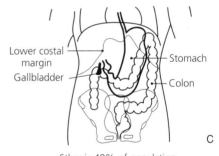

Sthenic 48% of population

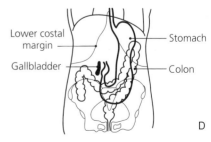

Hyposthenic 35% of population

Fig. 1.7 Body types (after Mill).

- ascites or free fluid also enhances the image of structures behind or within the fluid, especially the retroperitoneal structures such as the kidneys and abdominal aorta.

The idea behind using acoustic windows is to place the probe over the acoustic window in order to scan the deeper structures and avoid scanning through image-degrading structures such as gas-containing bowel.

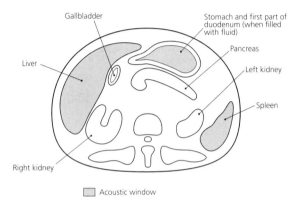

Fig. 1.8 Transverse section of upper abdomen demonstrating acoustic windows (liver, spleen and fluid-filled stomach).

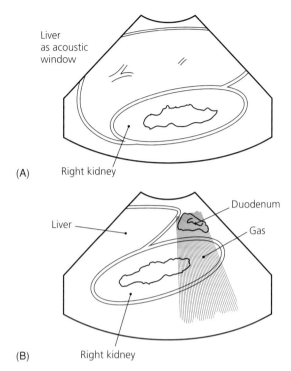

Fig. 1.9 (A) Section through liver and right kidney showing good use of acoustic window. (B) Similar section: scanning with transducer in lower position uses less acoustic window and allows gas in duodenum to obscure lower pole of kidney.

Avoiding scanning through gas

The patient should be scanned in such a way that no gas or air appears between the probe and the organs under examination. If this happens, most of the sound will be reflected back to the probe, leaving no information seen behind the gas (Fig. 1.9). Instead, scan through an acoustic window, scan behind the anterior gas-filled stomach and bowel, either through the left or right flanks or with the patient prone, or move the patient onto one side or another so that the gas-filled bowel moves and the gas rises away from the mid-region of the patient. When it is safe to do so, gentle-to-firm pressure can be used to displace intestinal gas that would normally obscure the image.

Scanning positions – general abdomen

The flexibility of ultrasound allows for scanning patients in a variety of positions, all of which are used for convenience, preference and for reasons of accessibility to the various structures.

SUPINE

In this position:

- the patient is usually most comfortable
- abdominal muscles are relaxed
- the abdomen flattens
- the patient can see the sonographer and the screen
- gas rises anteriorly; free fluid, if present, rests on the most posterior part of the peritoneum (in the hepatorenal recess or over the surface of the liver) or the posterior part of the structure containing the fluid; calculi, if present, lie on the most dependent portion of the gallbladder (Fig. 1.10).

LEFT POSTERIOR OBLIQUE 45° (LPO)

This position is:

- best for scanning the gallbladder and proximal common duct

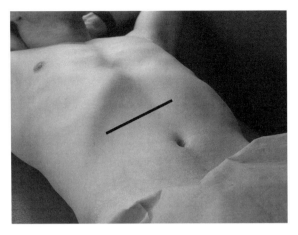

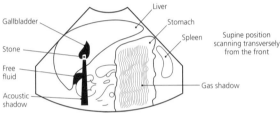

Fig. 1.10 Supine position – effect on gas and stone shadowing.

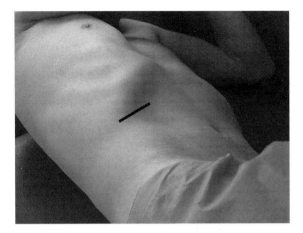

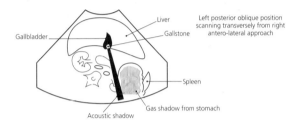

Fig. 1.11 Left posterior oblique – effect on gas and stone shadowing.

- good for scanning structures in the right upper quadrant

- used in scanning oblique coronal views of the inferior vena cava (IVC) and abdominal aorta and for the right adrenal gland (Fig. 1.11).

RIGHT POSTERIOR OBLIQUE 45° (RPO)

This position is:

- used in scanning oblique views of the IVC and abdominal aorta and for the left adrenal gland

- used for scanning the spleen and left kidney (Fig. 1.12).

LEFT LATERAL DECUBITUS (LLD)

In this position:

- the liver descends more into the abdomen

- the right kidney and IVC are better visualized

- gas rises to the right side away from the patient's midline

- gallstones, if present, fall to the fundus or left lateral wall of the gallbladder

- fluid falls to the left dependent part of the abdomen

- fat shifts to the level of the scanning couch away from the midline (Fig. 1.13).

RIGHT LATERAL DECUBITUS (RLD)

In this position:

- the spleen descends further into the abdomen

- there is better coverage of the left kidney, the abdominal aorta and the tail of the pancreas

- intestinal gas rises to the left side

- gallstones, if present, fall to the right lateral/fundal wall

- fluid falls to the right dependent parts of the abdomen

- fat falls to the right (Fig. 1.14).

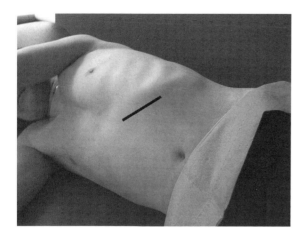

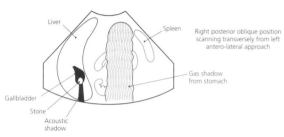

Fig. 1.12 Right posterior oblique – effect on gas and stone shadowing.

UPRIGHT

Positions help patients who have difficulty in breathing when lying down.

STANDING

In this position, the liver and gallbladder descend into the abdomen and the intraabdominal veins distend. Some sonographers prefer this position for scanning the pancreas.

SITTING

This position is better for scanning patients in wheel-chairs. It allows a substantial survey without having to move the patient onto the couch.

PRONE

Used for scanning kidneys, especially those of neonates and some younger paediatric patients, the psoas muscles and for renal interventional procedures.

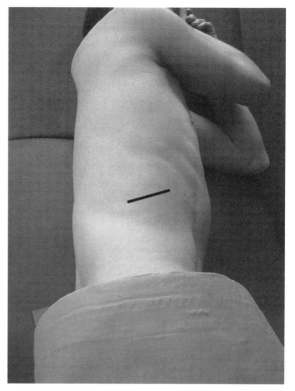

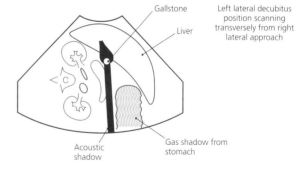

Fig. 1.13 Left lateral decubitus – effect on gas and stone shadowing.

Patient cooperation

Quiet breathing should be used when possible with instructions to stop breathing/breathe in and stop/breathe out and stop when necessary in order to obtain a clear image or insert a biopsy or drainage needle. Patients should also be told that they can continue breathing at the earliest opportunity! The use of the cine-loop facility can help obtain better images when patients cannot hold their breath or when they are breathing rapidly.

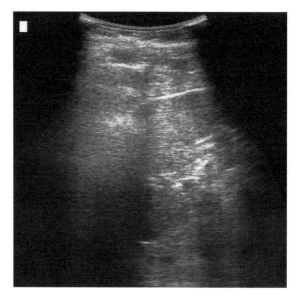

Fig. 1.15 Effects of inspiration on scanning the spleen.

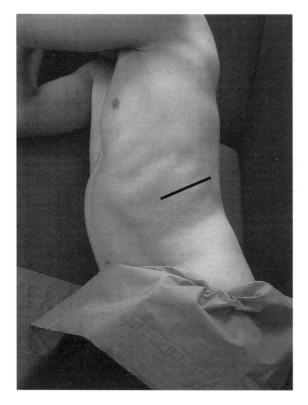

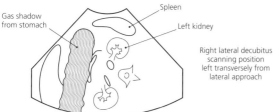

Gas shadow
from stomach

Spleen

Left kidney

Right lateral decubitus
scanning position
left transversely from
lateral approach

Fig. 1.14 Right lateral decubitus – effect on gas and stone shadowing.

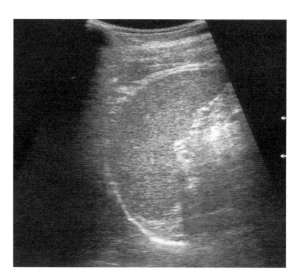

Fig. 1.16 The spleen on expiration.

Deep inspiration can help to lower the diaphragm and upper abdominal organs slightly but, conversely, this adds to the amount of intestinal gas present. Deep inspiration can also hinder attempts to scan the spleen and liver when approaching from the lateral positions by lowering the lateral aspect of the diaphragm between the probe and the organs.

Be patient with infants and young children when scanning their sides, especially the left side, as they tend to be very ticklish.

Cooperation from children is essential and can usually be obtained by means of patience and the use of a toy or two that should be kept in the ultrasound room for this purpose. Male sonographers can sometimes get better results by removing their white coat, if one is worn, as a fractious child may be remembering a previous, unpleasant hospital visit. A teddy bear or parent (or both) can be scanned to show what is going to happen and this may help to relax the child, especially when they can see their 'insides'. Parents should be encouraged to stay in the room with children and babies during the scan to help the sonographer and calm the child if anxious. This action should also eliminate any possible allegation of assault that could be made against the sonographer. Female sonographers should not feel exempt from this advice. In addition, it helps not to have too many other people in the scanning room watching the procedure; children are shy about their bodies, especially as they get slightly older, and should be given the respect and privacy afforded to adults.

References

1. ter Haar G, Duck FA (eds) 2000 The safe use of ultrasound in medical diagnosis. British Institute of Radiology, London

2. Anon 1992 The technology of ultrasound scanning gels. Diagnostic Sonar Ltd, Edinburgh

3. Spencer P, Spencer RC 1988 Ultrasound scanning of post-operative wounds: the risks of cross-infection. Clin Radiol 39: 245–246

4. Marshall REK, Steger AC, Delicata R, Wafula JMC, Brunell CL, Wyatt AP 1995 Does pre-scan oxygen improve ultrasonic imaging of the pancreas? Clin Radiol 50: 26–28

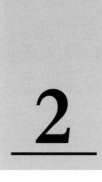

2

A BACKGROUND TO DOPPLER ULTRASOUND

Basics of Doppler ultrasound
Pulsed wave Doppler
Colour Doppler
Power Doppler
Doppler in the upper abdominal scan

Basics of Doppler ultrasound

There are many publications devoted to the use of Doppler ultrasound. The technique for scanning using Doppler ultrasound is outside the scope of this book, but Doppler is found in areas where its use contributes to the diagnostic procedure. Here, with no apologies, the physics of Doppler will be kept to less than a minimum.

Doppler ultrasound is used to study the behaviour of blood flow as Doppler signals are reflected off moving red blood cells. On B-mode real-time scanning, blood vessels that are patent or stenosed appear ultrasonically similar. The use of Doppler information can help to distinguish between the two. It can also differentiate between blood vessel and duct if an anatomical query arises.

The main forms of Doppler used are pulsed wave Doppler (PWD), colour Doppler (CD) and power Doppler (PD). Modern ultrasound equipment with CD facilities usually offers conventional B-mode real-time scanning, CD, which shows colour representation of blood flow towards and away from the probe, pulsed wave spectral analysis shown as waveforms above and below a baseline and often PD.

Pulsed wave Doppler (PWD)

This is used to detect the presence of flow in a vessel at a known depth. Sound is transmitted and received intermittently, using a sector, linear or curved linear probe as in conventional B-mode scanning. The Doppler signals from a vessel at a known depth are 'gated' and those signals from within the 'gate' or sample site are analysed. If the sample site is large, this increases the size of the volume of moving fluid to be sampled (the sample volume). In turn, this makes it easier to detect a vessel but harder to detect small amounts of flow.

A PWD signal can be superimposed on a B-scan real-time image so that the vessel in which the gate is placed can be seen (duplex scanning). If there are vessels in front of the one under investigation, they will not be analysed as only the gated vessel is being examined.

Direction of the flow of blood, important in the examination of portal hypertension, for example, can be determined by noting whether the signal is above or below the baseline. The pattern of flow can be assessed to differentiate between arterial and venous flow (Fig. 2.1).

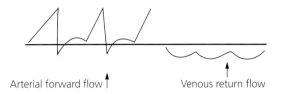

Arterial forward flow ↑   Venous return flow ↑

Fig. 2.1 Example of pulse wave signals.

By knowing the peak systolic flow frequency and the angle of the Doppler beam to the vessel, the velocity of the blood flow can be calculated from the change in frequency (returning frequency compared to the outgoing frequency) when the Doppler signal is reflected by the moving target. The Doppler signal increases as the blood flow velocity increases and as the ultrasound frequency increases. In practice, higher frequency transducers are more sensitive to low flow rates but as lower frequencies are often required to see deep abdominal vessels, low flow rates may not be seen. The angle of the sound to the vessel wall should be <60°; at 70° the velocity error is 25%. As it approaches 90°, the signal rapidly decreases until it may eventually be lost.

Velocity shift is sometimes preferred to frequency shift as the angle used is less critical and the frequency used does not alter the calculation. A stenotic vessel increases the velocity of blood through it; dilatation decreases the flow rate. The velocity of blood is greater in the middle of the vessel and slower near the vessel walls except where there are wall irregularities. Flow distortion can be seen by high velocities from blood passing through the stenosed part of the vessel and turbulence caused by the high velocity flow hitting flow from the normal lumen distal to the stenosis.

High or low resistance to arterial flow can also be detected. High resistance shows a typical pattern of a high systolic peak and a low diastolic flow. Low resistance shows as a double or biphasic systolic peak and a relatively high diastolic flow (Fig. 2.2).

The resistance is calculated by (the systolic frequency − the diastolic frequency)/the systolic frequency. This is the resistive index. High resistance to flow is seen in a number of renal pathologies such as hydronephrosis or renal transplant rejection.

Flow volume can also be calculated from knowing the width of the vessel and the rate of blood flow.

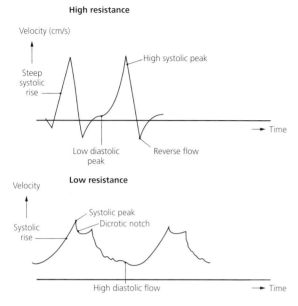

High resistance

Velocity (cm/s)

High systolic peak

Steep systolic rise

Time

Low diastolic peak

Reverse flow

Low resistance

Velocity

Systolic peak

Dicrotic notch

Systolic rise

High diastolic flow

Time

Fig. 2.2 High and low resistance shown as pulsed wave Doppler signal.

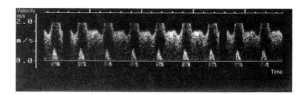

Fig. 2.3 Pulsed wave Doppler signal demonstrating aliasing.

Box 2.1 Advice

The angle of the Doppler signal to the vessel must be less than 60° for accuracy to be maintained. However, for B-mode scanning, advice has previously been given to scan at right angles to the interfaces of the structures under examination. In the case of Doppler ultrasound, it must be understood that the image quality must be forsaken for the accuracy of the Doppler signal angle.

PWD controls

POWER OUTPUT

This increases the Doppler sensitivity but also the patient exposure. The maximum must be <0.4 watts, as set in the American Institute for Ultrasound in Medicine (AIUM) guidelines.

DOPPLER GATE CURSOR AND SAMPLE VOLUME

The sample volume size controls the axial length of the Doppler sample so that unwanted areas are not considered. When obtaining a signal from a vessel, the Doppler gate cursor, shown on screen as either a box or two parallel bars, should be positioned within the centre of flow and parallel to the walls of the vessel. The size of the gate shows the volume of blood and the size of the area being investigated. The gate size can be enlarged or made smaller, ranging from about 2 to 20 mm. The larger the gate, the harder it is to see slower flow (Fig. 2.4).

BASELINE

The reflection of high-frequency sound waves from blood flow towards the transducer shows as a signal above the baseline while flow away from the transducer shows as signals below the baseline. As the flow to and from the transducer is dependent on the

Aliasing

The Doppler waveform is constructed from a series of samples. For a given sampling rate or pulse repetition frequency (PRF), there is a maximum frequency. Above this, the sampled waveform cannot be constructed accurately and a lower frequency signal is produced.

To sample a Doppler signal adequately, at least two samples must be taken on the shortest cycle for the correct frequency to be determined. This is called the Nyquist limit. This can also be expressed as the sample rate being at least 2 × maximum frequency in the Doppler signal. If the sample rate, controlled by the PRF, is less than the essential twice per cycle, then a phenomenon called aliasing occurs. Aliasing is the misinterpretation of the high frequencies above one half of the sampling frequency. Because the signal is not sampled quickly enough, it appears to wrap around itself and some of the signal appears below the baseline (Fig. 2.3). The PRF therefore should be at least twice the maximum value of Doppler frequency to be measured in order to avoid aliasing.

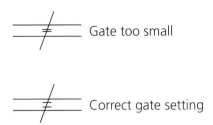

Fig. 2.4 Size of gate cursor within vessel.

position and angle of the transducer to the vessel, the signal can be inverted for easier viewing. The baseline level should be adjusted to make most use of the spectrum analyser.

DOPPLER RECEIVER GAIN CONTROL

The Doppler receiver gain control amplifies the received signal and alters the spectral waveform. Noise should be just visible in the background. If too low, flow that may be present may be missed and no clear outline to the signal seen; too high and directional information may be missed, noise is produced throughout the display and sometimes a mirror image of the display is seen on the other side of the baseline.

FREQUENCY SCALE

This needs to be increased if higher velocities are being set. Usually the PRF increases accordingly.

BEAM STEERING

The Doppler beam is electronically steered or offset from the imaging scan lines in order to improve the angle of incidence with the vessel.

ANGLE CORRECTION

This can improve the angle between the beam and the direction of flow.

WALL FILTER

Usually between 100 and 1000 Hz, this is used to filter out low-frequency, high-amplitude Doppler signals from patient respiration and movement of vessels (wall thump). With a low wall filter setting, more information is displayed. A high setting not only filters out movement artefact but can also filter out the signal; beware when looking for low blood flow.

SWEEP SPEED

Controls the rate at which the spectral information can be displayed, typically slow (25 mm/s), moderate (50 mm/s) or fast (100 mm/s). The faster the sweep speed, the more cycles can be sampled, although a slower sweep speed is easier to measure.

PULSE REPETITION FREQUENCY (PRF)

The number of pulses per given time emitted by the transducer is measured in KHz. The PRF is determined by the depth of the measuring site and decreases with the increase of depth at which it is sampling. Typically, at 5 cm the maximum PRF is 16.6 KHz, reducing to 5.5 KHz at 15 cm. Increasing the PRF increases the range of Doppler shift frequencies that can be displayed. Decreasing the PRF will increase the sensitivity of the system but will reduce the frame rate. There must be a fine balance between frame rate and sensitivity (Fig. 2.5).

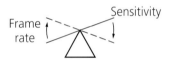

Fig. 2.5 Frame rate vs sensitivity.

Whatever combination of scanning systems is used, the more that is asked of the machine, the slower it will be, i.e. the frame rate will decrease.

Factors affecting sensitivity and frame rate in PWD systems

Sensitivity will be increased if:

- power output is increased

- transducer frequency is higher

- PRF is lowered

- angle of the Doppler beam to the vessel is optimum

- receiver gain is set to a level which will allow background noise to be just visible, while the sample volume is set to the full range of velocities within the vessel under examination.

The frame rate can be increased if:

- a higher frequency transducer is used

- width of the scan sector is decreased

- magnification of the B-mode image is increased

- single rather than double line density is used

- fewer things are asked of the equipment, i.e. use is made of B-mode and PWD (duplex scanning) rather than B-mode, PWD and CD (triplex scanning).

To obtain an optimum image with PWD:

- use the appropriate frequency transducer for the part under investigation

- magnify the image

- reduce the sector width to obtain a higher frame rate

- position sample volume before pulsed Doppler is used

- use the best angle (at least <60°)

- activate spectral Doppler and freeze B-mode if possible to obtain a clearer trace.

Colour Doppler (CD)

This technique combines conventional real-time B-mode scanning and real-time two-dimensional Doppler imaging. In a selected area of the image, the mean velocity and variance are estimated by analysing all sample volumes for Doppler shift signals. As this can be from a relatively large area, information is obtained at the expense of the grey-scale image. As it takes longer to obtain the Doppler information, the larger the area of CD sampled, the lower the frame rate and line density become. The colour area must be kept as small as possible to produce an optimum image.

With CD, blood flow images in colour can be placed over a real-time B-mode image. Velocity in each direction is quantified by allocating one pixel to each area. Each velocity frequency change is allocated a colour. The allocated colours are often red for flow towards the transducer and blue for flow away from the transducer (it should not be seen as red for arteries and blue for veins). Vessels can be distinguished from each other and from ducts in order to evaluate arterial supply and venous drainage of organs. Change of flow pattern can help to differentiate between normal variants and neoplasms.

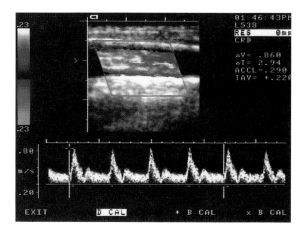

Fig. 2.6 Example of colour flow and pulsed wave Doppler.

> **Box 2.2   Advice**
>
> Although direction is clearly shown and areas of stenosis can be demonstrated by CD, an apparent lack of flow can sometimes be seen in a normal vessel if the Doppler beam is positioned at 90° to it. Careful angling of the probe relative to the vessel helps to eliminate this artefact.

Aliasing in CD

As CD is a sampling technique, the Nyquist limit still applies, as in PWD, and aliasing can occur if that limit is exceeded. Instead of a waveform wrapping around above and below the baseline, aliasing shows as a sudden change in a block of colour from one bright colour to another. An area of reversed flow can sometimes cause this appearance. As the velocity or frequency shift depends on the angle of the signal to vessel, a change in colour can be attributed to a change in angle that might be seen when scanning a tortuous vessel.

CD controls in addition to PWD controls

COLOUR GAIN

Amplifies the returning signals. If set too high, there is bleeding of colour into surrounding tissue. If too low, no or little colour is seen.

COLOUR BOX SIZE

Colour box size is important. It has a significant effect on frame rate, this increasing as the box is reduced to the area of interest. A frame rate of 10/s is acceptable. The width and depth of the box are important. The best images are produced when the width of the box is as small as possible.

WALL FILTER

Wall filter sets the lowest frequency or velocity that will be seen as a colour. An increase in the filter prevents a fill of colour to the edge of the vessel. Set to 50–100 Hz.

VELOCITY OR FREQUENCY SCALE

This controls the display of flow velocities. It must be adjusted so that the velocity is near to the top of the colour scale without aliasing.

BASELINE SHIFT

This helps to make better use of the velocity ranges for unidirectional flow by moving the baseline up and down the colour scale.

PACKET SIZE OR COLOUR SENSITIVITY

Controls the number of pulses used to create one line of colour information. The larger the packet, the greater the sensitivity but the lower the frame rate.

PERSISTENCE

Persistence controls the colour image average between the frames. Increased persistence increases the image's signal to noise ratio.

PIXEL SIZE

Only available on some equipment; increases spatial resolution at the expense of frame rate.

Factors increasing the sensitivity and frame rate of CD systems

Sensitivity will be increased if:

- the same factors as for PWD systems are used
- colour sensitivity is increased
- persistence (frame averaging, colour averaging or smoothing) is increased.

Frame rate will be increased if:

- the same factors as for PWD systems are used
- duplex rather than triplex scanning is undertaken.

To obtain an optimum image using CD:

- follow the steps used for PWD
- keep the colour box as narrow as possible
- set the colour gain so that the colour does not bleed outside the walls of the vessels
- adjust the PRF to allow colour to fill in the lumen as far as the walls.

When using CD and PWD together:

- find the vessel using CD
- superimpose the sample volume on the B-mode image of the vessel without using PWD
- obtain the optimum angle
- apply the PWD and freeze the B-mode and CD to obtain the best spectral trace.

Power Doppler (PD)

PD is an additional feature on many colour flow machines. The power or amount of sound energy reflected back to the transducer from each point or pixel is coded in colour. Red blood cells are about 1% of the wavelength of the sound and the power of the sound scattered back to the transducer increases as the fourth power of the frequency. The power scattered back is almost proportional to the number of blood cells at a point. The scattering of blood in several directions does not much affect the value as the Doppler shift is only used to detect movement.

PD gives no information about the direction of blood flow. Variations in colour represent different numbers of blood cells. PD displays energy rather than movement and is four times more sensitive to movement of slow blood flow rates than CD but frame rate and resolution are not as good. The images can be considered as variations in blood flow distribution rather than blood flow velocity. PD is less angle dependent than CD and so is better for vessels lying at right angles to the probe. A concise resumé of PD is given in Evans.[1]

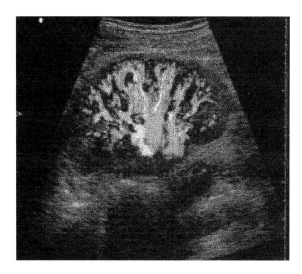

Fig. 2.7 Power Doppler image of kidney.

The use of Doppler as part of the upper abdominal scan

Doppler is now used to provide further information during an ultrasound examination and it is recommended that it is used as an integral part of the examination when it is appropriate to do so. It is especially useful when assessing blood flow in the patient with portal hypertension, the renal and liver transplant patient, abdominal aortic aneurysm graft follow-up, arterial stenoses and arteriovenous malformations and blood supply to tumours, with even more information revealed with the recent addition of ultrasound contrast media. However, there are still many aspects of abdominal diagnosis where colour is not required. Power Doppler is useful for looking at lower velocities (seen in the normal upper abdominal organs with low vascular resistance (Fig. 2.7)) although the improved quality of colour flow imaging has reduced the impact of PD. Below is a summary of the general applications of the use of colour in the upper abdomen.

Liver

- Differentiation of common duct from portal vein and hepatic artery.
- Differentiation of intrahepatic blood vessels from bile ducts.
- Observing hyperaemia in cholecystitis.
- Defining a vascular supply to tumours (Fig. 2.8).

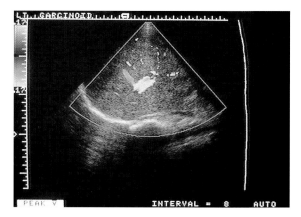

Fig. 2.8 Vascular supply to liver tumour.

- Defining and assessing transplant vessels.
- Defining hepatic veins assessing hepatic veins in liver transplants (Fig. 2.9) and in patients with the Budd–Chiari syndrome (Fig. 2.10).
- Helping to differentiate between haemangioma and malignancy (Fig. 2.11).

Gallbladder

Confirming the presence of varices in the gallbladder wall (Fig. 2.12).

Portal venous system

- Confirming portal vein patency.
- Assessing direction of portal vein blood flow in portal hypertension.
- Confirming presence of thrombus and stenosis/occlusion.

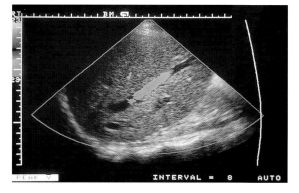

Fig. 2.9 Longitudinal section of liver showing hepatic vein.

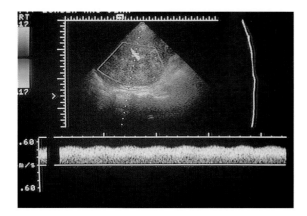

Fig. 2.10 Hepatic vein obstruction in Budd–Chiari syndrome.

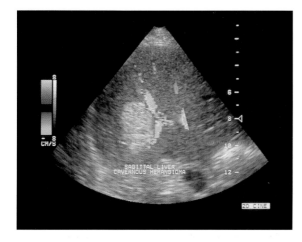

Fig. 2.11 Vessels bending around a haemangioma in the liver.

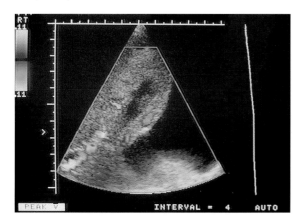

Fig. 2.12 Varices in a thick-walled gallbladder (note ascites).

- Confirming presence of varices in portal hypertension such as under left lobe of liver and around splenic hilum.

Mesenteric vessels

Identifying stenosis, occlusion, variations in normal appearance or aneurysmal formation.

Bowel wall

Identifying hyperaemia of appendix and bowel wall (indication of inflammation).

Pancreas

Differentiating the splenic artery from the duct.

Abdominal aorta

- Identifying stenosis, thrombus, aneurysmal formation and the position of other vessels of aortic origin relative to an aneurysm.
- Confirmation of dissection or dissecting aneurysm.

Inferior vena cava

- Identifying thrombus, tumour extension and occlusion.
- Confirming filter position.

Renal system

- Observation of ureteric jets (Fig. 2.13).
- Can help to confirm renal artery stenosis.

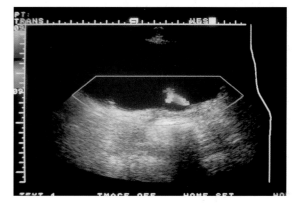

Fig. 2.13 Left-sided ureteric jet.

- Pre- and posttransplant assessment – vascular complications, arterial occlusion, renal vein thrombosis (Fig. 2.14).

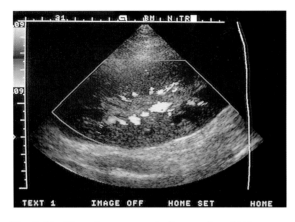

Fig. 2.14 Normal appearances in the transplanted kidney.

Colour Doppler is still not as useful in determining benign or malignant tumours as was hoped originally. It is not a good screening tool for renal artery stenosis as even with the use of contrast, its sensitivity is only about 75%. It is not useful in acute rejection of the post-transplant kidney and has little use in the assessment of the spleen. Its main use within the upper abdomen seems to be in the demonstration of the change of flow and the general appearance of vessels.

Reference

1. Evans DH 1998 Theory and application of power Doppler. Reflections 3: 8–10

3

THE LIVER

Main functions
Anatomy
Scanning
Normal ultrasound appearances
Pathology
Focal lesions
Benign focal lesions
Malignant focal lesions
Infective lesions
Trauma
Diffuse diseases
Portal hypertension
Vessel related pathology
The abnormal liver
Liver biopsy
Liver transplant

The liver is the largest organ in the body and also the largest acoustic window. It weighs 1.4–1.8 kg in the male and 1.2–1.4 kg in the female. It represents approximately one-fortieth of the total body weight in the adult compared with one-eighth in the foetus and neonate. It is roughly wedge shaped with the thin edge on the left.

Main functions

- Production of 700–1200 ml of bile every day, the removal of bilirubin formed from broken-down cells in the blood and its excretion in the bile. If bile cannot pass into the duodenum, serum bilirubin level rises and jaundice develops.

- Formation of most of the plasma proteins which are concerned with reabsorption of tissue fluid, a lack of which causes oedema.

- Prevention of intravascular clotting of blood by the formation of heparin.

- Regulation of blood clotting by the formation of prothrombin and fibrinogen.

- Formation of glycogen (used to maintain normal blood glucose) from excess carbohydrate, surplus protein and fat. Failure or removal of the liver can eventually lead to a fatal fall in blood glucose level (hypoglycaemia).

- Regulation of transport of fat stores.

- Storage of certain vitamins, minerals and sugars.

- Storage of antianaemic factor, vitamin B12, until required and vitamins A and D.

- Metabolism of alcohol and modification of some drugs so that they can be excreted by the kidneys.

- Removal of the nitrogenous parts of amino acids and their conversion to urea, ultimately excreted in the kidneys.

- Storage of iron.

- Formation of antibodies, production of immune factors and removal of bacteria from the blood-stream.

- Control of production and excretion of cholesterol.

- Formation of up to half of the body's lymph supply.

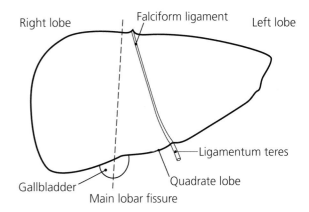

Fig. 3.1 Anterior aspect of liver.

Anatomy

The liver consists of five surfaces: superior, anterior, posterior, right lateral and inferior (visceral). The surfaces merge at the borders which are all rounded except for the inferior border between the anterior and visceral surfaces, which is sharply defined in the normal liver.

The majority of the liver is situated in the right hypochondrium, passing across (according to body shape) into the epigastrium and left hypochondrium. It is protected by ribs and costal cartilage. Its upper surface is smooth and curved and lies under the right hemidiaphragm. It consists of four lobes: a large right lobe and a smaller left lobe (one-sixteenth of the size of the right lobe) consisting of the smaller quadrate and caudate lobes in the inferior or visceral surface. The quadrate lobe is now usually referred to as the medial segment of the left lobe and, together with the lateral segment, forms the left lobe. The quadrate lobe or medial segment lies anteriorly and is bordered by the ligamentum teres on the left and by the gallbladder on the right. The caudate lobe lies posteriorly and is bordered by the ligamentum venosum on the left and the IVC on the right (Fig. 3.1).

The superior surface of the liver is smooth and is attached to the diaphragm by the coronary and right and left triangular peritoneal ligaments. The visceral surface is complex as it contains a hilum (also known as the porta hepatis or portal fissure) and numerous fossae and fissures for ligaments. The hilum allows passage of vessels and ducts in and out of the liver. These are the portal vein, the hepatic artery, the bile duct, sympathetic and parasympathetic nerve fibres and lymph vessels.

The fossae (indentations or impressions) caused by contact with adjacent organs are:

- right lobe:
  - colic impression from the hepatic flexure of the colon
  - right renal impression from the right kidney
  - right adrenal impression
  - duodenal impression
- left lobe: gastric impression from the stomach (Fig. 3.2).

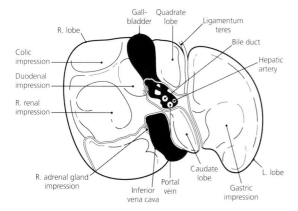

Fig. 3.2 Posterior aspect of liver.

The liver is traditionally divided into left and right lobes by the falciform ligament which releases the ligamentum teres (the obliterated remnant of the left umbilical vein) as it continues to the umbilicus and diaphragm anteriorly. It becomes the ligamentum venosum (the remnant of the ductus venosus) as it continues posteriorly towards the IVC. The liver is more usually divided into eight segments proposed by Couinaud in 1954. These segments are divided by the portal and hepatic veins and are used when planning surgery or describing the precise position of a tumour prior to treatment (Fig. 3.3).

The posterior surface has a deep concavity in the middle where the liver is in contact with the spine and a groove to the right where the IVC runs through. The anterior surface is attached to the anterior wall by the falciform ligament, a sickle-shaped double fold of peritoneum.

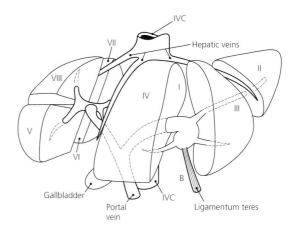

Fig. 3.3 Liver segments according to Couinaud.

Blood supply

The portal vein supplies the liver with approximately 80% of its blood, nutrients and other substances from the stomach, spleen, pancreas and small and large intestines.

The hepatic artery, originating from the coeliac axis at the upper anterior part of the abdominal aorta, supplies the other 20%.

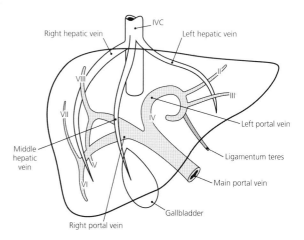

Fig. 3.4 Portal supply and hepatic drainage.

Blood drainage

The liver is drained by three main hepatic veins: the right, middle and left hepatic veins. They empty into the upper part of the IVC just below the diaphragm, the right separately and the middle and left joining to form a common trunk to empty into the anterior part of the IVC. Some short hepatic veins, the inferior group, drain parts of the liver in contact with the IVC and caudate lobe.

Bile drainage

The right and left hepatic ducts join in or just outside the liver to form the common hepatic duct through which bile flows en route to the gallbladder and duodenum. The hilum is bounded by the quadrate lobe in front and the caudate lobe behind.

Lymph drainage

Lymph vessels drain into the hepatic group of nodes which lie along the course of the hepatic artery and leave the liver via the hilum, passing through the hepatoduodenal ligament. Thus the hilum is a point of interest when lymph nodes enlarge.

Position of vessels

The portal vein lies posterior to the bile duct and hepatic artery, the bile duct lying anterolaterally and the hepatic artery anteromedially. As the portal vein enters the liver, it branches and the right branch veers to the right and soon divides into anterior and posterior parts. The left branch curves to the left and anteriorly and gives off branches to the rest of the right and left lobes. The branches of the hepatic artery and the bile ducts follow those of the portal veins.

Although the right and left lobes have been described as being divided by the falciform ligament, the distribution of the right and left vessels is different. The main lobar fissure separating the right and left lobes of the liver runs between the gallbladder bed and the IVC. The fissure runs approximately along the course of the middle hepatic vein. In effect, this makes the functional right and left lobes about equal in size and explains the equal size of the associated vessels. The left portal vein supplies the quadrate lobe and part of the caudate lobe as well as the left lobe.

The IVC itself lies within a groove on the posterior surface of the liver, to the right of the midline. It is sometimes enclosed by liver tissue. The abdominal aorta lies posterior to the caudate lobe of the liver in

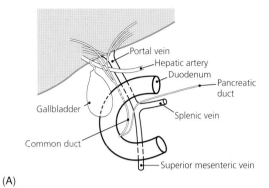

(A)

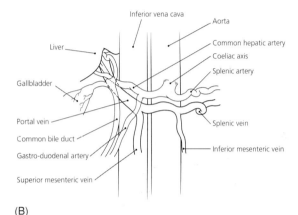

(B)

Fig. 3.5 (A) The hepatobiliary and portal vessels. (B) Vessels and ducts of the upper abdomen.

the retroperitoneum, just in front and to the left of the upper four lumbar vertebrae (Fig. 3.5).

Relations

- Superiorly and anteriorly – diaphragm and anterior abdominal wall.

- Inferiorly – stomach, bile ducts, duodenum, right colic flexure of the colon, right kidney and adrenal gland.

- Posteriorly – oesophagus, inferior vena cava, aorta, gallbladder, vertebrae, diaphragm.

Surface markings

The anterior surface is delineated superiorly by a line running from just below the right nipple (5th rib) through the xiphisternal joint to just below and medial to the left nipple in the mid-clavicular line. The right

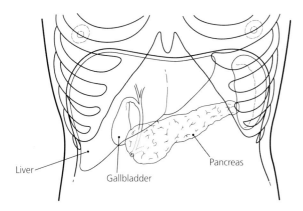

Fig. 3.6 Surface markings of the liver.

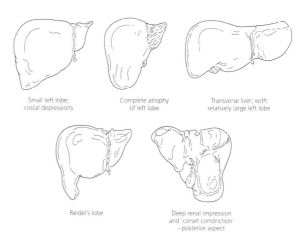

Small left lobe; costal depressions

Complete atrophy of left lobe

Transverse liver; with relatively large left lobe

Reidel's lobe

Deep renal impression and 'corset constriction' - posterior aspect

Fig. 3.7 Variations in liver shapes.

border extends to approximately 1 cm below the lower costal margin and the lower border is a line running from this point crossing the midline at the transpyloric plane and joining the lateral border of the left lobe below and medial to the left nipple (Fig. 3.6).

Variations in normal anatomy

- Reidel's lobes are tongue-like inferior projections of the right lobe lying anterior to the right kidney. They are often 2–5 cm long and irregularly shaped with a narrowing at the neck (almost pedunculated) or appear as an inferior extension. They are congenital anomalies often mistaken for an enlarged gallbladder, pancreatic or renal mass or hepatomegaly. Reidel's lobes usually accompany a smaller left lobe.

- The caudate lobe may be small or have a tongue extending inferiorly below the inferior border of the left lobe.

- The size of the left lobe may be reduced with compensatory hypertrophy of the right lobe with deep costal impressions.

- Absence of the left lobe is rare and results from occlusion of the left hepatic vein.

- There may be atrophy of the left lobe as a result of left portal vein compression.

- Alteration of the normal liver shape in females owing to tightly constrictive dressing has not been witnessed of late (Fig. 3.7).

- Complete or partial situs inversus is not unknown but is comparatively rare.

Palpation

With the patient supine, place the left hand behind the right lower ribs. The right hand is placed against the edge of the right rib cage and should press inwards and upwards. Ask the patient to take a deep breath in. The edge of the liver may be felt as the patient breathes in. Just by looking at the patient, the liver may be visible on respiration, especially if the patient is thin. A normal liver edge should be felt as a firm, sharp, smooth ridge. The fingertips of both hands may also be used as shown in Figure 3.8B.

Liver function and relevant tests – normal values

Serum α-fetoprotein (AFP)	<12 μg/l
Carcinoembryonic antigen (CEA)	0–2.5 μg/l
Serum bilirubin	<20 μmol/l
Alanine aminotransferase (ALT)	5–30 U/l
Aspartate aminotransferase (AST)	10–40 U/l
Alkaline phosphatase (ALP)	20–90 U/l
Serum albumin	35–55 g/l
Blood clotting time (prothrombin time)	12–16 s
γ-Glutamyl transpeptidase	11–50 U/l male, 7–32 U/l female

There is a wide variation of normal values according to age and sex. These are normally given in parentheses on the haematology forms. In the pathology section, raised and lowered test results will be indicated rather than definitive values.

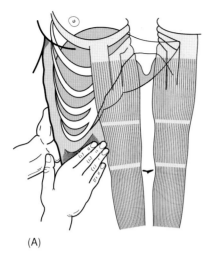

(A)

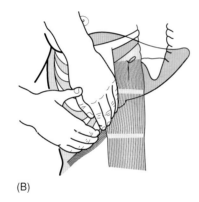

(B)

Fig. 3.8 (A, B) Palpating the liver.

Scanning

Patient preparation

The normal abdominal preparation is as follows.

- Fast for six hours in order to distend the gallbladder and use it as a landmark. Non-fizzy, non-fatty drinks may be taken but ensure no other tests on the same day require a nil-by-mouth preparation.

- Children can fast for four hours and babies can have a bottle of dextrose instead of the normal milky feed if the biliary system is being examined. Otherwise no preparation need be insisted upon for babies and children.

- Babies and diabetic patients should be placed first on the list for the scan.

Equipment required

Use a 3.5–5 MHz transducer (sector/curved linear) for an adult or child, 7.5 MHz for a baby. Adjust the power output, receiver gain and total gain control and focusing zone to obtain an even grey-scale image from the front to the back of the liver. A sector transducer with a small footprint is useful for intercostal scanning of the liver, although small curved linear transducers can be used when the choice is limited.

Suggested scanning technique

The possible position of the liver according to the patient type should be noted, as should the many barriers to scanning the liver. The barriers to scanning the liver are the lungs and diaphragm above and to the right, ribs to the side and in front, muscle and ribs at the back, gas-filled hepatic flexure and transverse colon below and the stomach and small bowel below and to the left.

The liver can be scanned with the patient in the following positions:

- supine
- left posterior oblique (LPO)
- left lateral decubitus (LLD).

Sections obtained when scanning the liver are traditionally:

- longitudinal
- transverse
- oblique.

Scanning approaches are:

- subcostally
- intercostally.

Patient positions

SUPINE

This should be done with quiet respiration or inspiration if necessary. It entirely depends on the patient.

Longitudinal sections

Place the transducer in the midline just below the xiphisternum. Angle the transducer up and down if necessary to view the diaphragm and the inferior border.

The inferior border should appear sharp (blunting of the inferior border suggests diffuse liver disease). Angle the transducer slowly as far left as possible until out of the left lobe. Look for the left lobe and left hepatic vein. Return slowly to the midline, see the portal vein and middle hepatic vein. Angle slightly towards the right to see as much of the right lobe as possible, again angling up and down. Look for the ligamentum venosum and the aorta and IVC in longitudinal sections.

Move the transducer to the right, still in the longitudinal position. Look for the right hepatic vein, portal vein and bile ducts. Angle upwards underneath the ribs to see the liver. Look for the right kidney and compare its texture with that of the liver. At this point you may start to hit colonic gas. Avoid this by asking the patient to breathe in deeply to force the liver down more under the ribs or, better, by turning the patient into the LLD position (described p 37). Before turning the patient, look for any free fluid that may be lying over the surface of the liver or lateral to it or in the sub-hepatic space.

If little can be seen subcostally, you will need to scan intercostally. Position the footprint of the transducer against an intercostal space in the axillary line so that the plane of the scan lies parallel to the intercostal space. If it does not lie parallel, shadows from the ribs will be apparent. The patient can raise their arms above their head to increase the intercostal space (inspiration will raise the ribs – the bucket handle effect). These sections will thus be longitudinal coronal views. Scans should also be made from different intercostal spaces. Intercostal scanning will better demonstrate the lateral aspect of the liver. You will probably have to scan at a higher intercostal space than you think; not too high though, remember that the diaphragm curves down laterally and will come between the transducer and the liver.

Transverse sections

Start with the transducer placed transversely in the subxiphisternal area. Angle to left and right as far as can be seen in order to show left and right lobes. Angle the transducer towards the head to see the diaphragm, as much of both lobes as possible, as much texture as possible and the confluence of the three hepatic veins into the IVC. Identify the ligamentum teres between the left and right lobes.

Oblique sections

Scan with the long axis of the ultrasound beam at right angles to the lower costal margin. This theoretically

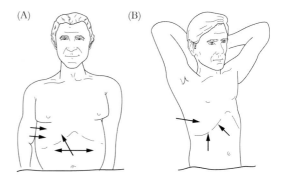

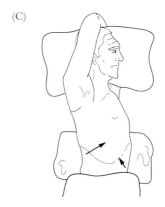

Fig. 3.9 Scanning positions. (A) Supine. (B) Left posterior oblique position. (C) Left lateral decubitus position.

should give the largest slice area of liver. Look carefully at the porta hepatis and the vessels entering the liver.

Having started by scanning the liver with the patient supine, gas will often be displaced and better images obtained by turning the patient into the LPO or LLD positions. The relationship of the transducer to the body surface is almost the same as when the patient lies supine.

LPO POSITION

Turn the patient 45° towards the left side and provide support so that the patient is comfortable. Raise the right arm to help raise the ribs. The liver should fall slightly inferiorly to allow better access and gas in the large intestine should rise up and away from the mid-portion of the abdomen.

LLD POSITION

Turn the patient a further 45° towards the left so that they are lying on the left side with hips and knees flexed slightly to encourage stability in this position. This is an alternative to the LPO position and allows an obese abdomen to fall away from the region of interest. It is expected that flexibility of technique and thought for the patient's condition will decide whether to turn the patient or not (Fig. 3.9).

Box 3.1   Advice

While scanning the patient's liver, all vessels should be traced and observed for size and regularity. Texture should be observed for normality. Adjacent organs and vessels should be noted for normality and any free fluid noted or excluded around the liver. It is essential that all the liver is seen, from diaphragm to inferior border. Subphrenic pathology can often be missed owing to poor technique.

It may be that the liver appears small yet the spleen is quite large. This may be a case of visceral transposition: check the vessels entering and leaving both organs.

Techniques for infants and neonates

A 5 MHz or 7.5 MHz sector or curved linear transducer, depending on the size of the subject, combined with careful focusing and gain control settings should be used for scanning the infant's and neonate's liver. The liver can be scanned from the front with the subject lying supine on the couch.

Suggested minimal sections

- Longitudinal sections – one of the left lobe to show the diaphragm and inferior border, vessels, texture and shape.

- Two of the right lobe – one including the right kidney to compare echogenicity.

- Transverse sections – three sections showing the hepatic veins and the confluence towards the IVC, the texture and the caudate lobe.

- Longitudinal oblique – one section to show the porta hepatis and portal vein, hepatic artery and common duct and a section at right angles to this to demonstrate a cross-section of the vessels.

Normal ultrasound appearances

Providing that the gain settings of the ultrasound equipment are correctly adjusted, a normal liver should appear as a sponge of mid-grey echoes, uniform throughout (homogeneous) and interrupted only by blood vessels, intrahepatic bile ducts (seen as branching, echo-free tubes) and ligaments. Normal liver texture should be a lighter shade of grey (higher reflectivity) than normal renal texture, darker than normal pancreatic texture (lower reflectivity) and approximately the same as that of the normal spleen (isoechoic).

The extreme left border of the left lobe and right border of the right lobe are difficult to visualize owing to their proximity to stomach and ribs respectively. The inferior border should have a sharp border as a blunt or rounded border usually indicates some form of diffuse liver disease (Fig. 3.10).

The hepatic vessels seen within the liver are as follows.

- Hepatic veins – these run superiorly and posteriorly, curving towards the IVC. Their walls are usually not discernibly echogenic as they are essentially sinusoids within the liver and have thin or absent walls. They are seen to taper, the widest part of the vessels (up to 10 mm) lying nearest to the IVC.

- Portal vein – this has a maximum diameter of approximately 13 mm and is usually about 10 mm in diameter. It has a bright, thicker, more highly reflective fibro-fatty wall. It enters the liver and branches laterally towards the right before dividing into anterior and posterior branches. The left branch curves anteriorly and to the left.

- Common duct (the common hepatic and common bile ducts are considered as one duct) – seen as a small tube with thin white walls. It lies anterolaterally to the portal vein, measures approximately 4–5 mm in diameter at a point where the hepatic artery crosses the portal vein. It is said to measure 1 mm for each decade of life. The normal intrahepatic bile ducts are too small to be seen, being a maximum of 2 mm in diameter.

- Hepatic artery – runs anteromedially to the portal vein then usually courses laterally, running between the portal vein and the common duct. There is a wide variation of positions in which the hepatic artery can lie, 10–15% lying anterior to the common duct (Fig. 3.11).

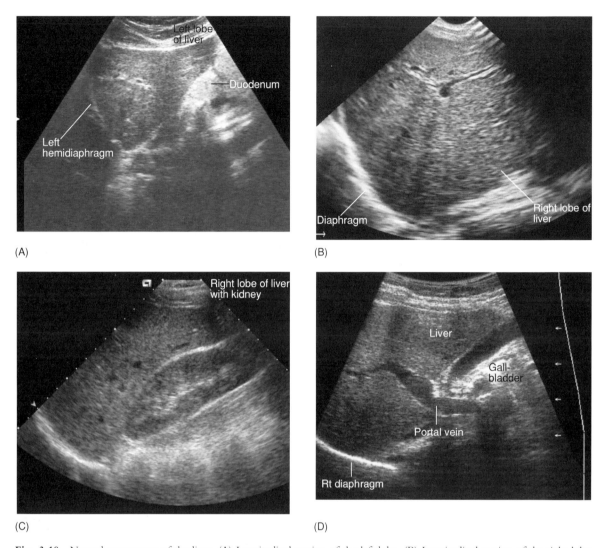

Fig. 3.10 Normal appearances of the liver. (A) Longitudinal section of the left lobe. (B) Longitudinal section of the right lobe. (C) Right lobe of liver with right kidney. (D) Portal vein entering the liver.

Other structures

The falciform ligament, containing the ligamentum teres, appears between the right and left lobes. This is a fibrous structure surrounded by fat and appears as a rounded, highly reflective mass in cross-sections of the liver and as a reflective band in longitudinal section (Fig. 3.11E).

The main interlobar fissure separates the left and right lobes and connects the gallbladder bed and the IVC.

The ligamentum venosum lying anterior to the caudate lobe causes this part of the liver to appear to be

of lower reflectivity than the rest of the liver and can appear like a liver mass (Fig. 3.12).

Normal sizes

The normal liver is considered to be approximately 10–13 cm long (although up to 15 cm has been reported) from diaphragm to inferior border in the right mid-clavicular line. The word 'approximately' is used here as there is much reported variation in normality. If the upper abdominal organs are normal,

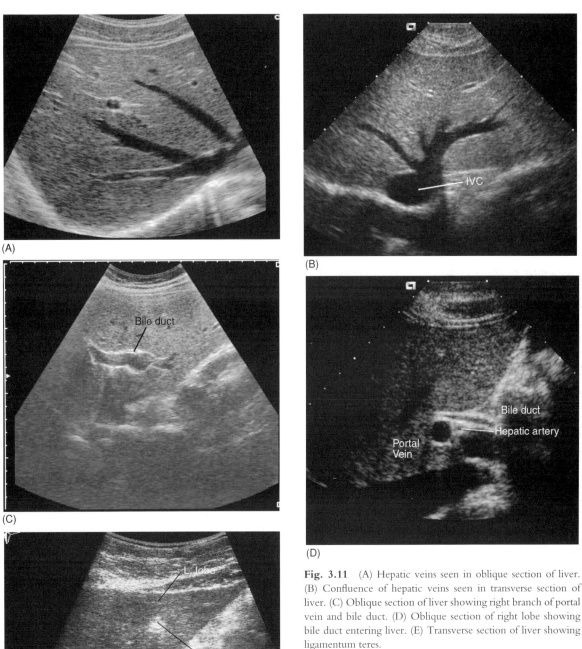

Fig. 3.11 (A) Hepatic veins seen in oblique section of liver. (B) Confluence of hepatic veins seen in transverse section of liver. (C) Oblique section of liver showing right branch of portal vein and bile duct. (D) Oblique section of right lobe showing bile duct entering liver. (E) Transverse section of liver showing ligamentum teres.

the liver is considered enlarged if the inferior border extends well below the right kidney. This rule cannot work if the kidney is situated close to the diaphragm, as is seen in hypersthenic patients.

The normal caudate lobe is less than two-thirds of the right lobe at the level of the portal vein.

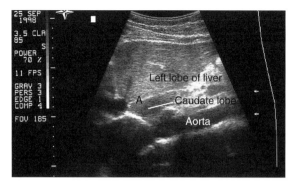

Fig. 3.12 Caudate lobe, normal size. A = Ligamentum venosum.

For sizes of the vessels within the liver, see above section on normal appearances.

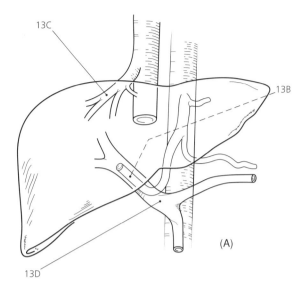

(A)

Box 3.2   Advice

There are reasons for apparent hepatomegaly as felt by palpation that are not necessarily caused by abdominal pathology.

- Flattened diaphragm from obstructive airways disease

- Pleural effusion

- Subphrenic mass/abscess

- Reidel's lobe – the liver usually has a small left lobe

- Low right kidney

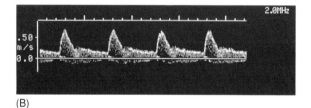

(B)

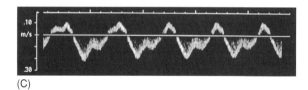

(C)

Normal pulsed wave Doppler

The hepatic artery demonstrates low resistance of the vessels in the liver characterized by a high diastolic phase (Fig. 3.13A). The hepatic veins are characterized by their triphasic waveform (Fig. 3.13B). The portal vein shows a continuous flow pattern modulated by respiratory variations with a mean velocity of about 15 cm/s (wide range of 12–20 cm/s) (Fig. 3.13C).

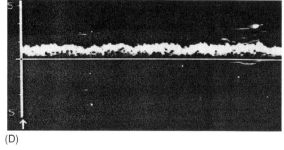

(D)

Fig. 3.13 (A) Hepatic vessels and their Spectral Doppler signals. (B) Normal spectral Doppler hepatic artery waveform. (C) Normal spectral Doppler hepatic vein waveform. (D) Normal spectral Doppler portal vein flow.

Pathology

Can be divided according to ultrasound appearances into focal and diffuse pathology.

Focal

- Cyst – simple and multiple
- Haemangioma
- Tumours – benign and malignant
- Infective lesions
- Trauma

Diffuse

- Hepatitis
- Fatty infiltration
- Cirrhosis
- Portal hypertension
- Congestive cardiac disease
- Vessel related pathology

Focal lesions

Focal lesions can be single or multiple, benign or malignant. It is sometimes hard to say definitely to which organ the lesion is attributable (hepatic/renal, for example), especially if the lesion is large. If it is hepatic in origin, the lesion will move with the movement of the liver on respiration or will often distort the vessels around it. When difficulties in identifying the origin of the tumour remain, other imaging modalities such as CT or MRI should be used to complement the ultrasound examination.

Lesions of the liver can cause hepatomegaly although there is a wide range of normal shapes and sizes. Diffuse and other malignant disease can cause rounding of the inferior border of the liver, although sometimes Reidel's lobes are present in a normal liver and give the appearance of a rounded free edge. Focal lesions or nodules can deviate the course of the hepatic veins or cause the appearance of lumps on the surface of the liver, seen especially in the presence of ascites. They can show as indentations on the surface of the diaphragm or on the wall of the larger intrahepatic blood vessels. Malignant disease, especially the more aggressive type such as primary hepatocellular carcinoma (HCC), can invade the portal and hepatic veins and eventually occlude them and in some cases invasion of the IVC can occur. Doppler examinations can be used to demonstrate lack of or reversed blood flow. Bile ducts can also be invaded and occlude causing intrahepatic duct dilatation. Jaundice rarely occurs with early malignant involvement because the liver is capable of compensating for one segment when excreting bile. Jaundice will only occur when the liver is extensively replaced by tumour.

ULTRASOUND APPEARANCES: GENERAL

Focal liver lesions can be divided into several ultrasonic patterns.

- Hyperechoic – the tumour is more highly reflective than the normal liver texture surrounding it, e.g. haemangiomas, fat.

- Hypoechoic – lesion is of lower reflectivity than the surrounding normal liver texture and is homogeneous, e.g. small hepatocellular carcinomas.

- Target (bull's eye) lesion – isoechoic to or more highly reflective than the normal texture with a hypoechoic rim or halo around it. Thin rims (1–2 mm) are seen with expansive hepatocellular carcinomas; thick rims (3–5 mm) are often seen with metastatic lesions.

- Mixed echo lesion – hyper- and hypoechoic areas within the lesion are usually seen where bleeding or degeneration occurs within a hyperechoic mass.

- Mosaic pattern lesion – seen rarely in large (4 cm+) tumours such as hepatocellular carcinomas. Echo-poor septations produce a 'tumour within tumour' pattern.

- Lesion with central necrosis (cystic) – a central anechoic area is seen, especially in metastases from malignancies of female reproductive system.

- Calcified lesions – uncommon; show as highly reflective with distal acoustic shadowing. Seen in metastases from mucin-producing primary cancers of the stomach or colon.

- Diffuse infiltrative lesion – seen when a multi-nodular hepatocellular carcinoma enlarges; the contour is indistinct.

- Cystic lesions – have few, if any, internal echoes and demonstrate posterior enhancement. Mostly benign.

> **Box 3.3 Advice**
>
> It is extremely difficult to correlate ultrasonic appearances to the nature or type of lesion. The role of ultrasound is to:
>
> - investigate the reason for a patient's liver being enlarged and to confirm or exclude focal lesions as being the cause, or
> - discover that a low-lying kidney, a renal tumour, grossly enlarged lymph nodes, an enlarged gallbladder, diffuse liver disease or a Reidel's lobe is in fact the reason for an apparent hepatomegaly.

Benign focal lesions

Simple cyst

CLINICAL INFORMATION

Cysts are often congenital developmental failures of the biliary tree; they are more common in the middle-aged and elderly and in women more than men. They can also form as a result of trauma or abscess. They do not often cause pain and are not palpable. Liver biochemistry is not changed.

ULTRASOUND APPEARANCES

Cysts are smooth, thin walled and well circumscribed. They contain clear fluid and therefore have no internal echoes but demonstrate acoustic enhancement posteriorly. Occasionally they have thin internal septations which are not considered to be a cause for concern (Fig. 3.14).

> **Box 3.4 Advice**
>
> Ensure no other lesion is hidden by the acoustic enhancement behind the cyst: change direction of the ultrasound beam. Acoustic enhancement is not seen if the cyst is anterior to other highly reflective structures such as the diaphragm.
>
> Intrahepatic gallbladders or high choledochal cysts have been mistaken for cysts. If irregular walls and/or internal echoes are present, this may indicate abscess, tumour degeneration, haematoma or necrotic metastasis. (Ensure internal echoes are not produced by incorrect gain settings.) Patients are often referred for guided aspiration and cytological analysis of the cyst content if any doubt exists.

Multiple cysts – polycystic disease

CLINICAL INFORMATION

The liver is often enlarged because of the presence of cysts. Cysts in the liver are most commonly seen in patients with polycystic disease (seen in approximately 40% of patients with polycystic renal disease). Sixty percent of patients with polycystic liver disease (an inherited defect in the formation of bile ducts) have associated renal cysts.

ULTRASOUND APPEARANCES

Cysts are of differing sizes and shapes and may present as one or two cysts positioned at random within the liver substance or as almost all the liver being taken up by cystic material. The acoustic enhancement behind multiple cysts can produce an abnormally bright liver pattern.

Polycystic disease involving the liver often causes hepatomegaly because of the amount or size of the cysts. These can produce discomfort or pain if haemorrhage or if infection occurs in any of the cysts. These cysts are clinically insignificant and do not interfere with the liver function (Fig. 3.15).

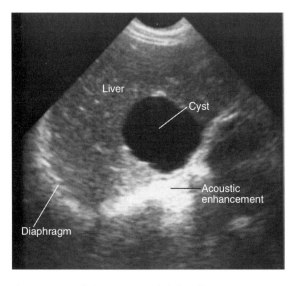

Fig. 3.14 Single liver cyst in right lobe of liver.

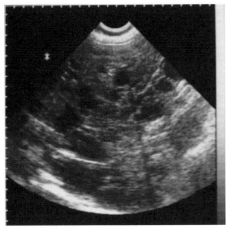

(A)

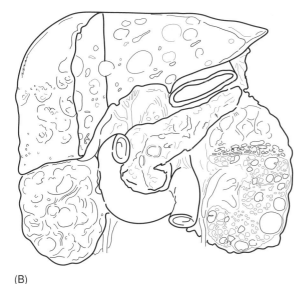

(B)

Fig. 3.15 (A) Hepatic involvement in polycystic renal disease. (B) Upper abdominal organs involved in polycystic renal disease.

Box 3.5   Advice

It is difficult to ensure that other pathology is not being masked by acoustic enhancement. Try to scan from other directions.

Multiple cysts can appear like multiple echo-poor metastases and grossly dilated intrahepatic duct dilatation, both of which can produce similar appearances of echo-poor areas with acoustic enhancement.

Haemangioma

CLINICAL INFORMATION

The cavernous haemangioma is the most common benign liver tumour; 70–95% are seen in women, the frequency increasing with age. Haemangiomas can also be seen in children who can present with hepatomegaly, cutaneous haemangiomas and congestive cardiac failure (CCF). There is often an increase in morbidity/mortality in these cases. Haemangiomas can rupture into the peritoneum but can also regress spontaneously. Neonates with haemangiomas may be very sick and require urgent treatment.

ULTRASOUND APPEARANCES

The majority of haemangiomas are small (<2 cm in diameter), well defined, highly reflective from multiple small blood vessels and are homogeneous in appearance. They are more common in the right lobe, tend towards a peripheral location near the hepatic capsule or near to blood vessels and are more frequently solitary but are sometimes multiple. Larger haemangiomas may develop a slightly lobular margin. Occasionally the larger haemangiomas produce a faint distal acoustic enhancement, probably related to their vascularity, but usually they do not enhance. As they undergo degeneration and fibrous replacement, their reflectivity becomes more heterogeneous.

Cavernous haemangiomas appear as focal lesions with increased reflectivity, an irregular or lobulated wall and no distal enhancement. Hepatic veins draining the

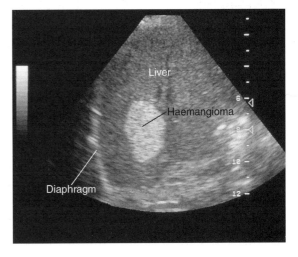

Fig. 3.16 Haemangioma.

lesion may be prominent and the coeliac axis and hepatic artery may be dilated while the aorta distal to the coeliac axis may be reduced in diameter. These vascular abnormalities suggest a benign vascular tumour as they do not occur with malignant liver disease (Fig. 3.16).

Box 3.6   Advice

It is difficult to tell the more heterogeneous type of lesion from other focal hepatic lesions. Large haemangiomas sometimes enhance distally. With smaller isolated heterogeneous echogenic lesions and no known history of malignancy, it is safe to assume that the lesion is a haemangioma. Magnetic resonance imaging is more sensitive in detecting haemangiomas. Fine needle biopsy has been performed with success where doubt exists but there is always the chance of haemorrhage when biopsying a vascular lesion.

Hepatic adenoma

CLINICAL INFORMATION

Hepatic adenomas are quite rare. They occur much more in women as there is a close association with the high oestrogen oral contraceptive pill (OCP). Patients present with right upper quadrant (RUQ) pain, a palpable mass and haemorrhage either into the tumour or from rupture into the peritoneum. Tumours can regress if the patient stops taking the OCP. Treatment is usually by surgery and is usually urgent. It is rare in children, with increased incidence in those with glycogen storage disease.

ULTRASOUND APPEARANCES

Hepatic adenomas are smooth, solitary masses, well circumscribed, rounded, solid and completely or partially encapsulated. They can be quite large (5–20 cm diameter). Appearances are similar to focal nodular hyperplasia (see below). Ultrasound appearances change if and when haemorrhage into the tumour has occurred (60% have haemorrhage in the tumour).

Hepatic adenomas are seen as cold nodules on radionuclide imaging (RNI) scans.

Focal nodular hyperplasia (FNH)

CLINICAL INFORMATION

This is quite rare, being found typically in women aged 20–40 years, but can be seen in the whole population. FNH is very rare in childhood. It is mostly asymptomatic. A small amount (6%) may haemorrhage. FNH is usually treated conservatively.

ULTRASOUND APPEARANCES

FNHs are usually solid, well circumscribed but not encapsulated, usually homogeneous and can be either of higher or lower reflectivity than the normal liver.

Box 3.7   Advice

Lesions 2–8 cm with no cold spots on isotope scan suggest FNH. Contrast-enhanced CT scans show a lesion with a central stellate scar.

Clinical presentation is more helpful than ultrasound for differentiating between hepatic adenoma and FNH.

Focal fatty tumours

CLINICAL INFORMATION

Fatty infiltration is a common occurrence; it arises from nutritional disturbance or toxic insult. Changes can be seen within a few weeks and may regress within days.

ULTRASOUND APPEARANCES

Box 3.8   Advice

Fatty infiltration may appear similar to other focal lesions. It has sharp, angular boundaries and does not displace venous structures as other lesions often do. Guided biopsy can often help differentiate fatty from other lesions although care must be taken to ensure that fatty lesions are not highly vascular lesions which then must be handled with care.

When most of the liver is infiltrated with fat, there is often focal sparing of small areas of normal liver which can appear like echo-poor

---

Malignant focal lesions

Hepatocellular carcinoma (HCC)

CLINICAL INFORMATION

Primary liver cancer (hepatocellular carcinoma or HCC) is a major malignancy, especially in the Far East and Saharan Africa. It is more common in males. Amongst others, causes include carcinogens (aflatoxins), haemochromatosis, schistosomiasis and the banned radiographic contrast medium Thorotrast. Seventy-five to 80% of HCC patients in the West and the Far East have associated cirrhosis and malignant primary tumours are also found in those who have had hepatitis B. HCC and adenocarcinoma arising from the intrahepatic bile ducts (cholangiocarcinoma – see page 85) both have a poor prognosis, most patients being dead within six months of diagnosis. Both primary cancers are rare in infancy where they peak at one year and 13 years.

The normal value of α-fetoprotein (AFP) is <12 kU/l. Serum levels rise in chronic liver disease. A specific diagnosis of HCC is made when the level of AFP is >400 kU/l. However, with some small HCCs, AFP does not always rise to a diagnostic level so a combination of AFP and ultrasound is essential.

Portal vein invasion is more frequently detected by ultrasound (71%) than by CT (29%) or angiography (15%). Seventy-five percent of liver lesions are malignant, either primary or secondary.

ULTRASOUND APPEARANCES

HCCs can appear nodular with single or multiple nodules. Their contour is regular, their boundary well defined. They can be large (5 cm+). They can also be diffuse where the boundary with normal liver tissue is vague. The mass is indistinct in this case; large areas of liver can be invaded by tumour and the liver may demonstrate either increased or decreased reflectivity. Mostly all types of reflectivity are demonstrated:

hypoechoic, hyperechoic, isoechoic with normal liver texture and mixed echo patterns. A halo is often seen around small nodules. Highly reflective patterns (from necrosis and haemorrhage within the tumour) are found in about half of all HCCs. Of the small HCCs (1–3 cm in diameter), 77% tend to be poorly reflective. It is thought that the smaller hypoechoic lesions grow more slowly than those larger tumours with a halo, but this has not been fully substantiated (Fig. 3.17).

DOPPLER STUDIES

HCC often invades the portal venous system. Pulsed wave and colour Doppler examinations show a

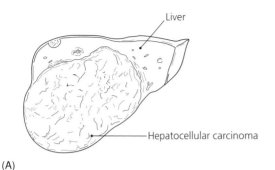

(A)

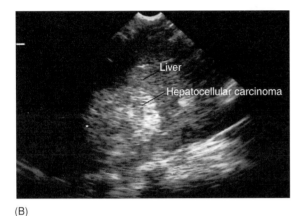

(B)

Fig. 3.17 (A, B) Hepatocellular carcinoma.

characteristic ring of vessels at the periphery of the mass. Arterial signals have been seen in all 3 cm+ HCCs and in 76% of those smaller than 3 cm. Power Doppler is more sensitive than CD and so is more often used in detecting low levels of blood flow.

Hepatoblastoma

CLINICAL INFORMATION

Seven percent of all malignant liver tumours are hepatoblastomas. They occur in children up to three years of age (50% before 18 months). Tumours are often large and can occupy substantial lobes/segments of the liver, occupying 75% the right lobe. There is an associated increase in AFP in 67–90% of cases. Liver enzymes are usually normal. Hepatoblastomas may occlude the portal vein and invade the hepatic vein and the IVC. They are treated with chemotherapy to shrink the tumour prior to surgery. The lesion often calcifies or becomes cystic.

ULTRASOUND APPEARANCES

Hepatoblastomas are solitary or multiple lesions, poorly defined, of slightly higher reflectivity than the normal liver and occasionally contain some calcification.

Metastases

CLINICAL INFORMATION

Metastases are almost always multiple and appear as described in the section on ultrasound appearances of liver tumours (see page 41). They have a range of sizes and are randomly distributed. As they have so many varying appearances, they often overlap with the appearances seen in benign tumours, resulting in a lack of specificity. Liver metastases are on the whole not particularly vascular. The smallest viable metastases measure only a fraction of a millimetre in diameter and therefore cannot be seen by imaging techniques.

The liver is the second most common metastatic site after regional lymph nodes. The incidence of metastases is 20 times greater than that of primary carcinoma.

The liver is often enlarged with a hard and craggy feeling on palpation. Any tumours causing active necrosis of liver cells will usually result in an increase in the levels of ALT, carcinoembryonic antigen, ALP and AFP.

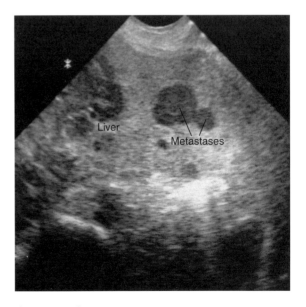

Fig. 3.18 Echo-poor metastases.

ULTRASOUND APPEARANCES

Liver metastases can be grouped under the following generalization: 25% hyperechoic, 37.5% hypoechoic and 37.5% of mixed echogenicity.

Echo-poor metastases are quite well defined and are derived from any type of primary cancer (typically from breast or bronchus). It is the most common metastatic appearance (Fig. 3.18).

Box 3.10   Advice

Malignant lymphomas can appear in this way but there tends to be a diffuse appearance in this condition. Therefore scan the spleen carefully and look for evidence of enlarged lymph nodes.

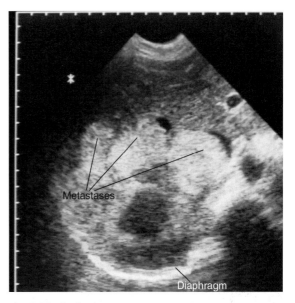

Fig. 3.19   Reflective metastases.

Highly reflective metastases (Fig. 3.19) are usually quite well defined and relatively easy to see, depending on size. They tend to originate from primaries of the gastrointestinal and genitourinary tracts. Acoustic shadowing or enhancement is rarely seen. Small, highly reflective lesions seen throughout the liver can suggest hepatic tuberculosis (TB).

Cystic metastases demonstrate little, if any, posterior acoustic enhancement They are seen in necrosis of all types of metastases and from mucin-secreting primary tumours such as ovary, stomach, colon, pancreas and breast.

Calcified metastases (Fig. 3.20A & B) are most often seen from colorectal or stomach primaries and may produce some acoustic shadowing. Colorectal metastases are often solitary. A solitary metastasis must be distinguished from the appearance of the ligamentum teres.

Target lesions (Fig. 3.21) are usually seen in larger metastases and, although generally non-specific, are often seen with bronchogenic carcinoma. Target lesions can be highly reflective with echo-poor haloes or sometimes echo poor with an echogenic halo.

Necrotic metastases (Fig. 3.22) tend to be larger lesions, irregular in shape with thick irregular walls containing centres of mixed echogenicity. Necrotic metastases can appear like abscesses but with no local tenderness and history of fever.

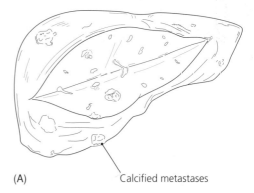

(A)   Calcified metastases

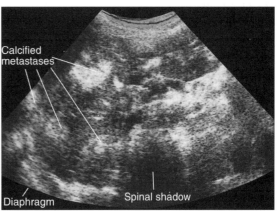

(B)

Fig. 3.20   (A, B) Calcified metastases.

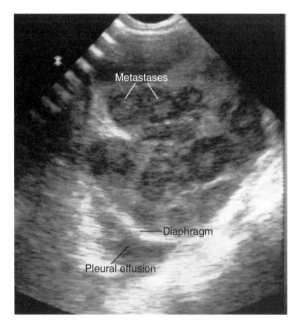

Fig. 3.21 Target metastases.

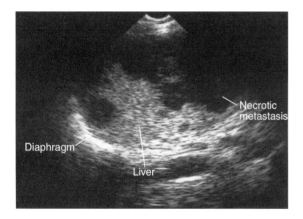

Fig. 3.22 Necrotic metastases.

Box 3.11   Advice

Malignant lymphomas can appear like metastases but they tend to be quite diffuse. Scan the spleen carefully and look for evidence of enlarged lymph nodes in the abdomen.

Focal metastases can become extensive and confluent and the liver can appear patchy, making it difficult to tell which is normal and which is abnormal liver texture.

Metastases may be small (1 mm diameter) and appear as diffuse disease. This appearance is difficult to differentiate from fatty infiltration and early cirrhosis when spread uniformly throughout the entire liver.

Metastases can cause hepatomegaly and change the shape of the inferior border of the liver from a sharp to a rounded appearance. Liver enlargement without any accompanying features of cirrhosis may suggest a metastatic disease.

Metastases can have a nodular appearance (Fig. 3.23) if near to the surface of the liver (they are then easier to see in the presence of ascites). The muscle of the diaphragm has been known to form into thickened bundles indenting the superior border of the liver. This should not be confused with nodular metastases indenting the diaphragm.

Metastases can displace or occlude hepatic vessels which is why it is essential to examine the hepatic vessels for normal appearances when searching for metastases.

Hyperechoic metastases tend to be hypervascular; hypoechoic metastases tend to be hypovascular.

Infective lesions

Abscess

CLINICAL INFORMATION

Abscesses may arise from the spread of infection into the liver via the portal veins, hepatic artery or biliary tree or by a penetrating injury. Pyogenic abscesses often arise from complications of intraabdominal infection found in places such as the biliary tract, colon and appendix, from previous abdominal surgery, trauma, neoplasm or bacteraemia. Rapid diagnosis and prompt treatment are necessary owing to the high morbidity and mortality from untreated abscesses. Patients present with fever, pain, nausea and vomiting.

An abscess requires a fine needle aspiration for confirmation, the sample being taken from the inflammatory capsule of the abscess rather than the purulent portion which may itself be sterile.

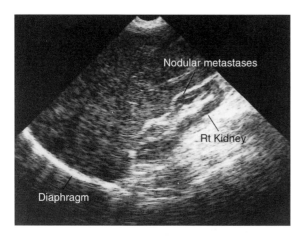

Fig. 3.23 Nodular metastases indenting the right kidney.

ULTRASOUND APPEARANCES

These depend on the age of the abscess.

- Early (within a few days) – the abscess appears diffuse, ill defined with areas of low reflectivity from local oedema and inflammation.

- Later – the lesion has better definition although irregular in shape and still of low reflectivity. It may have an echogenic rim surrounding it.

- Later still – a thick-walled irregular capsule develops. The centre shows mixed echogenicity from tissue necrosis, gas formation and debris. It may calcify if chronic. Gas and calcification show as brightly echogenic areas with posterior acoustic shadowing. Acoustic enhancement can be seen posterior to areas of low reflectivity (the pus).

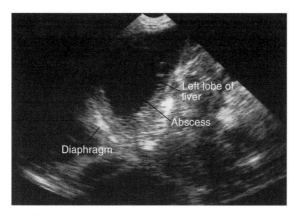

Fig. 3.24 Abscess.

Box 3.12   Advice

Abscesses tend to form either in the subphrenic space or in the subhepatic space. These are the most dependent parts of the peritoneal cavity. Much of the pelvis and lower abdomen is in direct communication with these spaces via the right paracolic gutter. Therefore when scanning patients with symptoms of abscess, very careful attention should be paid to the renal and diaphragmatic areas.

Abscesses can be mistaken for complicated hepatic cysts or necrotic tumours (although these often have thicker walls).

Amoebic abscess

CLINICAL INFORMATION

Caused by the protozoan parasite *Entamoeba histolytica* and spread by infected food or water. Trophozoites digest their way through the colonic mucosa and can enter the liver by way of the portal venous system. Patients may be asymptomatic but can have RUQ pain. Liver function tests are usually normal.

Amoebic abscesses are most common in the right lobe of the liver and close to the diaphragm. They are usually solitary.

ULTRASOUND APPEARANCES

Amoebic abscesses have no significant wall echo, are symmetrically round or oval and are of lower reflectivity than the normal liver with homogeneous echoes – this is not pus but necrotic liver tissue. They can exhibit some distal acoustic enhancement.

Box 3.13   Advice

Aspiration not usually carried out. Diagnosis is confirmed by haemoglutination levels and response to metronidazole therapy. After therapy, the lesion should decrease in size and contents lessen in reflectivity. Aspiration cannot be carried out as although contents appear as fluid, they are in fact semi-solid and cannot be aspirated. Complete resolution can take up to two years.

Amoebic abscesses can appear similar to a pyogenic abscess.

Hydatid cyst (echinococcal cyst)

CLINICAL INFORMATION

Hydatid cysts are a parasitic infection found particularly where sheep and cattle graze. There is a high incidence in the Middle East. They can be passed on to humans when in contact with infested dogs which have access to sheep and cattle carcases.

ULTRASOUND APPEARANCES

They are found most commonly in the right lobe of the liver and appear as a solitary cyst 1–20 cm in diameter, similar to congenital liver cysts. In endemic areas, any cyst must be considered to be hydatid until proven otherwise. There may be some hydatid sand (particles of imperfectly formed daughter cysts) seen as low-level echoes within the cyst and layering out. Sometimes the two layers of the cyst wall can be seen.

There can be separation of the membrane. Sometimes the membrane is seen to separate and the inner layer detaches and collapses, floating in the cyst fluid or lying in the dependent portion of the cyst. This produces the ultrasound 'waterlily' sign (Fig. 3.25).

DAUGHTER CYSTS

In well-developed disease, the inner lining of the hydatid cyst membrane produces daughter cysts; these give an ultrasound appearance of multiple small cysts within a cyst, characteristically described as a cartwheel or honeycomb cyst.

MULTIPLE CYSTS

Continued infestation of the liver can lead to multiple primary hydatid cysts producing hepatomegaly. If there is no evidence of membrane separation or daughter cysts, the appearance may be similar to necrotic metastases, polycystic disease, haematomas or simple cysts.

Box 3.14   Advice

Successful fine needle aspiration has been recorded but this must be undertaken with great care as hydatid cysts can disseminate.

Trauma

Haematoma

CLINICAL INFORMATION

Significant liver trauma occurs in 3–12% of all admissions to major centres and it is second only to the spleen as the organ most often injured. Liver haematoma can result from blunt trauma to the abdomen, rupture of an adenoma or haemangioma or a needle biopsy. Blunt abdominal trauma is relatively common in children as their rib cage is more flexible than that of the adult and they have less of a protective layer of fat around them.

Trauma of the liver can be divided into three main categories.

- Rupture of the liver and the capsule – CT is often the best imaging modality to demonstrate the extent of the injury. However, usually the patient is very ill and will proceed to immediate laparotomy. Liver rupture often requires immediate surgery while most haematomas require minimal intervention and are usually scanned serially to monitor resolution.

- Subcapsular haematoma.

- Central haematoma.

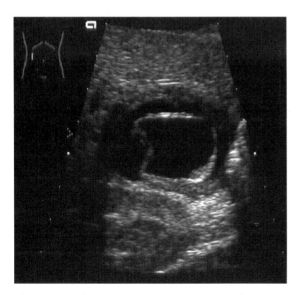

Fig. 3.25 Echinococcal cyst. (Image courtesy of Acuson, a Siemens Company.)

Haematomas change their ultrasound appearance according to how recent they are. They tend to be echo free when fresh but within a few hours highly reflective echoes appear within the haematoma caused by fibrin and erythrocyte deposits. Within a few days the clot undergoes liquefaction and decreases in reflectivity. The haematoma may increase in size at this stage. Over the next few months the haematoma can appear cystic with internal reflective strands. Fibrous scarring or a small cystic space may remain for a long time.

A subcapsular haematoma can appear as an echo-poor rim under the hepatic capsule. It is sometimes difficult to visualize small subcapsular haematomas as they can almost appear like normal liver texture. Larger subcapsular haematomas are easier to see when fresh owing to the larger amount of blood present.

Diffuse disease

Diseases of the liver usually result in failure of the main functions to detoxify and synthesize. The development of jaundice is common as a result. If the liver function is critically impaired through damage to the majority of liver cells, acute liver failure develops from which 80% of patients die.

Features of acute liver failure are:

- jaundice from failure of bilirubin metabolism

- coma from failure to detoxify nitrogenous compounds

- tendency to bleed from failure to synthesize protein (depleted factors 2, 7, 9 and 10)

- renal failure from a shock-induced low glomerular filtration rate.

Main causes of liver disease are:

- toxins (drugs, alcohol)

- infections (viruses, parasites, bacteria)

- bile duct or hepatic blood vessel pathology

- tumours.

Liver disease can be categorized as:

- acute hepatitis – seen in diseases causing necrosis of liver cells with associated inflammation

- chronic hepatitis – seen when there is continued liver cell inflammation, often resulting in fibrosis

- cholestasis – resulting from damage to the bile ducts

- cirrhosis – a result of long-standing liver cell destruction where the liver develops extensive scarring and nodules of regenerated liver cells. This can lead to distorted liver architecture and back pressure in the portal vessels (portal hypertension).

No study of the liver can be conducted without setting up the gain controls correctly at the beginning of the examination. Every examination must include an assessment of echogenicity of the liver compared with the right kidney at the same depth (see page 37).

Normal liver is of higher reflectivity than renal parenchyma, providing that the kidney itself is normal. A kidney with higher or lower reflectivity than normal caused by a pathological process can alter the subjective appearance of the liver; in other words, if the kidney is darker than usual, the liver may look bright in comparison.

It is also essential to compare the portal vessel walls with the liver texture as a liver showing very prominent portal vessel walls (in other words, very bright walls as a contrast to a dark liver texture) suggests a liver with reduced reflectivity. Conversely, a liver where the texture is almost the same brightness as the portal vessel walls, making them difficult to see, is a liver with increased reflectivity.

Normal liver echoes should be uniform in size and even throughout the liver (homogeneous). A diffuse disease can alter the texture so that the echoes appear fine or coarse and patchy. It may make the liver appear dark or bright and may or may not alter the normal size of the liver.

The patchy appearance of the liver is often caused by a bunching of focal lesions that have been described previously:

- focal fatty change

- multiple abscesses

- multiple metastases

- macronodular cirrhosis (considered below under the relevant section on cirrhosis).

Very generally, diffuse liver disease falls into two categories: dark and bright.

- Dark – conditions within the liver produce extra fluid, exaggerated contrast occurs between the liver texture and vessel walls (see above) and the portal vessel walls show up markedly (called the 'starry sky' appearance). The liver tissue is also isoechoic with normal renal tissue (so do not compare with a kidney in a patient with known glomerulonephritis, for example).

- Bright – liver tissue has an echogenicity equal to the vascular walls and the ligamentum teres and lack of prominent vascular markings gives a uniform, ground-glass look. The normal right renal texture appears dark in comparison and the bright collecting system of the kidney may be isoechoic to the liver.

Pathology that causes diffuse liver disease can be considered under the following main categories:

- hepatitis
- fatty infiltration
- cirrhosis
- congestive cardiac disease
- portal hypertension.

Hepatitis

CLINICAL INFORMATION

Hepatitis can be acute or chronic and can be caused by viral infections, drug reactions, alcohol and auto-immune disorders.

Patients can present with nausea, anorexia, low-grade pyrexia and general malaise. The liver can be palpably enlarged and tender. Jaundice (yellow discolouration of skin and sclera) can appear seven days after the onset of symptoms, peaking at 10 days after. It generally regresses after between three and 10 weeks.

Acute viral hepatitis (hepatitis A, B, C, D, E)

CLINICAL INFORMATION

- Hepatitis A is a virus contracted from sewage-contaminated water or from eating seafood contaminated by sewage. It is transmitted by the faecal–oral route and is detected in the stools of patients. Biopsy is rarely performed.

- Hepatitis B is transmitted by blood, saliva, semen and through breaks in the skin, by sexual contact and by sharing of unsterile needles by IV drug abusers. It can progress to chronic hepatitis and patients have a greater risk of developing hepatocellular carcinoma.

- Hepatitis C is transmitted in a similar manner to hepatitis B, incubates over about two months and produces the usual hepatitis symptoms. Recovery often follows within a further two months for half of those infected; the other half will have persistently abnormal liver function tests for the next year, being in remission and then relapsing. Of this half, 75% will recover in time, the other 25% will progress to chronic hepatitis, some to cirrhosis and the associated hepatocellular carcinoma.

- Hepatitis D causes disease only in the presence of hepatitis B. It is transmitted in the same way as hepatitis B, increases the severity of chronic hepatitis and can lead to the development of fulminant hepatitis and its associated massive necrosis of liver cells.

- Hepatitis E is similar to hepatitis A, being transmitted by the same route. It has an incubation period of about one month, causes a mild infection with jaundice and does not progress to chronic hepatitis.

In acute viral hepatitis, bilirubin levels are greatly increased; clinical jaundice is evident when serum bilirubin >50 µmol/l (approximately 2.5 times normal level). Both ALT and AST levels are very high early in the disease process, reflecting cell necrosis, and fall with clinical recovery. Serum albumin is generally normal.

Blood clotting time (prothrombin) may be abnormal, demonstrating severity of disease; this is why clotting time is always checked prior to liver biopsy.

ULTRASOUND APPEARANCES

Ultrasound is of use in excluding obstructive jaundice. The liver appears dark compared to the portal vessel wall reflectivity. The wall of the gallbladder is often thickened (>3 mm). Sometimes some ascites may be present.

Acute alcoholic hepatitis

CLINICAL INFORMATION

Acute alcoholic hepatitis varies between mild and aggressive, can be reversible but may progress to cirrhosis. Liver function tests are raised. Alcoholic liver damage can lead to a fatty liver; the amount of fat in the hepatocytes can decrease with abstinence from alcohol. If alcohol consumption continues, fibrosis develops around the central veins, possibly leading to cirrhosis.

ULTRASOUND APPEARANCES

The liver is almost always enlarged and of increased reflectivity with increased attenuation distally. The inferior border can appear rounded or blunted.

Chronic hepatitis

CLINICAL INFORMATION

Chronic hepatitis is defined as inflammation of the liver persisting for more than six months. There are three types.

- Chronic active or aggressive hepatitis (CAH) – where there is continued necrosis of liver cells; the main complication is the development of cirrhosis.

- Chronic persistent hepatitis (CPH) – where inflammation is confined to the portal tracts; necrosis of liver cells is not seen.

- Chronic lobular hepatitis (CLH) – where there is inflammation of the portal tracts and patchy inflammation of the hepatic parenchyma.

Liver function tests (alkaline phosphatase, AST and ALT, bilirubin, albumin and prothrombin time) vary according to the type of chronic hepatitis. With CPH, all are normal except AST and ALT which are 2–5 times normal. CLH and CAH have normal to slightly increased levels of alkaline phosphatase, 5–20 times normal levels of AST and 5–30 times normal levels of ALT, mild to moderate increases of bilirubin and normal levels of albumin. Prothrombin time is mildly increased with CLH and often increased with CAH.

ULTRASOUND APPEARANCES

There is usually increased reflectivity and sometimes altered echo patterns. Distal attenuation occurs only sometimes, depending on how much fatty infiltration, necrosis and fibrosis are present. Fatty infiltration will attenuate ultrasound distally, making the diaphragm hard to see, whereas fibrotic infiltration will allow through transmission of sound.

Fatty infiltration (steatosis)

CLINICAL INFORMATION

A fatty liver can be caused by toxins (alcohol, corticosteroids, tetracyclines), nutritional disorders (obesity, starvation) and metabolic disorders (glycogen storage disease). It can be seen in patients with diabetes, Cushing's disease, obesity and ulcerative colitis, those on steroids, and those with acute fatty liver of pregnancy (AFLP). It is usually reversible after treatment.

AFLP occurs in between 1/14 000 and 1/16 000 cases. Patients can present with lethargy, nausea and vomiting, restlessness, mild jaundice and itching and symptoms can progress to severe headache, convulsions and coma. Liver failure leads to hypothrombinaemia and disseminated intravascular coagulation, resulting in haematemesis, spontaneous bleeding and multiple organ failure. ALP, ALT and serum bilirubin levels are often markedly raised. A case report by Allen et al involving AFLP is helpful.[3]

ULTRASOUND APPEARANCES

The abnormal accumulation of fat (considered to be more than 7% in total) in the liver leads to the ultrasound appearance of a bright liver, caused by interfaces produced by multiple fat droplets. The liver is usually enlarged (75% have hepatomegaly). The fat attenuates the sound distally; sometimes, however, this does not occur. Efforts have to be made in the former case to scan from another direction to exclude concurrent metastases in the 'hidden' area (Fig. 3.26).

Ultrasound is very sensitive in the detection of fatty infiltration, being in the region of 86% in mild cases to 100% in moderate to severe cases. Patchily affected regions of fat can appear like focal metastases although vessels are seen to pass through fat rather than around metastases. Similarly, when only a few areas of liver are spared the fat infiltration, these can appear to be the abnormal areas of tissue and can produce pseudometastatic appearances. The clinical details must be understood to avoid making a misdiagnosis. With AFLP, the ultrasound appearances can be normal so AFLP cannot be excluded even when the ultrasound appearances are normal.

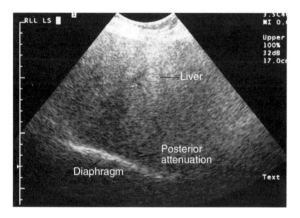

Fig. 3.26 Fatty liver.

Cirrhosis

CLINICAL INFORMATION

Failure of the liver to metabolize causes clinical signs. As the condition is more prevalent in males, failure by the liver to metabolize oestrogens results in gynaeco-mastia (breast development) and testicular atrophy. Patients with cirrhosis often present with weakness, weight loss and fatigue. The liver is palpably enlarged and firm with a blunt or nodular edge. Of all cases of cirrhosis >65% are alcohol related.

Patients can present with mild jaundice at first, which increases in severity. Biochemically, AST and ALT levels are usually elevated, AST more than ALT. The level is proportional to the amount of liver cell destruction. Serum albumin level is low because of the failure of the liver to synthesize. Prothrombin time is longer because coagulation factors are not synthesized.

Cirrhosis is an end result in several conditions such as hepatitis, carcinogens, parasites and alcohol. Patho-logically, it appears as the destruction of normally functioning liver cells and their replacement by nodules separated by bands of fibrous tissue. Two types can be considered: micronodular (nodules <3 mm diameter), often seen after chronic, long-term alcoholism, and macronodular (nodules 3 mm to >2 cm diameter) (Fig. 3.27). There is a higher inci-dence of HCC with this type. Cirrhosis results in liver failure and portal hypertension. In association with portal hypertension, it can cause ascites (the accumula-tion of fluid in the peritoneal cavity). Cirrhosis may also develop as a consequence of long-standing biliary obstruction (see Chapter 4).

Micronodular liver

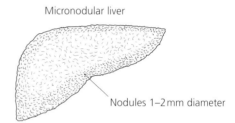

Nodules 1–2 mm diameter

Macronodular liver

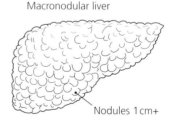

Nodules 1 cm+

Mixed nodular liver

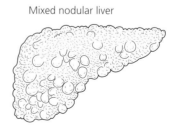

Fig. 3.27 Types of nodular cirrhosis.

ULTRASOUND APPEARANCES

The cirrhotic liver appears normal in one-third of cases and abnormalities are seen in two-thirds. The abnormal appearance shows as a liver with a higher reflectivity than normal, resulting in the loss of portal vessel wall detail. Echo pattern is described as coarse and irregular. There is no increase in sound attenuation distally, unlike that accompanying the fatty liver, but in alcohol-related disease the liver can have cirrhotic and fatty attributes, confusing the appearance. A grainy appearance may be seen in micronodular cirrhosis while macronodular cirrhosis can be seen as a nodular 'rippling' on the inferior surface, contrasting against the relatively smooth surface of the right kidney and gallbladder and seen especially well in the presence of ascites.

The liver size may be normal at first but tends to shrink in the more advanced stages of the disease. The right lobe of the liver may shrink while the caudate lobe retains a larger proportion of the liver volume. If a transverse scan of the liver is made at the level just below the portal vein bifurcation, a normal liver should show a ratio of caudate lobe to right lobe as being <0.6. If >0.65, this is considered 100% specific of cirrhosis. The caudate lobe and left lobe of the liver are thus usually spared shrinkage and hypertrophy may even occur. This is thought to be caused by the siting of the hepatic veins.

Box 3.17   Advice

Large nodules may mimic tumours. As hepatomas are not infrequently seen accompanying macronodular cirrhosis, a careful check must be made to ensure that the large nodules are not tumours and a Doppler examination should be carried out if doubt persists. A blood supply to the mass will confirm the presence of a hepatoma.

There are other signs associated with cirrhosis, both ultrasonically and clinically, that suggest portal hypertension which will be seen under the relevant section.

Portal hypertension

CLINICAL INFORMATION

Portal hypertension is the increased pressure of blood flowing into the liver from the portal vessels owing to the rigidity of a nodular or fibrosed liver. It can be caused:

- intrahepatically by cirrhosis (because of the disturbance and obstruction to blood flow through the liver), HCC, hepatitis and alcoholic liver disease

- suprahepatically by hepatic vein obstruction (from thrombosis, tumour, constrictive pericarditis)

- infrahepatically by portal vein thrombosis and by portal vein compression from pancreatic carcinoma or pancreatitis. In these cases, the segments of the vessels proximal to the obstruction dilate.

In portal hypertension, the liver damage produces other clinical signs in addition to those described above under cirrhosis.

- Bruising can occur from failure to synthesize clotting factors.

- Ascites can occur, caused by a low level of serum albumin. It can be diagnosed by abdominal percussion, a technique used to differentiate between gaseous distension or ascites, resulting in a dull sound in the flanks with a hollow sound in the mid upper zone, compared to gas which makes the abdomen sound hollow all over. In extreme cases it produces an enlarged, taut abdomen.

- Enlarged veins may, in addition, be seen on the abdominal surface around the umbilicus (the caput medusae).

ULTRASOUND APPEARANCES

The spleen may be grossly enlarged. Extrahepatic portal vessels may enlarge. Intrahepatic vessels often do not enlarge as they are constricted by the hepatic nodules and fibrosis. Studies involving ultrasound have shown a wide variation of measurements of portal vessels involved in portal hypertension.

Collateral vessels joining the high-pressure portal vessels and the lower pressure systemic circulation (portosystemic anastomoses) may become dilated which is highly specific of portal hypertension. These varices may appear as small tortuous vessels looking like a bag of worms in the region of the splenic hilum (see page 118), porta hepatis, pancreatic bed, gastric fundus (not seen usually owing to gas) and oesophagus (difficult to see). There can be large pathways between the splenic varices and the left renal vein, which help to relieve the portal hypertension and even lead to the reversal of blood flow in the splenic and portal veins.

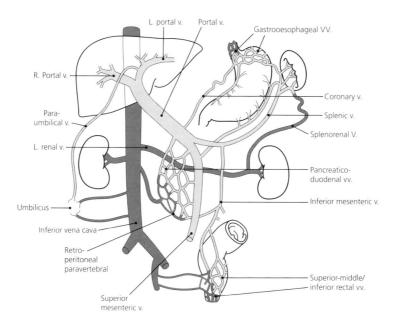

Fig. 3.28 Sites of portosystemic venous collaterals.

Ascites may help outline a nodular liver. On ultrasound, uncomplicated ascites (that is, non-malignant or non-infected ascites) is seen as echo-free, mobile fluid within the peritoneum which, in extreme cases, allows loops of bowel to float freely within it and in minimal cases can show as it settles in dependent portions of the abdomen such as over the surface of the liver, the subhepatic space and in both paracolic gutters (see chapter 15). The right kidney may appear more reflective than usual because of the acoustic enhancement from the ascites. The gallbladder wall in a starved patient can thicken in the presence of ascites.

The paraumbilical vein, a notable portosystemic collateral, may appear within the ligamentum teres, showing on a transverse ultrasound scan of the liver as an echo-free circular structure in the middle of the highly reflective round ligament. (Do not confuse this appearance with the normal left branch of the portal vein.) If it exceeds 3 mm diameter and has a typical portal venous flow, this is highly suggestive of portal hypertension.

It is generally accepted that the range of measurements of normal portal vessels is as follows.

- Normal portal vein diameter 10–13 mm maximum.

- Normal splenic vein diameter 8–10 mm.

- Normal superior mesenteric vein diameter 5–10 mm.

- Dilatation of the portal vein (13 mm–>15 mm diameter) has been seen in 56% of patients with portal hypertension caused by cirrhosis. A portal vein diameter of 17 mm+ is an indication of the presence of large varices and a splenic vein diameter of 20 mm is a specific sign of portal hypertension. A normal portal vein diameter, however, does not exclude portal hypertension as portal vessels often reduce in size when collaterals form. It must be emphasized that there is no hard and fast rule regarding portal vessel measurements and their correlation with pathology.

Box 3.18   Advice

Portal vessels can change according to respiration (suspended inspiration can dilate the portal vein), posture (portal vein dilates) and whether the patient has recently eaten (portal vein dilates). Therefore all measurements should be taken with the patient breathing quietly, lying in the supine position and in a fasted state. In patients with portal hypertension, as there is increased pressure inside the liver, the portal vessels do not tend to increase with suspended inspiration (the Valsalva manoeuvre).

ABNORMAL PULSED WAVE DOPPLER

Portal vein

Doppler is needed to confirm portal vein flow. Colour Doppler is best for this. If the portal vein is thrombosed, this can be seen by absent flow in the portal vein and high-frequency flow from the hepatic artery as it takes over all the blood supply to the liver. Doppler is very sensitive in this respect. A decrease in flow velocity down to around 8 cm/s is frequently seen. Reversed (hepatofugal) flow is seen in over 8% of cases with liver cirrhosis.

Hepatic vein

The triphasic pattern is lost or markedly reduced in liver cirrhosis with portal hypertension in up to 50% of cases, probably due to liver stiffness. There can be variations in velocity from respiration.

Congestive Cardiac Disease

CLINICAL INFORMATION

Patients are at risk with some or all of the following: high cholesterol, hypertension, diabetes, obesity. Smokers are especially at risk They present with fluid retention (selling of ankles and knees; fluid in abdomen and lungs) shortness of breath, weight gain, loss of appetite and nausea

ULTRASOUND APPEARANCES

The liver is often slightly enlarged and of lower echogenicity than normal. The hepatic veins appear dilated with a dilated IVC sometimes seen. With mitral valve disease the triphasic flow of the hepatic veins becomes highly pulsatile.

Vessel-related pathology

Budd–Chiari syndrome

CLINICAL INFORMATION

Budd–Chiari syndrome is a rare disorder in which the hepatic veins are obstructed. The liver is usually enlarged and tender. In cases of complete and rapid venous obstruction, patients usually die from acute liver failure.

ULTRASOUND APPEARANCES *often spared*

The liver is often enlarged, the caudate lobe is enlarged as the inferior hepatic veins are spared, the hepatic veins are not seen or are dilated and irregular, the confluence of the hepatic veins into the IVC is not seen and the IVC is often obstructed or stenosed. Some ascites can be present. The spleen size is usually normal at first, enlarging as the disease progresses. Thrombus can sometimes be seen in major hepatic veins. There is often reverse flow in the portal vein. Chronic conditions can reveal small areas of high reflectivity with distal acoustic shadowing within the liver.

The Budd–Chiari syndrome can be seen on pulsed wave Doppler as reversed flow in the lower part of the IVC or as flow in the normal direction but with a lost triphasic pattern suggesting partial obstruction. Steady flow suggests upper IVC or hepatic vein obstruction but this is also found with cirrhosis so the specificity is poor.

Suggested minimal sections for imaging the abnormal liver

Solitary lesions

- Longitudinal sections and transverse sections through the lesion with measurements.

- One or two sections to show effect of mass on surrounding tissue, biliary tree or circulation.

- Sections to show pathology in related organs or lymph nodes.

Multiple lesions

- Longitudinal sections and transverse sections showing pathology.

- Sections showing extent of pathology in related organs.

- Sections showing effects of pathology such as ascites or biliary obstruction.

- An oblique section through the porta hepatis showing the presence or absence of enlarged lymph nodes and a measurement of the common duct.

Diffuse liver disease

- Longitudinal sections and transverse sections through the liver.

- A section through the porta hepatis to show the portal vein, common duct and hepatic artery.

- Sections showing pathology in other organs.

- A section showing a comparison between the hepatic and renal parenchyma.

Obstructive jaundice

- Sections of the liver demonstrating dilated bile ducts.

- A section through the porta hepatis to show the portal vein, common duct (measured), enlarged lymph nodes if present and the hepatic artery.

- Longitudinal sections and transverse sections through the gallbladder.

- Sections showing the cause and level of obstruction such as pancreatic tumour or bile duct stone.

- Sections through the pancreas with special attention to the head of pancreas, bile and pancreatic duct appearances.

Liver biopsy

Equipment used for ultrasound-guided biopsy of the liver, technique undertaken and protocols employed will vary from department to department. There are several accounts of biopsies undertaken but a general overview such as the chapter on interventional techniques by Holm *et al* is a useful reference.[4]

Indications for liver biopsy

- Confirmation and typing of tumours (primary and secondary)

- Unexplained hepatomegaly

- Some cases of jaundice

- Persistently abnormal liver function tests

- Cirrhosis

- Diffuse disease

- Tumours – primary and secondary

Contraindications

- Prolonged prothrombin time (3× normal)

- Low platelet count

For a fine needle biopsy (where the outer diameter of the needle is less than 1 mm) no blood tests such as prothrombin time or thrombocyte count are required and the patient can have the biopsy performed as an outpatient. Similarly, no postprocedural observations need take place.

If a larger bore needle is used or the patient has a coagulation disorder, the person must be treated as an inpatient: coagulation factors and platelet count must be adequate and a minimum of 1000 ml blood available for transfusion. However, recent studies have suggested that fine needle liver punctures appear to be safer than previously believed in patients with severe clotting defects.[5]

Cytological specimens are obtained by aspiration and should sample several regions around the periphery of the lesion as the centre may contain haemorrhage and lead to a non-diagnostic specimen; this allows a good evaluation of cellular detail.

Histological fine needle biopsies are prone to breaking up when in the laboratory if a 0.6 mm diameter needle is used but this is rarely a problem when one of 0.8 mm diameter is used. The biopsy gives good structural information used to diagnose benign and malignant lesions, and many sections can be made from one biopsy core.

There is a theoretical risk of spreading tumour cells along the needle tract into blood or lymph when performing a fine needle biopsy of a suspected malignancy. However, studies and clinical impressions have concluded that there is little risk of spreading tumour cells with this technique and even if some cells are spread to lymph nodes or along the needle tract, the immune response of the patient will eliminate those cells.

Equipment required for cytological fine needle aspiration biopsies:

- 0.6–0.8 mm needle (no stylet)

- guide needle 1.2 mm

- 10 ml syringe

- sterile scalpel

- sterile or covered needle guide to affix to transducer

- sterile gel

- sterile fenestrated drape.

The guide needle is inserted through the skin only 1–2 cm and then the fine needle is inserted through the guide and along the visualized path shown by the transducer until it penetrates the lesion. Suction is applied to the syringe and it is withdrawn and advanced into the lesion 2–3 times as the suction is applied. After withdrawal, the specimen is ejected from the needle by disconnecting the syringe, filling it with air, reconnecting and expelling it onto a glass slide. NB: A scalpel can be used to make a small incision for the guide needle if the skin resistance is too great.

Equipment required for histological fine needle aspiration biopsies:

- 0.6–0.8 mm cutting needle
- guide needle 1.2 mm
- 10 ml syringe
- sterile or covered needle guide to affix to transducer
- sterile gel
- sterile scalpel
- piece of sterile paper
- sterile fenestrated drape.

The cutting needle is inserted as above but only so that the needle tip is just outside the lesion. The plunger is retracted, the needle inserted into the lesion and a tissue core cut into the needle. After withdrawal, the tissue core is dislodged onto the sterile paper which is then placed into a specimen pot partially filled with formalin. Up to three needle passes can be performed at one time.

Coarse needle biopsies (outer diameter of needle 1 mm(+), usually 1.2–2 mm diameter are available and are used especially in biopsying diffuse disease.

Full informed consent for any interventional procedure must be obtained from the patient after discussion with the physician.

Liver transplant

Orthotopic liver transplantation is a way of treating:

- irreversible liver damage or livers not responding to conventional treatment
- end-stage liver disease (80% with cirrhosis and primary cholestatic disease; the survival rate after five years is 65–90%)
- biliary atresia
- malignant liver tumours (<5% in total; the prognosis is better if the tumour is <2 cm diameter and solitary)
- liver failure.

The role of ultrasound in a liver transplant is as follows.

PRIOR TO TRANSPLANT

- To exclude extrahepatic malignancy.
- To guide biopsies to confirm a correct diagnosis prior to transplant.
- To confirm or exclude other anomalies (as with biliary atresia).
- To investigate spread of disease.
- To confirm intra- and extrahepatic portal vein patency.
- To exclude tumour invasion of portal and hepatic veins in HCC.
- To identify the position of a tumour which may alter the patient management to resection rather than transplant.
- To measure the spleen prior to transplant as post-operative portal vein thrombosis can increase the size of the spleen.

DURING TRANSPLANT (INTRAOPERATIVE ULTRASOUND)

- To scan the donor organ if too large for the recipient. The major vessels of the donor liver can be identified to help reduce the time of the operation.
- To monitor the hepatic and portal blood flow after the surgical anastomoses prior to the end of the operation.

POST OPERATION

- Ultrasound and Doppler ultrasound are used to monitor the hepatic and portal blood flow in the recovery period. A blocked hepatic artery results in ischaemia and is therefore an emergency.
- The IVC is also monitored. It can narrow at the sites of anastomosis and blood flow can be turbulent at these sites. In addition, the portal vein should be

normal size or slightly larger with normal flow into the liver. Sometimes air is seen postoperatively in the portal vein.

- The common bile duct should also be measured to confirm normal size as any increase in size suggests obstruction or stenosis. Surgical clips may also be seen as bright artefacts with reverberation artefact posteriorly.

- New malignancies must be excluded from the liver, especially after the patient has been immuno-suppressed.

For a fuller account of the role of ultrasound in liver transplants, refer to Meire & Farrant.[6] The use of ultrasound-guided liver transplant biopsies in paediatric patients has been reviewed in a paper by Don et al.[7]

Although relatively old, there is a useful account of the hepatic vein anatomy, essential when identifying liver segments and the position of liver lesions, by Cosgrove et al.[8]

References

1. Calliada F, Campani R, Bottinelli O et al 1998 Ultrasound contrast agents: basic principles. Eur J Radiol 27: Suppl 2: 5157–5160

2. Cosgrove DO 1994 Ultrasound contrast enhancement of tumours. Adv Echo-contrast 3: 38–45

3. Allen AL, Feely A, McInnes E 1997 Reflections on the need for sonographer awareness of possible consequences of liver disease in pregnancy. BMUS Bull 5(4): 45–47

4. Holm HH, Pederson JF, Torp-Pederson S et al 1993 Interventional techniques. In: Cosgrove D, Meire H, Dewbury K (eds) Abdominal and general ultrasound, vol 1. Churchill Livingstone, Edinburgh, pp 97–126

5. Caturelli E, Squillante M, Andriulli A et al 1993 Fine-needle liver biopsy in patients with severely impaired coagulation. Liver 13: 270–273

6. Meire H, Farrant P 1993 Liver transplants. In: Cosgrove D, Meire H, Dewbury K (eds) Abdominal and general ultrasound, vol 1. Churchill Livingstone, Edinburgh, pp 327–349

7. Don S, Kopecky KK, Pescovitz MD 1994 Ultrasound-guided paediatric liver transplant biopsy using a spring-propelled cutting needle (biopsy gun). Pediatr Radiol 24: 21–24

8. Cosgrove DO, Arger PH, Coleman BG 1987 Ultrasonic anatomy of hepatic veins. J Clin Ultrasound 15: 231–235

Further reading

A general overview of colour flow and power Doppler examinations related to hepatic disease can be found in:

Meire HB, Farrant P 1994 Colour flow and power Doppler in liver disease. BMUS Bull 2: 15–20

Robinson PJ 2000 Imaging liver metastases: current limitations and future prospects. Br J Radiol 73(867): 234–241

4

THE BILIARY SYSTEM

Main functions
Anatomy
Scanning
Normal ultrasound appearances
Pathology of the gallbladder
Pathology of the bile ducts

The biliary system consists of the gallbladder and cystic duct, right and left hepatic ducts, common hepatic ducts and common bile duct.

Main functions

Gallbladder

- Stores bile manufactured in the liver; capacity 40–70 ml.
- Absorbs water and electrolytes in order to concentrate the bile. When bile accumulates in the gallbladder, water and electrolytes are absorbed and bile salts and pigments become between five and 10 times more concentrated than when secreted by the liver.

Bile ducts

Transport the 600–1000 ml of bile produced daily in the liver to the gallbladder and duodenum.

Anatomy

Gallbladder

The gallbladder is a thin-walled, pear-shaped structure which lies in the gallbladder fossa on the underside of the liver between the quadrate and right lobes. It contains a rounded fundus inferiorly and a curved body which tapers to the infundibulum and then to the neck where the fibromuscular tissue of the gallbladder wall is thickest. It is connected to the liver by areolar connective tissue containing lymphatics and veins. It joins to the common hepatic duct (CHD) near the porta hepatis via the cystic duct.

Bile ducts

The bile ducts start from the microscopic intercellular canaliculi which anastomose to form the intrahepatic bile ducts running alongside the branches of the portal vein. These form the left and right hepatic ducts, draining bile from the left and right lobes, and lie anterolateral to the portal vein branches.

The left and right intrahepatic bile ducts join just outside the porta hepatis or sometimes just inside the liver and become the CHD, which runs down for about

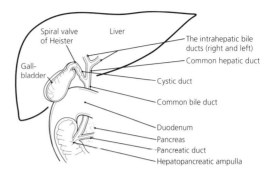

Fig. 4.1 Basic anatomy of gallbladder and bile ducts.

2.5 cm in front and to the right of the portal vein and to the right of the hepatic artery. The cystic duct of the gallbladder joins the CHD and at this point it becomes known as the common bile duct (CBD) which runs down for 7.5–10 cm behind the first part of the duodenum and passes through a groove in the posterior part of the head of the pancreas. Sometimes the CBD is completely enclosed in pancreatic tissue. At this point, the CBD often lies in the same sagittal plane as the inferior vena cava (IVC).

The CBD turns right, meets the pancreatic duct and enters the second part of the duodenum at the hepatopancreatic ampulla (ampulla of Vater). The sphincter muscle in the papilla (the hepatopancreatic ampullary sphincter or the sphincter of Oddi) controls the flow of bile and pancreatic secretion into the duodenum. This is the narrowest part of the common duct (CBD) (Fig. 4.1).

Bile flows freely in and out of the gallbladder via the cystic duct. When no fat has been consumed, the gallbladder distends and stores bile as the sphincter closes at the duodenal papilla. Fat and protein in the gut stimulate the release of cholecystokinin which in turn causes contraction of the gallbladder (in addition to increased flow of pancreatic juice) and the opening of the sphincter, allowing bile to flow freely into the duodenum.

The cystic duct is short, 2–4 cm in length, and extends from the neck of the gallbladder to the CHD which at that point becomes the CBD. The cystic duct contains spiral valves (of Heister), these being mucosal folds rather than proper valves. The cystic duct is rarely seen clearly on ultrasound and therefore the demarcation line is vague. The CHD and CBD is conventionally referred to as the common duct (CD) on ultrasound.

Blood supply

This is from the cystic artery, a branch of the hepatic artery.

Blood drainage

A complex of small veins run towards the liver bed and eventually drain into the portal vein.

Lymph drainage

This is via small lymphatic channels into the gallbladder bed of the liver to the coeliac group of nodes.

Nerve supply

The gallbladder receives nerve fibres from the sympathetic and parasympathetic nervous system. The nerve supply to the gallbladder is via the hepatic plexus which is joined below the liver by branches from the left trunk of the vagus. The afferent fibres in the hepatic plexus include some pain fibres, which explains the referral of pain to the epigastric or right hypochondrial areas.

Relations of the gallbladder

- Anteriorly – the abdominal wall.
- Superiorly – the right lobe of the liver.
- Left – the pylorus of the stomach.
- Posteroinferiorly – the second part of the duodenum, transverse/hepatic flexure of the colon.
- Posteriorly – the first part of the duodenum.

Relations of the CD

- Anteriorly – the first part of the duodenum (upper CD), the pancreatic head (lower CD).
- Right – the second part of the duodenum (lower CD).
- Inferiorly – the third part of the duodenum (lower CD).
- Left – the pancreatic duct (lower CD).

Surface markings

The gallbladder fundus projects from under the anterior border of the liver in the angle between the tips of the ninth and 10th costal cartilage and the outer border of the rectus abdominis muscle. It can be situated very close to the anterior abdominal wall. The position of the gallbladder varies enormously, especially from one body type to another (Fig. 4.2).

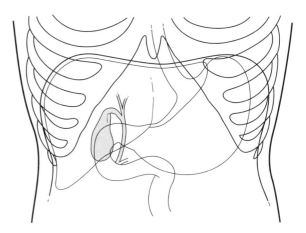

Fig. 4.2   Gallbladder and common duct – position in body.

Variations in normal anatomy

POSITION

The gallbladder can be found in a deep fossa in the liver or actually enclosed in liver tissue – the true intrahepatic gallbladder. This can imitate a solitary hepatic cyst on ultrasound at first sight.

It can be very mobile if suspended on a long mesentery and can lie in the pelvis, especially in the asthenic types.

There can be a congenital absence of the gallbladder or it can be situated on the left side. A paper by Naganuma et al considered anomalous positions of the gallbladder.[1]

SHAPE

- Phrygian cap. The fundus can be folded over, resembling a Phrygian cap and appearing similar to a septate gallbladder on ultrasound. This is a fairly normal variation. Unfolding the Phrygian cap can be attempted by an extra period of starvation in order to fill the gallbladder as much as possible, if this is felt necessary (Fig. 4.3A, B).

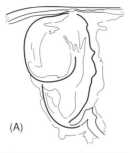

(A)

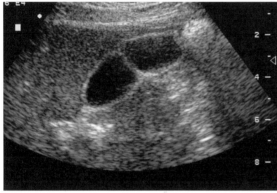

(B)

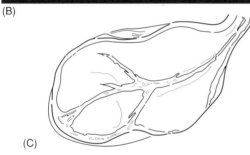

(C)

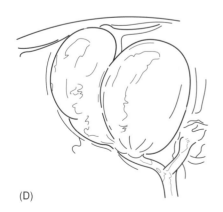

(D)

Fig. 4.3 Variations in gallbladder appearances. (A) Phrygian cap or folded gallbladder. (B) In some positions, the folded gallbladder can appear to have a septum dividing it in two. (C) Septate gallbladder. (D) Double gallbladder.

- Hourglass gallbladder – a bulge is seen at the neck of the gallbladder. Hartmann's pouch is an asymmetrical bulge close to the neck of the gallbladder. It is thought to be found in gallbladders with pathological conditions, rather than a normal variation.

- Septate gallbladder – septa may partly or totally divide the gallbladder (Fig. 4.3C), leading in some cases to an almost double gallbladder.

- The double gallbladder is rare (Fig. 4.3D).

- The choledochal cyst – a congenital cystic dilatation of the CD found at any age. The amount of dilatation varies.

Palpation

The tip of the gallbladder lies against the parietal peritoneum of the RUQ and can be palpated when the patient is very thin and the gallbladder is superficial or if the gallbladder is enlarged.

Relevant tests

Serum bilirubin	<17 µmol/l
Alkaline phosphatase	20–90 U/l
Aspartate aminotransferase (AST)	10–40 U/l

Scanning

Patient preparation

Has the patient still got a gallbladder? Look for scars, read the patient's history, ask if the patient has pain, talk to them.

A period of starvation is required for any ultrasound examination involving the biliary system. Six to eight hours fasting is recommended for patients aged around 12 to adult, four hours fasting for younger children. If the patient is not starved, food taken contracts the gallbladder and increases the thickness of the walls, imitating pathology.

Suggested preparation regime – fast for six to eight hours. Non-fizzy, non-fatty drinks may be taken. Ensure that no other tests such as barium studies are to take place on the same day that may cause artefacts when scanning. The patient should also refrain from smoking as this causes the bile ducts to contract, but some people find this hard to do.

Children can fast for four hours. Babies can have a bottle of dextrose instead of the normal milky feed or be scanned just before the normal time for a feed. If fractious, the baby can be fed at the time of the scan. Babies and diabetics should be placed first on the list for the scan.

Equipment required

A sector probe enables good intercostal scanning and avoidance of rib shadowing. It also allows good subcostal scanning with cephalic angulation – a small head allows the operator to push up under ribs. Often there is little choice and a curved linear probe is all that is available. The choice of transducer frequency is variable as the gallbladder lies at varying depths within the abdomen and can be very superficial or deep under the liver. Usually, it is 3.5–5 MHz for adults and 7.5 MHz for children.

A frequency appropriate to the depth of the gallbladder must be used. The focusing zone must be set for the appropriate depth and the gain settings must be low enough to avoid reverberation artefacts and false echoes in the superficial gallbladder.

Suggested scanning technique – gallbladder

The liver is usually used as an acoustic window to image the gallbladder owing to its position anterior and lateral to it. If distended and in the normal position, the gallbladder should be relatively easy to find. It is seen as an echo-free, pear-shaped organ on the inferior aspect of the liver.

SUPINE POSITION

Start by scanning longitudinally in the mid-clavicular line. Use the subcostal approach at first. When the echo-free gallbladder is seen, alter the scanning angle until the longest axis is seen. Scan from right to left sides of the gallbladder, ensuring that the neck to the fundus is well visualized. Once the lie of the gallbladder has been established, turn the probe 90° and scan from the neck to the fundus.

If there are any small masses on the lateral walls of the gallbladder, longitudinal scans alone will not reveal them as the longitudinal scan images the middle and largest part of the gallbladder in this section. The gallbladder may be superficial and false echoes may appear within the lumen caused by reverberation artefacts in the near-field. To avoid this, it is necessary to select a higher frequency probe and choose the appropriate focusing zone. When scanning the gallbladder, note the size, shape, wall thickness and smoothness of the gallbladder.

Frequently, and especially in hypersthenic patients, the gallbladder lies too high up under the liver to visualize subcostally. Colonic gas acts as a barrier between the transducer and the gallbladder. An intercostal approach may be required. Place the probe in an intercostal space on the right side (this may be quite high up) and use the liver as an acoustic window. The whole of the gallbladder is better visualized this way in this type of patient, especially the fundus.

With the hyposthenic type, the gallbladder may lie low in the pelvis and be hidden by gas from intestinal loops. In this case it may be necessary to tilt the patient in a Trendelenburg position (head down, feet up) in order to help the gallbladder ascend to the upper abdomen closer to the liver.

LEFT POSTERIOR OBLIQUE (LPO) POSITION

With an average build, better images of the gallbladder can often be obtained by turning the patient halfway towards the left. The weight of the bile in the gallbladder pulls it medially and inferiorly where it may be more easily scanned subcostally. Turning the patient into the LPO position will help to reveal any hidden stones. The gallbladder neck will stretch slightly and help reveal any stones in that area. Gas should also rise away from the gallbladder area in this position.

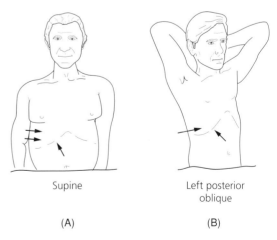

Supine

Left posterior oblique

(A)

(B)

Fig. 4.4 Scanning positions. (A) Supine. (B) Left posterior oblique.

LEFT LATERAL DECUBITUS POSITION

This is a variation on the above.

ERECT

This position is used to help lower the position of the gallbladder. It is often useful to scan extremely obese patients intercostally when they are in the erect position.

Suggested scanning technique – bile ducts

The acknowledged best position in which to scan the bile ducts, taking into consideration the position of the ducts, is with the patient in the LPO position. The right side is raised 45° from the couch. This allows the bile duct to move slightly medially and lie anterior to the portal vein. Position the transducer so that the sound beam is at right angles to the lower costal margin. It may be necessary to angle the transducer towards the head. On quiet respiration, follow the line of the CD. As the lower part of the CD is usually hidden by gas in the first part of the duodenum, it is necessary to assess the lower part of the duct by scanning transversely at the level of the head of pancreas where the bile duct is seen as an anechoic rounded area in the posterior part of the head of pancreas (see Chapter 5).

The intrahepatic bile ducts will only be seen if enlarged or if the liver is of lower reflectivity than normal. When measuring the CD, the image should be enlarged as much as possible to ensure an accurate measurement and the duct measured at the level of the porta hepatis. The diameter should be measured from inner to inner walls of the duct.

Technique for children and neonates

The technique follows broadly the same method as that for adults except that less movement of the patient should be used. The liver is proportionately larger in the infant than in the adult and so the acoustic window is relatively larger. The infant must be kept warm at all times.

Suggested minimal sections

- Longitudinal section through the gallbladder.
- Transverse section through the gallbladder.
- Any pathology observed.

- A measured section of the CD at the porta hepatis, longitudinal and transverse.
- A view of the lower CD through the head of the pancreas.
- A section through the liver to show the intrahepatic bile ducts plus one more to show dilatation if present.

Normal ultrasound appearances

GALLBLADDER

The gallbladder is recognized when scanning longitudinally and following the white interlobar fissure outside the liver. It appears as a pear-shaped organ, black with thin white walls. If it is tense and rounded it is probably pathological. The walls should be the same thickness all round and should measure no more than 3 mm thick when the patient is prepared by starving, except for nearer the neck of the gallbladder where the wall becomes thicker.

The bile is seen as a black area as the acoustic impedance of bile is about the same as water. Attenuation of ultrasound by bile is very low so there is acoustic enhancement posterior to the gallbladder. The cystic duct is often fairly tortuous and is seldom seen clearly. Some acoustic shadowing is often seen which sometimes gives rise for concern as stones can lie here and also be a source of acoustic shadowing.

The gallbladder wall thickens after eating, when it is inflamed, and in the presence of ascites so check whether there is pathology present or whether the patient has not followed the preparation instructions clearly. In babies and young children, the gallbladder appears almost triangular in cross-section when the child has been starved and, if circular, this often suggests a degree of abnormal distension. In neonates, small air bubbles can occasionally be seen owing to an immature hepatopancreatic sphincter (Fig. 4.5).

BILIARY TREE

The right and left main hepatic ducts appear as fine tubular structures with a diameter of between 1–2 mm in front of and parallel to the portal vein branches. At the porta hepatis the CD appears as a narrow tube running above and slightly to the right of the portal vein.

At this point, and when a gallbladder is present, the inner diameter measurement should be <5 mm; a diameter of 5–6 mm is equivocal and a 7 mm+ diameter measurement should be seen as abnormal in a

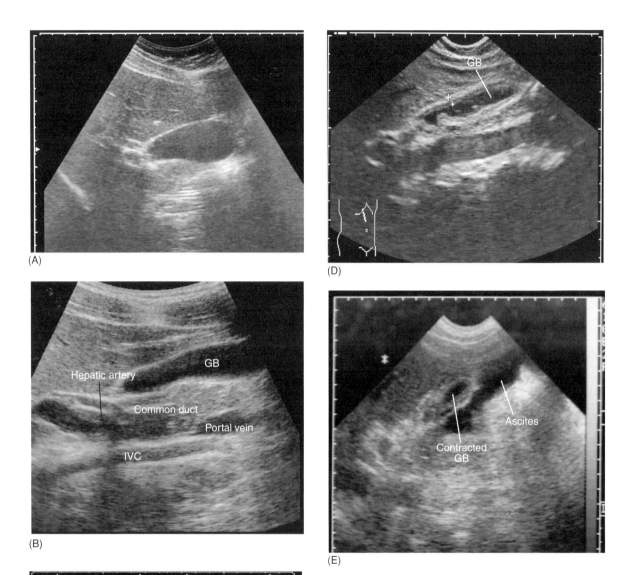

(A)

(B)

Hepatic artery

GB

Common duct

Portal vein

IVC

(C)

Liver   Duodenum   Liver   Gallbladder

Bile   Common
duct   hepatic duct

Hepatic   Infundibulum
artery

Portal vein   Portal vein

NO.48/48

F3

10:43:54

REVIEW

(D)

GB

(E)

Contracted
GB   Ascites

Fig. 4.5 (A) Normal gallbladder. (B) Normal gallbladder and associated vessels. (C) Gallbladder and cystic duct. (D) Gallbladder wall thickens after eating. (E) Contracted gallbladder with thick walls in the presence of ascites.

young subject. The CD enlarges with age and is said to increase by about 1 mm per decade of life. Anything more than 8 mm after a cholecystectomy should raise suspicion of an abnormality although the CD is said to take over some of the storage properties of the gallbladder. The appearance of the CD and portal vein is complicated by the position of the hepatic artery which lies medial to the CD. Identification of duct or

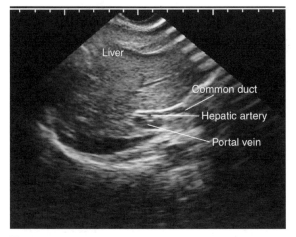

(A)

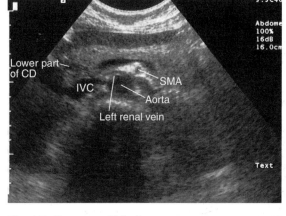

Fig. 4.7 Pancreas and bile duct.

Fig. 4.6 (A) Common duct relative to portal veins and hepatic artery. (B) Hepatic artery relative to portal vein and bile duct.

hepatic artery is determined by colour Doppler if required.

In approximately 85% of cases the right branch of the hepatic artery courses to the right between the portal vein and the CD, appearing as a cross-sectional tube between two linear tubes (the PV posteriorly and the CD anteriorly). There are variations to this: in 15% it crosses anterior to the CD (Fig. 4.6).

It is difficult to see the lower half of the CD as it passes behind the gas-filled duodenum. The lowest end of the CD is visualized by scanning the pancreas where it

is seen as a small, round, black shape situated in the posterior aspect of the head of the pancreas (Fig. 4.7).

Normal sizes

GALLBLADDER

The size of the gallbladder is variable, averaging 7–10 cm long and 4 cm in diameter maximum when distended after starving. Its capacity is approximately 45–70 ml, sometimes as much as 150 ml. The thickness of the wall when distended should be less than 3 mm all round. It is not so much the size but the shape which is important: the pear shape should be present, not a tense, rounded shape which probably indicates pathology.

Although the size of the gallbladder is variable, the 23 lb (10.4 kg) gallbladder removed from a 69-year-old woman in Maryland, USA, in 1989 after she complained of increased abdominal swelling could be considered as abnormal!

The size of the normal distended gallbladder in a starved adult is:

- length   7–10 cm (13 cm maximum, usually)
- diameter   3–4 cm
- wall thickness <3 mm

NB: The size of the gallbladder increases with age but the wall thickness is unaffected by age.

In the neonate, the gallbladder diameter is 0.5–1.6 cm (mean 0.9 cm).

Duct diameters in normal adults:

- intrahepatic ducts (only seen   1–2 mm maximum
  if liver is hypoechoic)
- upper CD (at the level of the   <4 mm
  portal vein branch)
- lower CD   <6–7 mm

Upper CD diameter in children is 3 mm up to 5 mm by late teens.

In neonates it is <1 mm.

NB: The duct diameter can be larger following chole-cystectomy, previous obstruction or with advancing age. There has often been a discrepancy over the size of the bile duct as measured on ultrasound compared with that on ERCP which, allowing for magnification factors, has traditionally been larger. Recent research has revealed that larger bile ducts in 70% of cases are oval and that the transverse diameter was larger than the anteroposterior measurement and correlated more with the ERCP measurement.[2]

GALLBLADDER VOLUME ESTIMATION

The volume of the gallbladder can be calculated by a number of methods, the quickest and nearest to reality being the ellipsoid method where:

$$\text{Volume} = 0.52 \,(\text{length} \times \text{width} \times \text{AP diameter})$$

Measurements may be taken after starving and compared to those after the administration of a fatty meal in order to assess the function of the gallbladder.

Box 4.1   Advice

- The gallbladder might be low lying (common) or on the left (rare).

- It may not be seen because it is obscured by gas (uncommon, you can usually find a way around this).

- It may have been removed by surgery: ask the patient, read the notes, look for the scar.

- It may be hard to see as an incorrect frequency and focusing zone may have been used. A stand-off gel block may have to be used with a superficial gallbladder.

- Gross obesity may cause problems when the gallbladder is beyond the penetrative depth of even a low-frequency probe.

Pathology of the gallbladder

- Gallstones
- Biliary sludge (viscid bile)
- Polyps
- Carcinoma
- Adenomyomatosis
- Porcelain gallbladder
- Acute cholecystitis
- Complications of acute cholecystitis
  - Gangrenous cholecystitis
  - Emphysematous cholecystitis
  - Empyema of the gallbladder
- Chronic cholecystitis
- Diffuse wall thickening
- Micro-gallbladder
- Non-visualized gallbladder
- Biliary ascaris

Gallstones

GENERAL INFORMATION

The prevalence of gallstones in developed countries is thought to be about 10% and as many as two-thirds are asymptomatic. The probability of developing biliary symptoms in the asymptomatic group of gallstone carriers is about 18% in 24 years. The number of gall-stones found within the gallbladder can range from one solitary stone to the impressive number of 23 530 removed from an 85-year-old woman in West Sussex in August, 1987.

Stones can range in size from less than 1 mm in diameter to that belonging to an 80-year-old woman which, on removal at the Charing Cross Hospital, London, on December 29th 1952, weighed 6.29 kg (13 lb 14 oz). Gallstones are seen in young and old alike (and have been noticed on fetal scanning), not just in the fair, fertile, fat, flatulent, 40-year-old female, as was always thought.

Gallstones are formed in several ways.

- An increase in concentration of cholesterol in the blood (hypercholesterolaemia) can lead to an increase in the bile and its subsequent precipitation. This occurs in obesity, diabetes and pregnancy.

Cholesterol stones are formed which are hard and radiolucent on X-ray examinations. The incidence of pure cholesterol stones is small.

- An increase of bilirubin in the blood (hyperbilirubinaemia) found in patients with haemolytic anaemia. Pure bilirubin stones are soft, small, brown and irregularly shaped. Calcium salts precipitated in the gallbladder usually contribute to the composition of these stones and make them radioopaque.

- Biliary stasis caused by faulty or non-emptying, a malformed gallbladder or obstruction to cystic duct leading to stagnant bile in the gallbladder. In turn, high concentrations of cholesterol and bile pigment are formed because of excessive water absorption. This leads to the formation of mixed cholesterol and bile pigment stones, the most common type. They are of variable size and are faceted if multiple. There is sufficient calcium in the stones to make them radioopaque. Stones can be so small as to appear as gravel (see Biliary sludge).

- Inflammation of the gallbladder mucosa. This allows bile acids to be absorbed and reduces the solubility of cholesterol. Protein oozes from the surface to provide a nucleus for stones and calcium salts diffuse into the bile in large amounts to add calcium bilirubinate to the developing cholesterol stone.

CLINICAL INFORMATION

Stones can be found at any point in the biliary tree, although the majority are found within the gallbladder.

There is an increased incidence of stones with cirrhosis, Crohn's disease, diabetes, pancreatic disease and hyperparathyroidism. In addition, 60% of children with sickle cell disease show evidence of biliary calculi by the age of 12 and 30% of children with cystic fibrosis develop bilirubin stones (Fig. 4.8).

Large stones can lead to acute and chronic cholecystitis. Multiple small stones can cause biliary obstruction as they can pass through the cystic duct and into the common bile duct and obstruct the narrower distal end. Often, the obstruction is incomplete or the stone is expelled into the duodenum, relieving the obstruction. Severe colicky pain, characteristic of a cholelithiasis attack, can be a result of spasm of the gallbladder as it tries to force a stone down the cystic duct or spasm of the pancreatoduodenal ampulla or of the ductal muscles, to a lesser degree. The spasm is caused by irritation of the gallbladder mucosa or by impaction of a stone in the cystic duct or CD.

Patients present in severe pain, sufficient to cause them to double up. The pain is constant and unremitting although seldom lasting for more than two hours. It is relieved only by strong analgesia. The patient is often frightened by the intensity of the pain and there is often a strong reluctance to be palpated in order to find a positive Murphy's sign. The enlarged gallbladder will appear beneath the tip of the right ninth rib. It is smooth, moves with respiration and is continuous with the edge of the liver (see section on Acute cholecystitis for additional information on physical examination).

Small stones may produce a partial obstruction, perhaps causing a mild jaundice, but are often passed into the duodenum which can account for the report of stones

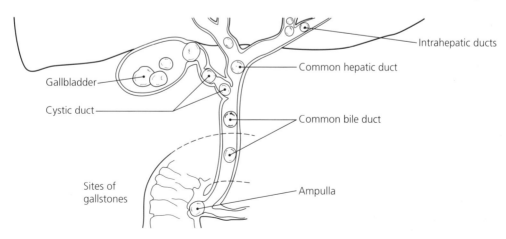

Fig. 4.8 Sites of biliary calculi.

being seen in the gallbladder at the time of the scan but not found at the time of the cholecystectomy. Ten percent of gallstones are seen on plain X-ray. Serum bilirubin, alkaline phosphatase and aspartate amino-transferase levels are often all slightly raised.

GALLSTONE ILEUS

When acute cholecystitis is accompanied by an obstruction of the cystic duct by a stone that is too large to be passed, a pericholecystitis may occur, developing into an abscess which can cause the gall-bladder to be attached to the duodenum. When the abscess ulcerates, a fistula can form which can allow the stone to pass into the duodenum. As a result, the stone can pass towards the terminal ileum where it is narrower and can obstruct, producing the 'gallstone ileus'. The obstructed small bowel and subsequent gas overload can make visualization of the pancreas diffi-cult. Less common are fistulae from the gallbladder to the stomach, large bowel and CD (Fig. 4.9).

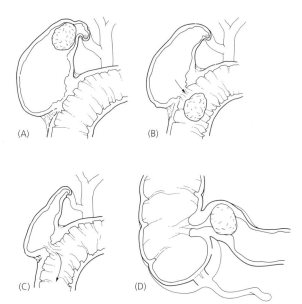

Fig. 4.9 Fistula between gallbladder and duodenum allowing stone to pass into the gut. (A) Inflamed gallbladder adheres to duodenum. (B) Fistula forms, stone passes into duodenum. (C) Gallbladder contracts after stone has passed into the duodenum. (D) Gallstone impacts at terminal ileum.

TREATMENT OF GALLSTONES

Cholecystectomy is a common method of treatment for biliary calculi. Half a million cholecystectomies are carried out in the USA each year. The gallbladder is not essential to life and bile continues to be produced and flows directly to the duodenum, having little or no effect on the digestion. It is a relatively safe operation except for the general risk of any form of surgery. Surgery may not alleviate the gas, bloating, pain or nausea suffered before, however.

Apart from surgery or endoscopic removal, there are other methods of treatment for gallstones. Patients will often ask if gallstones can be dissolved by chemicals. This is possible in some cases where there is no obstruction to the flow of bile and where the stones are composed of a higher degree of cholesterol.

Before the treatment, the type and composition of the calculi have to be assessed. Traditionally, oral chole-cystograms or CT have been used to assess the chemical composition of the stones and the function of the gall-bladder. Research into the ultrasound appearances of stones to exclude those unsuitable for dissolution has been carried out.[3] Dissolution therapy involves the bile acids chenodeoxycholic acid and ursodeoxycholic acid which increase cholesterol solubility in bile. They only dissolve radiolucent stones in a functioning gallbladder and not stones coated with calcium or bile pigment stones, making only about 10% of patients suitable for therapy. This can take from six months to two years depending on the size of the stones and after completion of therapy it is said that 50% of gallstones recur. Patients are advised to continue the dosage for three months after the radiological disappearance of the stones. Chenodeoxycholic acid can sometimes cause diarrhoea.

Ultrasound-guided lithotripsy is useful for treating non-calcified stones in a functioning gallbladder, after which the patients have dissolution therapy.

ULTRASOUND APPEARANCES

Gallstones are seen as highly reflective structures within the gallbladder, casting a clean acoustic shadow posteriorly if about 3 mm or more in diameter. This size allows the gallstone to fill the width of the ultra-sound beam. No shadow is seen if the stone is smaller than the beam width or if it is a larger stone lying partially outside the beam or if it is outside the focal zone of the beam.

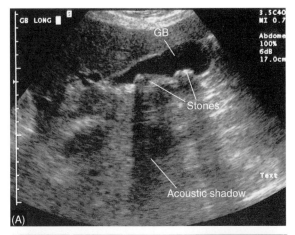

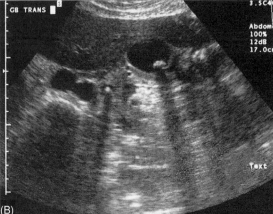

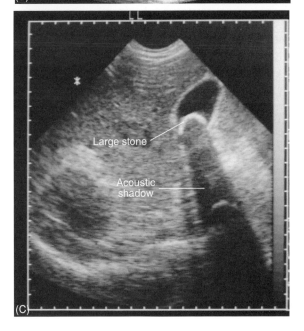

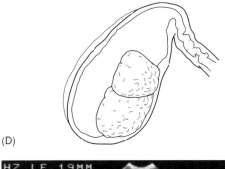

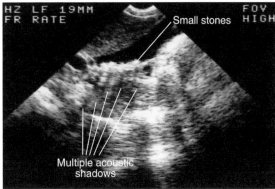

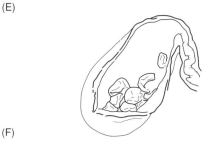

Fig. 4.10 Typical appearance of calculi in the gallbladder. Note posterior acoustic shadowing. (A) Longitudinal section. (B) Transverse section. (C & D) Large calculi. (E & F) Multiple smaller calculi.

The stones move with gravity: as the patient moves position, the stones should fall slowly to rest on the dependent portion of the gallbladder.

The acoustic shadows, caused by absorption and reflection of sound by the stone, should be sharp. They are not affected by the shape or composition of the stone. Shadowing from bowel gas is caused only by reflection and is less well defined. Shadowing is dependent on the relationship of the beam to the stone. In order to produce acoustic shadowing, use as small a beam width as possible by selecting the appropriate focusing zone and using the highest frequency transducer possible. When all features are present, the diagnostic accuracy is 100%.

> **Box 4.2   Advice**
>
> By moving the patient into the LLD, LPO or erect position, the gravity dependency of stones can be demonstrated and stones that are hidden in the neck of the gallbladder often reveal themselves. As calculi are often found in association with carcinoma of the gallbladder (see p. 75), any soft tissue mass or focal wall thickening must be excluded if calculi are seen.
>
> Small calculi may group together, forming a larger shadow than would otherwise be seen from very small stones that are separated from each other.

Biliary sludge (viscid bile or echogenic bile)

CLINICAL INFORMATION

Biliary sludge is a collection of very small particles of mainly calcium carbonate granules with some cholesterol crystals. Sometimes the granules and crystals group together and form sludge balls. It is thought that sludge balls may be precursors to biliary calculi but this is speculation at present. It may be seen when there is biliary stasis after pathological obstruction or after prolonged deliberate fasting or in patients on parenteral nutrition, e.g. those fed intravenously on the ITU and after gastrointestinal surgery. After a return to normal diet, the sludge often disappears.

ULTRASOUND APPEARANCES

Biliary sludge appears as a collection of non-shadowing, gravity-dependent echoes of relatively higher reflectivity than normal bile. It can be caused by pus or blood in the bile from trauma or infection. The diagnosis can be confirmed from the patient's history and other specific ultrasonic features.

After movement, it is usually slow to settle into position and therefore it is essential to wait and scan

other regions before returning to the gallbladder. Violent moving of the patient can spread the viscid bile and make it harder to identify. As it settles, it may not always demonstrate a straight bile–sludge level. There may be accompanying gallstones that may float if small enough and show as an echogenic line between the sludge and the bile (Fig. 4.11).

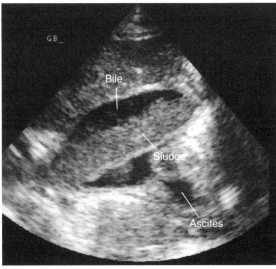

(A)

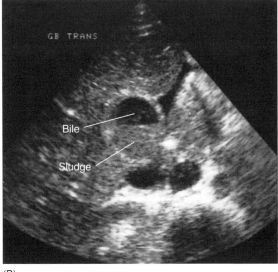

(B)

Fig. 4.11 Biliary sludge. (A) Longitudinal section of gallbladder showing bile–sludge level. (B) Transverse section.

Polyps

CLINICAL INFORMATION

This is a general term covering inflammatory polyps, cholesterol polyps and adenomyomas. These are usually incidental findings and are relatively common. The most common is a solitary benign adenoma; 10% of benign adenomas are multiple and 10% demonstrate evidence of a carcinoma *in situ*. Larger polyps, those more than 1 cm diameter, may tend towards malignant degeneration.

ULTRASOUND APPEARANCES

Polyps appear as small, rounded, highly reflective structures fixed to the wall of the gallbladder and projecting into its lumen. As they are fixed they do not move to a different location with the effect of gravity. They do not cast an acoustic shadow but may demonstrate some reverberation artefact posteriorly.

It is essential to scan the gallbladder in transverse section from neck to fundus in addition to the longitudinal sections otherwise a polyp may be missed (Fig. 4.12).

Gallbladder carcinoma

CLINICAL INFORMATION

Gallbladder carcinoma is highly malignant and

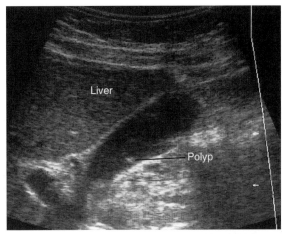

(A)

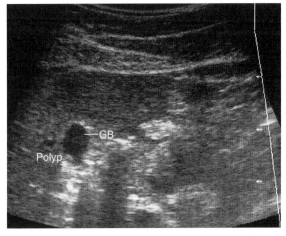

(B)

Fig. 4.12 Polyps. (A) Longitudinal section of gallbladder. (B) Transverse section.

metastasizes early and therefore the condition has a poor prognosis. Carcinoma near the neck of the gallbladder tends to invade hepatic hilar tissue and the common hepatic and common bile ducts. Carcinoma at the fundus tends to spread to the liver or peritoneum. Spread to the adjacent lymph nodes occurs quickly. Its prevalence increases with age to a peak between 60 and 70. It affects four times as many females as males; 80–90% have associated gallstones and there is a high correlation with chronic cholecystitis, suggesting a connection between inflammation and neoplastic change. The mean survival rate is less than five months from the time of detection and it has been seen that where the rate of cholecystectomy for cholelithiasis has increased, mortality from gallbladder carcinoma has decreased. Few patients survive one year. Metastases in the gallbladder commonly arise from malignant melanomas and the appearances will look similar to primary cancers there.

ULTRASOUND APPEARANCES

Carcinoma of the gallbladder appears as an irregular mass of mixed echoes attached to the wall of the gallbladder and so does not move with patient movement. It is usually an unexpected finding. There are often associated gallstones present. The gallbladder wall thickens focally at the region of the mass, as is seen with adenomyomatosis. Spread from carcinoma of the gallbladder can enlarge lymph nodes in the region of the head of the pancreas, causing the CD to obstruct and imitate carcinoma of the pancreatic head (Fig. 4.13).

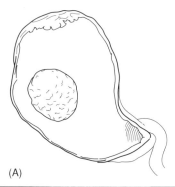

(A)

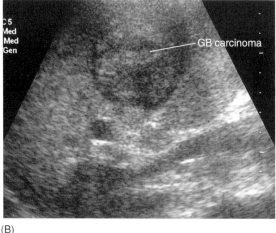

(B)

Fig. 4.13 (A) Fundal carcinoma and large calculus. (B) Advanced gallbladder carcinoma. (Reprinted from Clinical Ultrasound, Bates, p 49, Fig 3.17a, 1999 by permission of the publisher Churchill Livingstone.)

Adenomyomatosis

CLINICAL INFORMATION

Adenomyomatosis is the term given to hyperplastic changes in the wall of the gallbladder. It can occur in the absence of either gallstones or inflammatory infiltrates. It causes mild recurring RUQ pain and occurs mainly in those over 35 years old in a ratio of 3:1, females:males.

ULTRASOUND APPEARANCES

There may be diffuse or focal thickening (segmental wall thickening) of the gallbladder wall, multiple polyps and multiple septae within the gallbladder. Segmental wall thickening may provide a localized narrowing of the gallbladder lumen which may give it an hourglass appearance.

There can also be multiple comet-tail or reverberation artefacts resulting from small stones or cholesterol crystals (bile concretions) in the Rokitansky–Aschoff sinuses; these are the intramural diverticulae caused by the lining epithelium of the gallbladder extending as a downgrowth between the muscle bundles, giving rise to deep gland-like structures. The cholesterol in the Rokitansky–Aschoff sinuses can give a so-called 'diamond ring' appearance on transverse sections (Fig. 4.14).

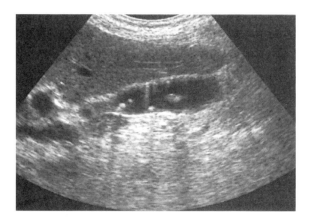

Fig. 4.14 Comet-tail artefacts in a gallbladder with adenomyomatosis.

Porcelain gallbladder

CLINICAL INFORMATION

Porcelain gallbladder, a rare condition, is the name given to calcification of the gallbladder wall. In cases of chronic cholecystitis, the entire wall of the gallbladder can consist of fibrous scar tissue which can in turn calcify. A rate of between 10% and 61% of patients with this condition develop or have associated carcinoma and this lesion may be hidden by the acoustic shadowing from the calcified anterior wall. Eighty percent of patients are female and 90% of porcelain gallbladders are associated with gallstones.

ULTRASOUND APPEARANCES

A normal gallbladder cannot be seen. However, in the gallbladder area there is a highly reflective curvilinear anterior wall which produces heavy posterior shadowing from the anterior surface of the calcified gallbladder wall. This will occur in any position of the transducer relative to the gallbladder.

Box 4.4   Advice

A porcelain gallbladder can appear like a contracted gallbladder around a line of stones. It is important to differentiate between this and a porcelain gallbladder because of the 25% association with carcinomas of the gallbladder. Try to find a non-calcified gallbladder wall anteriorly to confirm stones. A carcinoma can be detected by focal or diffuse thickening of the gallbladder wall external to the calcified area, a mass extending from the gallbladder wall or other signs such as biliary obstruction, enlarged lymph nodes around the porta hepatis or pancreas, or liver metastases.

Acute cholecystitis

CLINICAL INFORMATION

Acute cholecystitis usually presents in the age group 30–60, more in females than in males (75%). The symptoms are pain in the right hypochondrium radiating through the trunk to the right shoulder blade. Pain is continuous, made worse by breathing and movement so the patient breathes shallowly in order to avoid pain. The patient feels nauseated and often vomits; the abdomen often feels distended. Tachycardia of 90–100 beats/min and a pyrexia of 38–39°C is often noted. There is mild jaundice in 20% of cases.

The inflamed gallbladder can be felt as a large, very tender mass below the liver edge. Confirmation of acute cholecystitis can be made by placing the left hand on the lower costal margin and the thumb over the gallbladder with moderate pressure. On inspiration, if the inflamed gallbladder touches the thumb and the patient catches their breath, this is considered to be a positive sign of acute cholecystitis (the positive Murphy's sign).

ULTRASOUND APPEARANCES

There is no single sign for the diagnosis of acute cholecystitis. Studies have shown that ultrasound is 81–95% sensitive and 64–100% specific in acute cholecystitis.

Signs to look for are:

- a gallbladder with an echo-poor rim of oedema around it – the 'halo sign' (seen in 70% of cases)

- a positive sonographic Murphy's sign (where the area of maximum tenderness is directly under the probe). A positive sonographic Murphy's sign in addition to stones in the gallbladder is 92% specific for acute cholecystitis

- gallstones, especially in the cystic duct or neck of gallbladder; 90% of cases of acute cholecystitis are secondary to cystic duct/neck of gallbladder obstruction by an impacted gallstone although 5–10% contain no gallstones (acalcular cholecystitis) (Fig. 4.15)

- a gallbladder with a thick, echogenic wall after the patient has fasted (typically 5 mm+ when the normal thickness of the gallbladder after fasting is usually 3 mm at most)

- a large gallbladder (hydrops) that has a tense, rounded shape with an anteroposterior diameter of often more than 5 cm and a length of up to 20 cm.

NB: Cystic duct/neck of gallbladder obstruction leads to distension and inflammation which is often mild and can subside quickly. The bile is reabsorbed and the epithelium changes to a mucin-secreting pattern filling the gallbladder with clear mucus – a mucocoele. The gallbladder is palpable and there is mild discomfort.

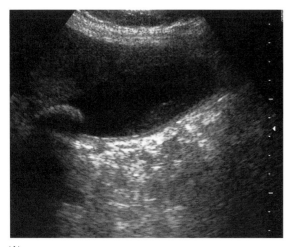

(A)

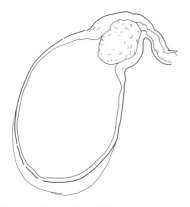

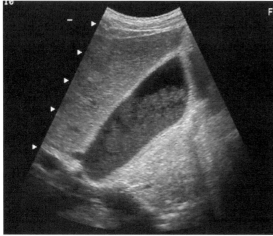

(B)

Fig. 4.15 (A) Impacted stone in neck of gallbladder causing obstruction. (B) Acalcular cholecystitis. Note sludge in the gallbladder.

Box 4.5   Advice

Acoustic shadowing can be seen posterior to stones although stones in the neck of the gallbladder or cystic duct are harder to see owing to the lack of bile around the stones in these areas. Shadow artefact can occur from folding over of the cystic duct and can mimic a stone. It is important to turn the patient into a LPO or LLD position in order to stretch out the cystic duct and help reveal any hidden stones or to exclude stones in that area.

COMPLICATIONS OF ACUTE CHOLECYSTITIS

Gangrenous cholecystitis

Acute cholecystitis may progress to gangrenous cholecystitis which may perforate, resulting in a pericholecystic abscess or peritonitis. Gangrene is seen usually in the older age group. Morbidity and mortality are higher with gangrenous cholecystitis. It is important to look for signs which may indicate the need for urgent surgery.

Gangrenous cholecystitis shows as membranes within the gallbladder from fibrinous strands of exudate and sloughing of the mucosa. Only 33% of gangrenous gallbladders have a positive sonographic Murphy's sign. Look for an echo-poor fluid collection around the gallbladder from localized peritonitis or perforation.

Emphysematous cholecystitis

Gas can form in the Rokitansky–Aschoff sinuses of the gallbladder wall or possibly in the gallbladder itself.

It is seen as highly reflective areas within a thick oedematous wall with distal shadowing and reverberations which can look like a loop of bowel. Although this is quite rare, it has a strong association with gangrene and perforation of the gallbladder. The diagnosis of emphysematous cholecystitis on ultrasound has an important role in the management of the patient with symptoms of acute cholecystitis.[5]

Empyema of the gallbladder

This occurs when bacterial infection arises from secondary infection and invades the gallbladder, the content becoming purulent. The cystic duct is usually occluded by a stone or from scarring or by inflammatory oedema.

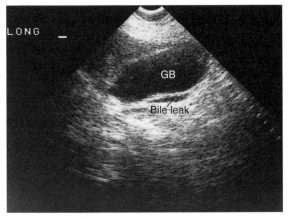

(A)

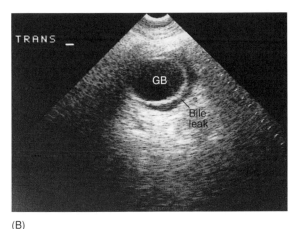

(B)

Fig. 4.16 Empyema of the gallbladder with leak of bile into peritoneum. (A) Longitudinal. (B) Transverse.

On ultrasound, there may be a leakage of bile through the gallbladder wall and fine echoes (pus) are seen in the gallbladder (Fig. 4.16).

Chronic cholecystitis

CLINICAL INFORMATION

Chronic cholecystitis is very frequently associated with gallstones. Patients are usually female between 30 and 60, although there is a wide variation on this. Symptoms are indigestion or pain after eating (especially fatty foods) and usually appear gradually 15–30 minutes after eating, lasting 30–90 minutes. Belching can occur after eating (flatulent dyspepsia). ALP, AST and ALT values are often raised.

ULTRASOUND APPEARANCES

The wall of the gallbladder is often thickened, measuring more than 3 mm. The gallbladder itself is often fibrosed and the size is normally reduced; it may be so small that it is difficult to see on ultrasound. It can, however, be distended. Stones within the gallbladder will produce acoustic shadowing posteriorly (Fig. 4.17).

Box 4.6   Advice

In chronic cholecystitis, the gallbladder either does not contract or contracts minimally in response to cholecystokinin. The size of the gallbladder therefore should be measured in longitudinal and transverse dimensions or the volume calculated if the equipment offers this facility so that the amount of contraction after giving the patient a fatty meal can be measured.

A contracted gallbladder with stones can be confused with bowel appearances, especially when little or no bile lies around a line of stones. Look for a wall-echo-shadow complex representing the reflective anterior wall of the gallbladder, the thin echo-poor rim (the bile) and the shadow from the anterior surface of the gallstones.

It is necessary to look for evidence of peristalsis and hazy shadowing posteriorly to confirm bowel. It is also necessary to find out if the patient has eaten prior to the ultrasound examination as if this has occurred, the gallbladder will be smaller and the wall thicker and this can mimic the appearances of chronic cholecystitis.

Diffuse wall thickening

A normal gallbladder wall thickness should be no more than 3 mm after fasting. The wall may be thicker if the patient has eaten or has:

- ascites
- cholecystitis (acute or chronic)
- hepatitis
- congestive heart failure
- AIDS.

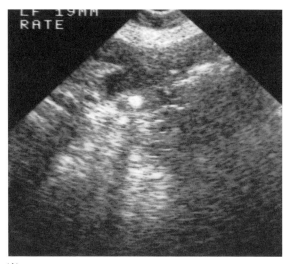

(A)

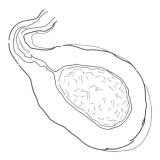

(B)

Fig. 4.17 Chronic cholecystitis. Gallbladder contracted around stone, no bile inside. Note that it is hard to find the gallbladder contracted around the calculus.

Micro-gallbladder

When the gallbladder is less than 3 cm × 1 cm after fasting, this is considered to be a micro-gallbladder; 30% of patients with cystic fibrosis have micro-gallbladders. There is an increased incidence of gallstones in patients with cystic fibrosis. The cystic duct often atrophies or is occluded by mucus in these cases.

Non-visualized gallbladder

The gallbladder is often not able to be identified if it is:

- fibrosed
- contracted around stones
- contracted through disease
- a porcelain gallbladder
- on the left side

and certainly not if it has been removed (look for scar).

Biliary ascaris

CLINICAL INFORMATION

Worms and parasites can enter the biliary system from the duodenum. It is rarely seen in Europe and North America but biliary infestation by worms is often encountered in many other countries. Sizes of 30 cm in length and 5 mm in diameter have been quoted. It causes biliary colic, recurrent pyogenic cholangitis, pancreatitis, hepatic abscesses and septicaemia.

ULTRASOUND APPEARANCES

The gallbladder is usually enlarged and contains many overlapping linear tubes similar to strands of spaghetti. Movement can sometimes be seen. The parasites may cause an acoustic shadow if dead and calcified. A recent paper has presented the appearances of intra- and extrahepatic biliary ascariasis.[6]

Pathology of the bile ducts

- Obstruction by stone (choledocholithiasis)
- Obstruction by tumour (cholangiocarcinoma, papilloma, cystadenoma)
- Choledochal cyst
- Biliary atresia
- Primary sclerosing cholangitis
- Klatskin tumour
- Caroli's disease
- Air in the biliary tree

Obstruction – general

CLINICAL INFORMATION

The CD is generally considered to be abnormally wide in adults if it measures 7 mm or more in diameter at its lower end although it can be up to 10 mm after undergoing a cholecystectomy and enlarges in the elderly and in pregnant patients. The size of the bile ducts can confirm normality of the ductal system or the severity of an obstruction if one is present.

Obstruction is caused by a blockage in the ducts somewhere in between the site of bile manufacture and the entry of bile into the duodenum through the ampulla. This blockage within the biliary system can cause surgical jaundice as distinct from medical jaundice which concerns pathology at a cellular or biochemical level. Adult patients do not become visibly jaundiced until their serum bilirubin level reaches 30 μmol/l.

Jaundice is seen in 90% of neonates, usually between days 2 and 8. However, a pathological reason for this jaundice is suggested if:

- it appears within 24 hours
- the serum bilirubin level is >200 μmol/l
- the bilirubin level continues to rise after day 8 and
- the jaundice persists.

The most likely pathology in the neonate is likely to be biliary calculi or a choledochal cyst, rather than tumour.

The main reason for scanning a patient with jaundice is to determine whether the jaundice is surgical (obstructive) or medical. In addition, ultrasound can help to determine the size of the ducts, the extent of gallbladder dilatation and the level of obstruction.

The bile ducts may be obstructed at any point, either extrinsically by a mass or intrinsically by stones, masses or fibrosis.

- If the common hepatic duct is obstructed, bile may build up proximally, causing the intrahepatic bile ducts to dilate. The patient will become jaundiced and the gallbladder will be small (Fig. 4.18B).

- If the cystic duct is obstructed, usually by a gallstone and rarely by intrinsic or extrinsic carcinoma, the patient will probably not become jaundiced as bile can still flow into the duodenum. The gallbladder may well contain mucus or pus as well as bile.

- If the common bile duct is completely obstructed (by whatever reason: stone, carcinoma of the head of the pancreas, cholangiocarcinoma, ampullary tumour, tumour infiltrate of the lower end of the

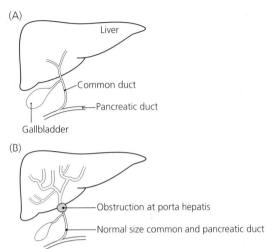

(A)

Liver

Common duct

Pancreatic duct

Gallbladder

(B)

Obstruction at porta hepatis

Normal size common and pancreatic duct

(C)

Dilated common hepatic duct

Obstruction below level of cystic duct

Normal size common and pancreatic duct

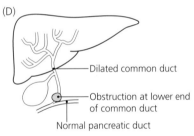

(D)

Dilated common duct

Obstruction at lower end of common duct

Normal pancreatic duct

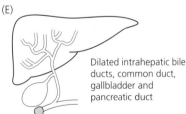

(E)

Dilated intrahepatic bile ducts, common duct, gallbladder and pancreatic duct

Obstruction at hepato-pancreatic ampulla

Fig. 4.18 Schematic drawing showing effects on bile ducts from obstruction at different levels. (A) Normal – no obstruction. (B) Dilated intrahepatic bile ducts – small gallbladder. (C) Dilated intrahepatic bile ducts – obstruction at outflow of bile from gallbladder. (D) Dilated gallbladder. (E) Obstruction at hepato-pancreatic ampulla.

CD or duodenal papillary tumour), the patient will become jaundiced and the gallbladder will dilate (Fig. 4.18D).

- An indication of level of the obstruction at the lower end of the duct can be inferred from ascertaining whether the pancreatic duct itself is obstructed (>2 mm diameter). Dilatation of the pancreatic duct as well as the CD implies an obstruction at the ampulla. This can be caused by both stone and tumour. Stones in the lower part of the CD can cause intermittent obstruction by what is known as the ball-valve effect where the stone causes blockage, moves, releases the flow of bile then moves again and obstructs (Fig. 4.18E).

Clinically, Courvoisier's law states that a palpable gall-bladder + jaundice = probable neoplasm at the lower end of the CD, causing obstruction and dilatation of the gallbladder (Fig. 4.19).

A non-palpable gallbladder + jaundice as a result of chronic cholecystitis suggests a small non-distensible gallbladder with an accompanying impacted stone and a stone in the lower part of the CD. The gallbladder does not dilate because of the impacted stone.

NB: There are exceptions: the distended gallbladder may be too deep to be felt in the presence of a carcinoma in the head of pancreas or there may be a tumour and calculi together. Calculi can act as irritants causing neoplastic change.

The accuracy of ultrasound in detecting duct dilatation is between 85% and 95%. It is also accurate in defining the level of obstruction but the cause of obstruction is only diagnosed in about 33% of patients. The main causes of obstructions are by stones in the CD, carcinoma of the head of the pancreas, tumour infiltrations of the lower end of the CD or congenital or acquired narrowing of the bile ducts.

ULTRASOUND APPEARANCES

With dilated ducts, the liver may show a variety of appearances related to the condition. Amongst these are:

- the double barrel shotgun sign where a cross-section through the portal vein and a dilated CD which is the same size or larger than the portal vein appears like the end of a double barrel shotgun. In longitudinal section, this appearance shows as two almost equal parallel channels

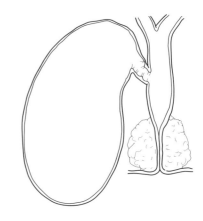

(A)

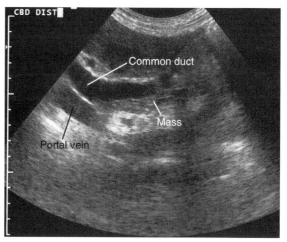

(B)

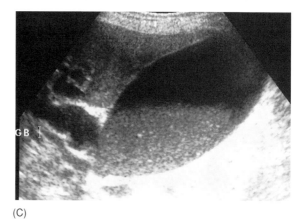

(C)

Fig. 4.19 Courvoisier's law.

- too many vessels in the liver where the normally unseen intrahepatic bile ducts become visible
- a stellate pattern of dilated ducts found near the porta hepatis, sometimes known as a monkey puzzle tree appearance
- acoustic enhancement distal to the dilated ducts, providing that the liver is not of higher reflectivity than normal such as a fatty liver, in which case the enhancement will be lost. If the liver is of normal echogenicity, the posterior enhancement can give the liver a patchy appearance and possibly mask small metastatic liver lesions that may be present

- a dilated extrahepatic CD seen as an anechoic tubular structure anterior to the portal vein. There may be too much bowel gas to see this structure clearly. If so, an estimate of the diameter of the duct can be made by scanning the head of the pancreas and viewing the CD in transverse section through the head, providing gas does not obscure this also. Care must be taken not to confuse the bile duct, which lies towards the posterior aspect of the head of the pancreas, with the gastroduodenal artery, which lies on its anterior surface (Fig. 4.20).

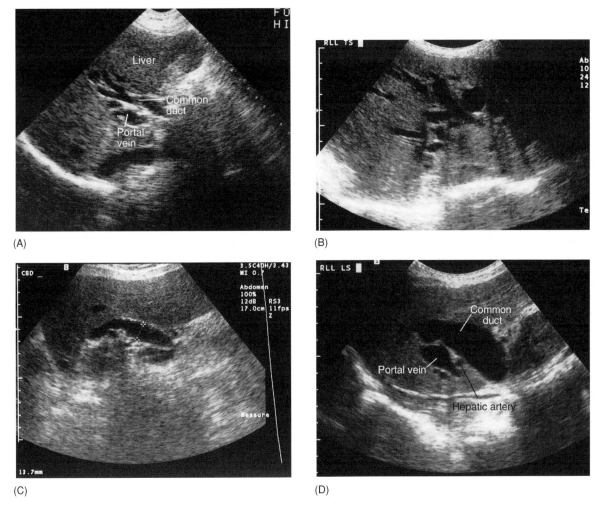

(A) (B) (C) (D)

Fig. 4.20 (A, B) Dilated intrahepatic bile ducts. (C) Dilated common duct measuring nearly 14 mm diameter. (D) Grossly dilated common duct – compare size with that of portal vein.

Box 4.7   Advice

If the patient is jaundiced and the clinical impression is one of surgical jaundice but the ducts are of normal calibre, it may be that the obstruction is very recent and the ducts have not yet had time to dilate, in which case it is best to rescan in a few days' time. Similarly, there may be obstruction without dilatation if the wall of the duct is fibrosed, as in sclerosing cholangitis, or where the liver is too rigid, from cirrhosis for example, to allow the ducts to expand.

If the intrahepatic ducts are dilated but the patient appears normal, this can be caused by obstruction by tumour of some branches and not others or by an intermittent relief of obstruction, allowing the bile to drain and preventing jaundice developing. This can happen when stones in the lower part of the CD exhibit a ball-valve effect or when a sloughing tumour of the CD obstructs, then breaks up and relieves the build-up of bile.

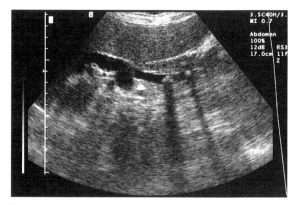

(A)

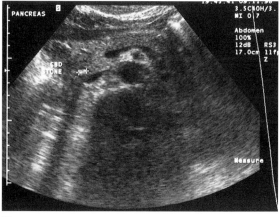

(B)

Fig. 4.21   Stones in the common duct. (A) Dilated common duct containing two stones. Note posterior acoustic shadowing. (B) View of pancreas showing stone at lower end of the common duct.

Obstruction by stone

CLINICAL INFORMATION

Sensitivity in diagnosing stones in the ducts (choledocholithiasis) by ultrasound is said to be between 75% and 80%. Choledocholithiasis can occur in about 15% of those patients with stones in the gallbladder. Clinically, patients present with Charcot's triad: biliary colic, jaundice and a spiking temperature, although one feature of this triad may be missing, depending on the individual degree of severity.

ULTRASOUND APPEARANCES

Stones are often not seen in the lower parts of the CD because of the proximity to bowel gas in the duodenal curve, lack of bile around the stone, lack of an acoustic shadow, because of the composition of the stone or because of technical factors. Acoustic shadowing posterior to stones must be sought although attenuation of the sound by gas can cause this appearance. Gas may also be present in the bile duct after an endoscopic sphincterotomy, making a search for retained stones very difficult. However, if the lower end of the duct is seen and appears dilated but no stone

is seen, the shape of the lower end of the duct can often suggest pathology. If, on magnification of the image, the end is rounded, this suggests the chance of there being an intrinsic mass such as a stone. If the end comes to a point, the probability of the cause of obstruction being extrinsic, i.e. a mass in the pancreatic head, is quite high.

Stones in the lower part of the duct can sometimes be seen by scanning the pancreas to view the duct as it passes through the groove in the posterior part of the head. If the duct is dilated, it can expand the head of the pancreas (Figs 4.21, 4.22).

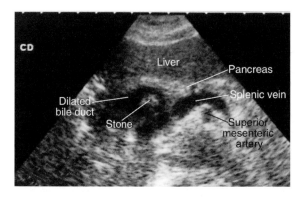

Fig. 4.22 'Stretching' of pancreatic head around dilated common bile duct.

Obstruction by tumour

CLINICAL INFORMATION

Malignant tumours of the bile duct (cholangiocarcinomas) can occur anywhere between the lower end of the CD and the liver, giving rise to jaundice. They tend to occur in males more than females and the incidence peaks between the ages of 50 and 60. When malignant tumours involve the confluence of the left and right hepatic ducts at the porta hepatis, they are called Klatskin tumours (see p. 88). Almost all tumours are adenocarcinomas. Carcinomas start as diffuse infiltration of the bile duct wall, later spreading to the surrounding tissue. The obstruction can be bypassed by means of a stent during a percutaneous transhepatic cholangiogram (PTC) or endoscopic retrograde cholangiopancreatogram (ERCP) or surgery may be attempted. The prognosis is poor, however.

Tumours of the bile duct around the ampulla of Vater, either of the ampulla itself, the CD or the pancreatic head, can sometimes be resected, giving a five-year survival rate of 40%. The tumour can be of the sloughing variety which can cause intermittent obstruction and relief, having a similar effect to a mobile stone as described previously.

ULTRASOUND APPEARANCES

Intrinsic carcinomas may develop anywhere in the ducts, appearing as rounded, ill-defined, heterogeneous lesions which can spread towards the liver and into the cystic duct. Sometimes all that can be seen is a local thickening of the bile duct wall. Lower situated carcinomas produce the typical obstructive picture of a dilated gallbladder with thin walls while carcinomas situated above the cystic duct level will tend to produce small collapsed gallbladders. Intrinsic carcinomas tend to produce a rounded, blunt-ended appearance to the duct while extrinsic masses often produce a narrower, more pointed end (Fig. 4.23).

BENIGN TUMOURS

These are much less common than malignant tumours.

Papillomas

These can grow to the size of a cherry and may obstruct biliary/pancreatic ducts, depending on position. They appear as solid masses and do not produce an acoustic shadow.

Cystadenomas

These appear as a multilocular cystic mass, occurring mostly in young females.

It is often difficult to determine whether the origin of the obstruction is from the bile duct, pancreatic duct or duodenum. It is important, though, to assess the level of obstruction from the appearance of the dilated ducts, exclude or confirm shadowing from calculi if present and assess the head of the pancreas.

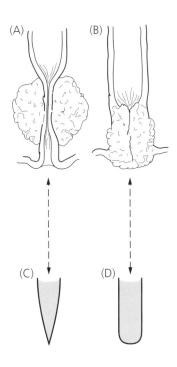

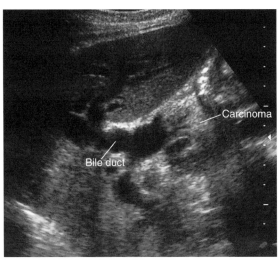

(E)

Fig. 4.23 (A) Extrinsic carcinoma at lower end of common duct. (B) Intrinsic carcinoma. (C) With extrinsic mass, lower end of bile duct runs to a point. (D) With stone or intrinsic mass, lower part of bile duct is rounded. (E) Intrinsic carcinoma of lower part of common bile duct.

Choledochal cyst

CLINICAL INFORMATION

A choledochal cyst is a congenital cystic dilatation of the extrahepatic bile ducts. Most present in children (60% under the age of 10) although the age is variable, some not presenting until early adult life. Patients with choledochal cysts usually present with an abdominal mass, pain, fever and, sometimes, jaundice. The jaundice is usually intermittent and the condition is treated surgically. There are several types of choledochal cyst (Fig. 4.24).

There is a link between choledochal cysts and pancreatic disease. In some patients there are anomalies of bile and pancreatic duct insertions into the ampulla. These may allow reflux of pancreatic juice into the bile duct, effectively scarring and stricturing the bile duct and allowing the proximal part to dilate (raised amylase has been found in samples of the cyst fluid).

Intrahepatic ducts are often of normal calibre but can sometimes be markedly dilated, giving an appearance similar to Caroli's syndrome (see below). Surgical correction of the choledochal cyst resolves the dilated intrahepatic ducts when present but there is no treatment that is effective for Caroli's syndrome.

ULTRASOUND APPEARANCES

The most common appearance is of a large spherical cyst lying below the liver in addition to the classic shape of the gallbladder. Usually the contents of the cyst are free of echoes; sometimes bile salts can be detected. It may be mistaken for the gallbladder in those who have an associated fibrosed, contracted gallbladder or post cholecystectomy although the latter would be rare as it would normally be noted either in the imaging lead-up to the operation or at the time of the operation itself.

Box 4.9 Advice

The pancreas should be carefully scanned and any pseudocysts noted. The presence of a pseudocyst at the head of the pancreas and a choledochal cyst at the lower end of the bile duct can be confusing.

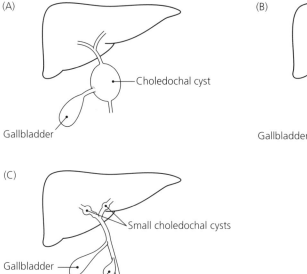

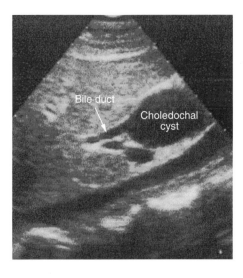

(D)

Fig. 4.24 Choledochal cysts – common types.

two years if undiagnosed. It is thought to be caused by an inflammatory process, the resulting scarring causing the atresia. It destroys most or part of the ducts and those parts not destroyed can fill with fluid and appear similar to a choledochal cyst. Those with biliary atresia have an increased incidence of congenital anomalies such as situs inversus, gut malrotation and perihepatic vascular anomalies. Fewer than 30% of patients with biliary atresia have a normal-looking gallbladder; the rest have gallbladders that are small, misshapen, thick-walled, intrahepatic or filled with mucus.

Of patients, 15% have a correctible condition where the proximal ducts are patent but the distal ducts are occluded. The remaining 85% are rarely correctible as the proximal ducts are occluded. Treatment in this situation is by a portoenterostomy which can extend the life expectancy to 10 years or more by providing a partial drainage, but liver transplant is the main alternative.

Biliary atresia

CLINICAL INFORMATION

Biliary atresia usually occurs in children from a few months to a few years old with a frequency of one in 10–15 000 live births. Biliary cirrhosis and death secondary to biliary atresia can occur within the first

ULTRASOUND APPEARANCES

If the liver has secondary biliary cirrhosis, imaging the portal vein and radicles is difficult owing to their compression by the liver tissue. Colour flow imaging, if available, can confirm portal patency, although it is important to note that a rapid arterial flow from quite large arteries can be present.

Primary sclerosing cholangitis

CLINICAL INFORMATION

This condition causes progressive obstructive jaundice, characterized by chronic inflammation and bile duct fibrosis. It affects males more than females and the incidence peaks at between 25 and 40 years. It is associated with inflammatory bowel disease and 60% of patients with primary sclerosing cholangitis have ulcerative colitis. Primary sclerosing cholangitis affects intra- and extrahepatic bile ducts. Over a period of 10 years the patient develops cholestatic jaundice, slowly progressing to cirrhosis. The chance of developing cholangiocarcinoma increases with this condition.

ULTRASOUND APPEARANCES

The larger ducts are seen to develop fibrous strictures in places, causing segmental dilatation and showing as an intermittent duct; medium ducts become fibrosed and more echogenic than usual and small ducts develop collagenous scarring and are difficult to see. Ultrasound is not able to exclude intrahepatic duct disease but is useful in diagnosing and monitoring primary sclerosing cholangitis.[7]

Klatskin tumour

CLINICAL INFORMATION

Klatskin tumours are usually relatively slow-growing malignant tumours (mostly adenocarcinomas) of the bile ducts involving the confluence of the right and left main bile ducts at the porta hepatis (see section on Obstruction by tumour, above). They comprise 10–25% of bile duct carcinomas. They are often linked with gallstones, inflammatory bowel disease and cystic disease of the biliary system.

ULTRASOUND APPEARANCES

Appearances are usually dilated intrahepatic bile ducts and normal extrahepatic ducts, with stones in the gallbladder. In addition, the pancreas is normal but the adjacent liver is invaded by the tumour. Nearly 80% are echogenic and just under 20% are hypoechoic.

Caroli's disease

CLINICAL INFORMATION

Caroli's disease is a congenital non-obstructive, saccular dilatation of the intrahepatic bile ducts. It is associated with an increased incidence of biliary calculi, biliary cirrhosis and cholangitis. It is seen mostly in adults and is more common in females than males.

ULTRASOUND APPEARANCES

Multiple cyst-like areas form within the liver tissue. The extrahepatic ducts are usually unaffected. Stones can form in the dilated ducts and give rise to cholangitis and pyogenic liver abscesses. The appearance can sometimes be mistaken for polycystic disease of the liver. However, these 'cysts' communicate with each other and with the main bile ducts whereas the polycystic cysts do not communicate. Colour Doppler is useful for evaluating the Caroli intrahepatic bile duct malformation.[8]

Air in the biliary tree

CLINICAL INFORMATION

Air in the biliary tree can occur after biliary surgery, endoscopic retrograde cholangiopancreatography (ERCP) or sphincterotomy and although it usually resolves quite quickly, it can persist for some time. It is not considered to be significant.

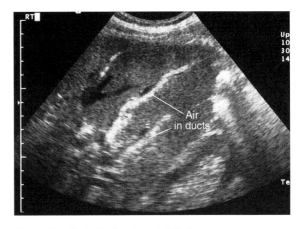

Fig. 4.25 Air in the intrahepatic bile ducts.

ULTRASOUND APPEARANCES

The normal course of the bile ducts, not usually seen in the liver, is outlined by highly reflective lines, sometimes casting a reverberation shadow posteriorly (Fig. 4.25).

References

1 Naganuma S, Ischida H, Konno K *et al* 1998 Sonographic findings of anomalous position of the gallbladder. Abdom Imaging 23: 67–72

2 Majeed A, Ross B, Johnson A 1999 The preoperatively normal bile duct does not dilate after cholecystectomy: results of a five year study. Gut 45(5): 637–638

3 Waschberg RH, Kim KH, Sundaram K 1998 Sonographic versus endoscopic retrograde cholangiographic measurements of the bile duct revisited: importance of the transverse diameter. Am J Roentgenol 170: 669–674

4 Kapoor BS, Agarwal AK, Khanna NN 1995 Prediction of gallstone composition by ultrasound: implications for non-surgical therapy. Br J Radiol 68: 459–462

5 Gill KS, Chapman AH, Weston MJ 1997 The changing face of emphysematous cholecystitis. Br J Radiol 70: 986–991

6 Schulman A 1998 Ultrasound appearances of intra- and extra-hepatic biliary ascariasis. Abdom Imaging 23: 60–66

7 Majoie CBLM, Smits N, Phoa S *et al* 1995 Primary sclerosing cholangitis: sonographic findings. Abdom imaging 20: 109–113

8 Kumakura H, Ichikawa S, Tange S *et al* 1994 A case of Caroli's disease: usefulness of color Doppler sonography for evaluating the malformation of the intrahepatic bile ducts. Radiat Med Imag Radiat Oncol 12: 75–77

Further reading

Bowie JD 2000 What is the upper limit of normal for the common bile duct on ultrasound: how much do you want it to be? Am J Gastroenterol 95(4): 897–900

Pandey M, Sood BP, Shukla RC *et al* 2000 Carcinoma of the gallbladder: role of sonography in diagnosis and staging. J Clin Ultrasound 28(5): 227–232

5

THE PANCREAS

Main functions
Anatomy
Scanning
Normal ultrasound appearances
Pathology
Focal disease
Diffuse disease

The pancreas is an exocrine and an endocrine gland and has important functions in the digestive cycle. It lies in the retroperitoneum.

Main functions

- The endocrine portion (2% of the pancreas) consists of hormone-producing cells, the pancreatic islets. It secretes insulin and glucagon, essential in carbohydrate metabolism and the regulation of blood glucose, via the splenic and superior mesenteric veins into the portal vein.

- The exocrine portion (98% of the pancreas) secretes pancreatic juice which drains into the duodenum via the pancreatic duct.

Anatomy

The pancreas consists of a head, neck, body, tail and pancreatic duct. It extends transversely across the posterior abdominal wall at the level of the first and second lumbar vertebrae. Greyish pink in colour, it weighs about 90 g and measures approximately 15 cm in length.

The pancreas lies in the epigastrium either transversely or up to 45° to the transverse, across the posterior abdominal wall from the second part of the duodenum to the spleen. The head lies in the C-shaped duodenal loop formed by the first, second and third parts of the duodenum, to the right of the midline. The head and neck lie anterior to the IVC and the body lies anterior to the aorta. The tail often abuts onto the hilum of the spleen. The head usually lies inferior to the tail. The uncinate process, a hook-like extension of the head, can extend posteriorly to the SMV and even the SMA. It is very variable in position.

The hepatic artery, arising from the coeliac axis, runs along the superior border of the pancreas. The hepatic artery gives rise to the gastroduodenal artery seen on the anterior part of the head of the pancreas. The main pancreatic duct (Wirsung's duct) tapers towards the tail of the pancreas. It joins the common duct to enter the duodenum as a single duct at the ampulla of Vater. The accessory duct (of Santorini), which is seen in up to 15% of the population, drains the head of the pancreas and opens into the accessory duodenal papilla (just proximal to the main duodenal papilla). The pancreas is fixed in position. It may be seen to pulsate owing to the position of the abdominal aorta posteriorly (Figs 5.1, 5.3).

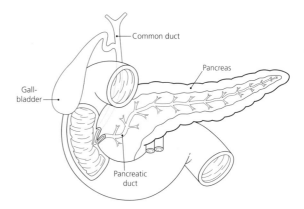

Fig. 5.1 Pancreas showing biliary and pancreatic ducts.

Blood supply

Branches of the splenic artery, the superior pancreatico-duodenal artery (a branch of the superior mesenteric artery) and the inferior pancreatico-duodenal artery (which branches from the gastroduodenal artery).

Blood drainage

Via the splenic vein and superior mesenteric vein into the portal vein. The splenic vein lies posterior to the pancreas and runs towards the portosplenic junction (junction of portal and superior mesenteric veins).

Lymph drainage

Head to pancreatico-duodenal and subpyloric nodes, body to coeliac nodes and tail to pancreatico-splenic and splenic nodes near the splenic hilum.

Nerve supply

Parasympathetic nerve supply from the coeliac plexus (increases pancreatic juice secretion); sympathetic nerve supply depresses the secretion.

Relations of pancreas

HEAD

- Anteriorly – transverse colon, liver.

- Posteriorly – superior mesenteric vein which in turn is anterior to the uncinate process if present, the lower common duct, the IVC, sometimes the right and left renal veins, L1 and L2.

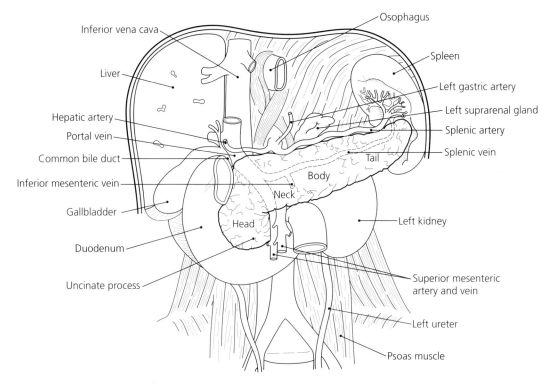

Fig. 5.2 Pancreas showing surrounding anatomy.

- Superiorly – the first part of the duodenum.

- Right lateral – the second part of the duodenum, bile and pancreatic duct confluence.

- Inferiorly – the third part of the duodenum.

BODY
- Posteriorly – L1 and L2, abdominal aorta and IVC, left psoas muscle and crus of the diaphragm, the left kidney, the splenic artery, the splenic vein.

- Anteriorly – the lesser sac, liver.

- Inferiorly – jejunum.

- Superiorly – stomach/pylorus, first part of duodenum depending on body type.

TAIL
- Left lateral – the spleen.

- Anteriorly – the stomach.

- Posteriorly – the left kidney (Fig. 5.2).

Surface markings

The head lies approximately on the transpyloric plane, 1–2 cm to the right of the midline.

The body runs upwards and to the left for about 10 cm until touching the spleen.

Variations in normal anatomy

- Pancreatic tissue can be found anywhere in the gut. The stomach wall, small intestine, spleen and gall-bladder can all contain pancreatic tissue.

- An annular pancreas can encircle the second part of the duodenum (50% within the first year); this can lead to obstruction.

- Pancreas divisum – this is a congenital abnormality involving 1–6% of the population; there are separate duct systems as dorsal and ventral anlagen have not fused. The small ventral pancreas drains through the main ampulla and the larger dorsal pancreas through an accessory papilla.

- The uncinate process is a hook-like extension of the

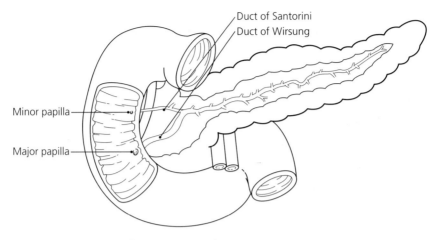

Fig. 5.3 Detail of pancreatic ductal system showing accessory duct.

head of the pancreas that can extend to the left behind the superior mesenteric vein and even the superior mesenteric artery.

- There may be an accessory duct of Santorini present that drains into a separate, more proximal part of the duodenum.

Palpation

The pancreas is not felt if normal.

Relevant tests – normal values

Serum amylase	50–300 U/l
Blood urea	2.5–6.5 mmol/l
Serum albumin	36–50 g/l
Serum calcium	2.1–2.6 mmol/l

Scanning

Patient preparation

A period of starvation is required for any ultrasound examination involving the hepatobiliary system. Six to eight hours of fasting are recommended for patients aged between 12 and adult; four hours fasting for younger children. Overnight fasting ensures an empty stomach and reduces peristalsis.

- Fast for six hours; non-fizzy, non-fatty drinks may be taken.

- Ensure no other tests on the same day require nil by mouth.

- Refrain from smoking as this causes the ducts to contract.

- Children can fast for four hours.

- Babies can have a bottle of dextrose instead of the normal milky feed or be scanned just before the normal time for a feed.

- Babies and diabetics should be placed first on the list for the scan.

Equipment required

5 MHz (7.5 MHz in children), 3.5 MHz in large patients. A sector or curved linear transducer can be used. A frequency appropriate to the depth of the pancreas must be selected, this often being relatively superficial. The focusing zone must be set for the appropriate depth.

Suggested scanning technique

The liver is usually used as an acoustic window to image the pancreas in the thinner body types. If the patient is hypersthenic, the stomach lies horizontally and gas lies close to the pancreas. In this type, the left lobe of the liver does not often extend far enough to the left of midline to offer a good acoustic window for the majority of the pancreas.

Owing to the position of the pancreas relative to the duodenum, intestinal gas prevents good visualization. The pancreas is frequently scanned first in order to obtain a gas artefact-free image before all is lost. If gas is obscuring the view, scan other areas and return to the pancreas afterwards. Methods of moving intervening bowel gas away from the pancreas have been developed. Firm pressure with the probe, providing that an abdominal aortic aneurysm or other large mass underneath has been excluded, can often be sufficient.

Use of positive pressure in the abdomen, pushing the abdomen up to meet the transducer without breathing in first and gently pressing down, is sometimes useful to rid the upper abdomen of gas, as is lying prone for a few minutes. Scanning the patient upright or moving them into the LLD or LPO position can often work by allowing bowel to fall away from the pancreas. Sometimes a water load of 500 ml of any non-gassy fluid may be needed. It should be given with the patient in the LLD position in order to fill the body of the stomach. The body and tail of the pancreas can sometimes be seen in this position. When the patient turns onto the RLD position, the water moves into the duodenum and the head of pancreas can be more clearly visualized.

Patient positions

Scan in quiet respiration, transversely in the sub-xiphisternal space. Alter the angulation of the transducer up to 45° to the horizontal as required. Use as much of the liver as possible as an acoustic window. Identify the landmarks of the splenic vein, SMV, SMA, liver, aorta in transverse section and the pancreas should lie anterior to these structures. Angle towards the head of the patient or down as necessary. Use water in the stomach to see the tail of pancreas, also scan through spleen to see the tail. Turn the patient onto the RLD position for a few minutes to allow fluid to run along the first part of the duodenum and to allow gas to move back to the stomach. Note the parenchyma and the duct size and normality of relations.

Turn the transducer at right angles to the long axis of the pancreas and scan longitudinally to obtain cross-sections through the pancreas, moving from the tail to the head. Observe the duct, pancreatic size and any masses, outline change or vessel disturbance.

The tail of the pancreas can be seen more clearly by scanning through the spleen or left kidney with the

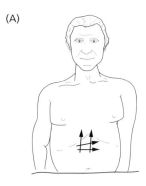

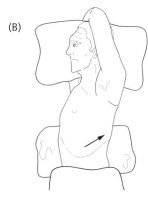

Fig. 5.4 (A) Scanning the patient in the supine position. (B) Scanning technique for obtaining pancreatic tail images – the right lateral decubitus position.

patient in the RLD or the prone position. The tail usually lies just anterior to the upper third of the left kidney. The pancreatic tail is more reliably seen on CT scan except in thin subjects (Fig. 5.4).

NB: Endoscopic ultrasound using a linear or transverse radial transducer at the tip has been used to investigate the pancreas. The endoscope is passed to the third part of the duodenum after the bowel has been distended with air. The air is removed and a balloon covering the transducer is distended with water to allow good through transmission of sound and proximity of the duodenal wall to the pancreatic head and uncinate process. Close proximity also allows a higher frequency to be used. As the endoscope is slowly withdrawn, the pancreatic body and neck can be examined through the gastric antrum and the tail of the pancreas through the body of the stomach. Some endoscopes allow a biopsy to be taken at the same time.

Suggested minimal sections

- Transverse pancreas sections showing the pancreas and splenic vein and the pancreatic duct (with measurement).

- Long axis sections to show the pancreas related to the aorta, the superior mesenteric artery, coeliac axis, IVC, splenic vein and superior mesenteric vein.

- The image should include head, body and tail (the head showing the gastroduodenal artery and the lower part of the common bile duct).

- An image demonstrating the tail of the pancreas.

Normal ultrasound appearances

The normal pancreas is a homogeneous structure. The average normal adult pancreas is usually of slightly higher reflectivity than the normal liver but the infant pancreas is of lower reflectivity than the liver compared with that of the adult. With the more obese patient and after 60 years old, when there is higher fatty infiltration, and in those on corticosteroids or with Cushing's disease, the pancreas becomes more highly reflective and blends in with surrounding retroperitoneal fat. This can make for overestimation of size when measuring. The pancreatic duct is sinusoidal and usually seen either as a parallel lined, tubular, echogenic structure within the middle of the pancreas, where it lies perpendicular to the sound beam, or as a series of '=' signs where the portion of sinusoidal duct lies under the ultrasound beam.

The pancreas is not always easy to identify for the student starting to scan. The easiest way is to identify the vessels lying posterior to the pancreas, i.e. the aorta, SMA and splenic vein. The pancreas usually lies anterior to the splenic vein. Seeing the pancreas in transverse section is even more difficult but can be accomplished by careful identification of the surrounding structures.

When scanning the long axis of the pancreas, two small anechoic rounded structures are often seen within the head of the pancreas: the gastroduodenal artery anteriorly and the slightly larger lower end of the common bile duct posteriorly.

In transverse section, the pancreatic duct can often be seen within the pancreatic tissue as as a small, anechoic structure (Fig. 5.5).

The ventrally derived part of the gland (the uncinate process and posterior part of the head) has less fat and is of lower reflectivity than the rest of the body in

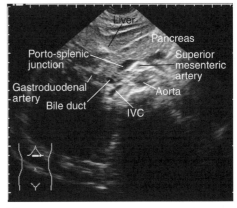

(A)

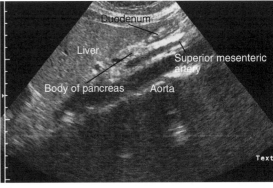

(B)

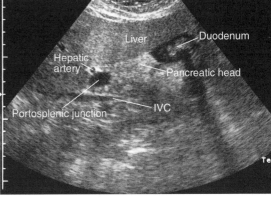

(C)

Fig. 5.5 (A) The normal adult pancreas: transverse scan of abdomen showing long axis of pancreas. (B,C) Longitudinal scans showing transverse sections through the pancreas.

approximately 28% of cases. The pancreas infiltrated by fat can be difficult to see and a CT scan is often required. In the elderly, the pancreas can shrink and become fibrosed. Children have a relatively larger, bulkier pancreas with lower reflectivity than that of the adult. The neonatal pancreas has an even lower reflectivity than that of the paediatric pancreas.

Box 5.1 Advice

- The uncinate process is sometimes thought to be a tumour. Look for normality of tissue.

- When comparing reflectivities with any other organ, remember that the other tissue may be abnormal.

- A horseshoe kidney can resemble the pancreas, as can the duodenum. The posterior duodenal wall and anterior pancreatic surface interface can look like a duct. Also the pancreatic duct can be confused with the hepatic artery, splenic vein and the gastro-duodenal mucosa.

- An annular pancreas is a congenital abnormality associated with duodenal atresia. It presents as a high intestinal obstruction in the neonate.

- The duodenum can be mistaken for part of the head of pancreas and the splenic artery for the pancreatic duct.

Normal sizes

The irregular shape of the pancreas makes the usefulness of measuring questionable. The pancreas is between 15 and 20 cm long from head to tail but becomes smaller in the elderly. In the neonate and small child, the pancreas often appears prominent with a bulky tail in comparison to the adult. Average anteroposterior measurements are as follows (sizes quoted in cm).

Age	Head	Body	Tail
Adult	2.5–3	5–2	1.5–2
10–19 years	2.0–2.5	1.1–1.4	2.0–2.4
1–10 years	1.7–2	1.0–1.3	1.8–2.2
1 month–1 year	1.5–2	0.8–1.1	1.2–1.6
<1 month	1–1.4	0.6–0.8	1–1.4

The duct should be visualized whenever possible. The inner to inner measurement should be a maximum of 2 mm although it may measure 3–4 mm shortly after a meal; another reason to starve patients prior to the scan. The duct increases in calibre with age and can be up to 6 mm wide in the elderly.

Pathology

Focal disease:

- carcinoma

- cyst

- pseudocyst

Diffuse disease:

- acute pancreatitis

- chronic pancreatitis

- fat infiltration

- cystic fibrosis

Focal disease

Carcinoma

CLINICAL INFORMATION

Cancer of the pancreas is more common in men than women (1.5 : 1) but the incidence of pancreatic carcinoma in women has recently increased. The incidence of pancreatic carcinoma has increased fourfold in the last 40 years. It is uncommon before the age of 45 but becomes increasingly common with age, especially over 70. It has been linked to smoking, possibly coffee drinking, and exposure to asbestos and chronic alcoholism, especially the consumption of spirits, has been implicated but not conclusively linked.

Patients commonly present with a long-standing epigastric pain, weight loss and progressive jaundice. More precisely, with carcinoma of the pancreatic head or ampulla, jaundice is present at first eventually with pain increasing in severity.

With carcinoma of the body and tail, the patient presents with weight loss and pain which feels as if it is boring into the back and this is often relieved by sitting forward.

From presentation to death, the mean survival time is approximately six months, only 1–2% surviving five

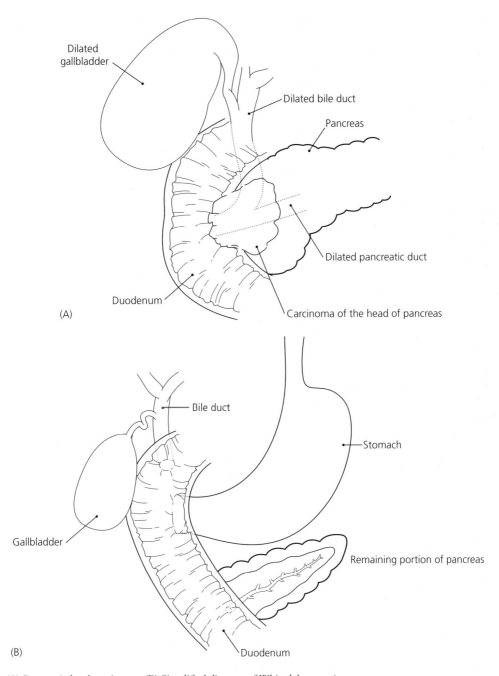

Dilated
gallbladder

Dilated bile duct

Pancreas

Dilated pancreatic duct

Duodenum

Carcinoma of the head of pancreas

(A)

Bile duct

Stomach

Gallbladder

Remaining portion of pancreas

Duodenum

(B)

Fig. 5.6 (A) Pancreatic head carcinoma. (B) Simplified diagram of Whipple's operation.

years. Excision of the tumour, the only cure, is only possible in 10% of cases. This can only be undertaken if the tumour is less than 3 cm in diameter, is sited in the head of the pancreas, has not invaded the portal system or retroperitoneum or metastasized. Removal of part of the pancreas (pancreatoduodenectomy or Whipple's operation) has a similar survival rate to a total pancreatectomy (20% mortality rate). Palliative relief of symptoms by use of a stent is useful in patients with pancreatic carcinoma (Figs 5.6, 5.8D).

- Ductal carcinoma is the most common, comprising 80% of pancreatic carcinomas; next most common is the giant cell carcinoma (5%) and adenosquamous carcinoma (4%).

- A ductal carcinoma tumour ranges between 1.5 and 5 cm in diameter. It tends to grow rapidly, taking 60 days to double its volume.

- Most pancreatic carcinomas (61–70%) occur in the head of the pancreas, 13% in the body and 5% in the tail, the remainder being found in a combination of sites.

ULTRASOUND APPEARANCES

Sensitivity in detecting a pancreatic mass by ultrasound is 90–98%. With a suspected mass, ultrasound should be the initial test.

Bile and pancreatic ducts often dilate with a pancreatic head carcinoma. The pancreatic duct is dilated in up to 97% of cases and bile ducts dilate in 80–90% of cases. In addition, a dilated gallbladder and palpable mass are found in 20% of cases. If bile and pancreatic ducts are obstructed, this helps confirm a diagnosis of pancreatic carcinoma. Some tumours do not obstruct, however, and as jaundice is not then present, the tumours are relatively large by the time the patient is investigated for any other related symptom (Fig. 5.7).

If the tumour is situated away from the head, it is usually more difficult to see and can often only be detected by a change in the normal outline. Most tumours are of low reflectivity and small tumours appear homogeneous as there are few irregular internal structures to cause multiple interfaces to the sound beam. Ultrasound has been shown to detect lesions as small as 1 cm. The larger the lesion, the more heterogeneous the lesion becomes as the internal structures become less well organized. Only 3% of pancreatic carcinomas are highly reflective.

Carcinoma of the pancreas often appears as an irregular enlarged mass at the head which can be lobulated or grape-like or smooth and well defined. A mass enlarging the head of pancreas can cause other effects. Depending on the shape and position of the mass, it can compress the IVC, displace the SMV anteriorly (if the uncinate process is involved) or downwards (if the head/body is involved) and if large enough, deviate the SMV and SMA to the left (Fig. 5.8).

If the biliary system is dilated without the presence of calculi, the gallbladder does not contract after a fatty meal and the pancreatic duct is dilated proximal to the head of pancreas, these appearances are extremely suggestive of the presence of a pancreatic tumour. Without a biopsy, the false-positive rate of pancreatic carcinoma is 25% as inflammatory masses often have the same appearance. With the use of mechanical cutting devices such as the Biopty Gun® using a Trucut needle fired by a spring-powered trigger, sensitivity for diagnosing adenocarcinoma of the pancreas has been quoted as 91.4%.

The role of ultrasound is to determine whether there is a mass or not and if there is an obstruction of the pancreatic and/or common bile ducts being caused by the mass.

A careful study should be undertaken to determine whether there is any portal vein invasion as tumour resection is extremely complex in this situation. Using

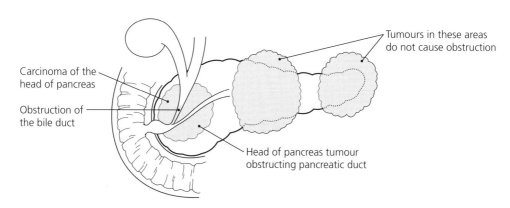

Fig. 5.7 Sites where pancreatic carcinoma is found.

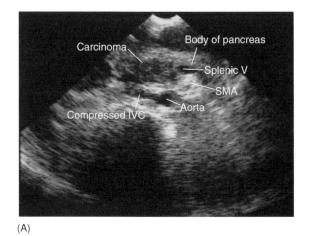

(A)

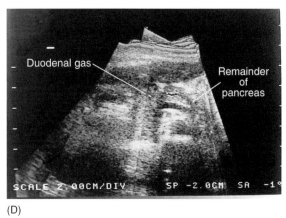

(D)

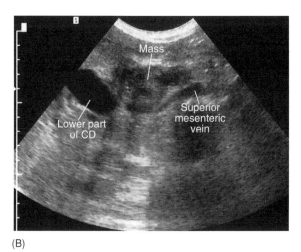

(B)

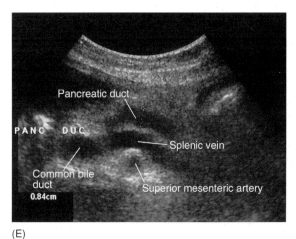

(E)

Fig. 5.8 (A) Pancreatic head carcinoma compressing the IVC. (B) Longitudinal section showing compression of superior mesenteric vein. (C) Ampullary mass causing grossly dilated pancreatic duct. (D) Appearance of pancreas after Whipple's operation. (E) Pancreas showing dilated bile duct and 8.4 mm diameter pancreatic duct.

(C)

a 20 MHz endoscopic transducer to demonstrate portal vein tumours, ultrasound showed a sensitivity and specificity of 100% compared with angiography (77%) and CT (65%), the latter two modalities not being able to differentiate subtle invasion from tumour compression. However, few ultrasound departments will have these facilities at present. Measurement of the head of the pancreas is important as anything more than 3.0–3.5 cm is suspicious. Lymph node involvement around the pancreas, liver and coeliac axis may be seen. Tumour can spread to the liver.

If the tumour is ampullary rather than pancreatic, the prognosis is considered to be better but the two tumours are difficult to differentiate. The diagnosis of ampullary tumour is better as symptoms appear earlier. The accuracy of endoscopic ultrasound in diagnosing ampullary tumours is 96% compared with CT (67%) and MRI (84%). It is especially good for tumours of less than 3 cm diameter. The five-year survival rate for ampullary tumours is 30–40%.

There are other types of malignant tumour seen in addition to ductal adenocarcinomas.

Types	Appearance
Mucinous cystic neoplasms	Mainly cystic, micro/ macrocystic. Macrocystic may be 2 cm+ and possibly premalignant (cysts form in inflammatory lesions)
Endocrine tumours (islet cell tumours)	Slow growing, low grade
Malignancy	Small, reflective capsule
Pancreatic lymphoma	Large, usually homogeneous, sometimes multifocal, ± lymphadenopathy

ABNORMAL PULSED WAVE DOPPLER

Flow in hepatic and gastric arteries may be affected by pancreatic masses. They can become surrounded by tumour leading to stenosis. The portal vein can become compressed, producing a high-velocity jet through the stenosis with turbulent flow distally. Portal vein occlusion impedes the flow but collaterals may be seen with colour Doppler around the occlusion. Doppler signals can be noted from some pancreatic tumours as well as the change in surrounding vessel flow. Vessels supplying the tumour are small and blood flows slowly, better seen with power Doppler.

ENDOSCOPIC ULTRASOUND

Endoscopic ultrasound has been shown to be helpful in diagnosing small tumours and bile and pancreatic duct disorders. Endocrine tumours not seen on thin slice sections on a CT scan have been found using endo-scopic ultrasound.

Box 5.2   Advice

The appearance of a mass at the head of the pancreas can be suggested by the following normal appearances:

- an uncinate process posterior to the superior mesenteric vein
- food in the duodenum (observe peristalsis)
- a pronounced caudate lobe extending medially
- an aneurysm of the splenic artery
- enlarged lymph nodes at the porta hepatis.

Areas of focal inflammation can also appear like carcinomas.

Cyst

CLINICAL INFORMATION

Cysts are rarely seen in the pancreas but are more common in patients with polycystic renal disease (approximately 10–15%), cystic fibrosis or von Hippel–Lindau disease.

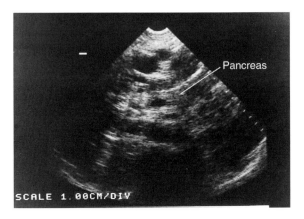

Fig. 5.9 Involvement of the pancreas in adult polycystic kidney disease.

ULTRASOUND APPEARANCES

Typical appearances as for a simple cyst: thin capsule, rounded, anechoic with posterior acoustic enhancement.

Pseudocyst

CLINICAL INFORMATION

A pseudocyst occurs as a result of acute pancreatitis (see below) in 50% of cases up to 2–3 weeks after a severe attack of pancreatitis, if blunt abdominal trauma or surgery has taken place and sometimes it occurs without a known cause. It is a collection of pancreatic secretions with a high amylase content surrounded by a fibrous wall on the surface of the pancreas or in a part or whole of the lesser sac of the omentum.

Patients can give a history of acute pancreatitis and present with epigastric fullness, pain, nausea and perhaps vomiting. The pseudocyst can become quite large. If infected, sweating and severe pain can occur.

The epigastrium contains a firm and perhaps tender mass with an indistinct lower edge, moving slightly with respiration and being dull to percussion. It is often difficult to palpate as it is mostly hidden beneath the costal margin. Most resolve within six weeks.

ULTRASOUND APPEARANCES

Pseudocysts show as anechoic areas anterior to and around the pancreas, occasionally containing internal echoes representing clot or necrotic tissue. They may appear for a short while and collections of less than 5 cm can be treated conservatively. They can be massive and fill the abdomen, sometimes dissecting into remote locations unless treated. Large pseudocysts can be treated surgically although they are often simply aspirated and followed up with ultrasound (Fig. 5.10).

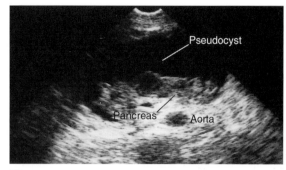

(A)

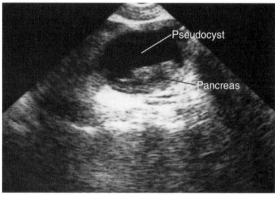

(B)

Fig. 5.10 Severe pancreatic pseudocyst. (A) Longitudinal section of pancreas. (B) Transverse section of pancreas.

Diffuse disease

Pancreatitis

CLINICAL INFORMATION

Pancreatitis is considered to be an acute condition presenting with abdominal pain and usually pancreatic enzymes in the blood or urine due to the inflammatory process. It is usually linked with disease caused by gallstones (60% in the UK), alcohol, obstruction of the pancreatic duct and a variety of lesser causes such as viral infections (e.g. mumps), trauma, iatrogenically (from ERCP), acute fatty liver of pregnancy and from unusual sources such as the bite from a brown recluse spider or a scorpion sting. Alcohol can cause acute pancreatitis but the pancreas has usually been damaged by alcohol already, so acute episodes of pancreatitis in heavy consumers of alcohol are often termed chronic relapsing pancreatitis.

Gallstones cause acute pancreatitis which sometimes recurs but the pancreas is rarely damaged and the

---

Box 5.3   Advice

- Pseudocysts can be mistaken for fluid in the bowel so look for evidence of peristalsis to exclude this.

- When pseudocysts lie close to the spleen they can cause splenic vein thrombosis and splenic infarction. Patency of the splenic vein must be confirmed with a Doppler examination. In addition, aneurysms of the splenic artery can develop (these appearing like pancreatic masses without the benefit of Doppler to differentiate).

pancreatitis is not a chronic condition. One-third of cases of pancreatitis have no link with alcohol or gall-stones. Unfused ducts of Wirsung and Santorini cause 21–45% of cases of pancreatitis.

Acute pancreatitis is a condition where pancreatic enzymes leak into the pancreatic substance and the pancreas starts the process of digesting itself. Obstruction of the pancreatic duct caused by duct anomalies or calculi raises the pressure within the ductal system. Above 60 cm H_2O, alveolar basement membranes rupture, allowing the enzymes into the interstitium. This can cause pancreatitis in itself but the action of the enzymes is accelerated by the presence of bile or duodenal contents, especially cholecystokinin (Fig. 5.11).

Pancreatitis ranges in severity from mild inflammation to acute haemorrhagic destruction of the whole gland, this being fatal in 50% of cases. In cases of acute interstitial pancreatitis mild acute pancreatitis – there is usually a rapid recovery to normal. A more severe pancreatitis – necrotizing pancreatitis – can present in a less severe form (where <50% of the pancreas is involved) to severe (>50% involvement of the pancreas). The severe type involves a much higher mortality rate (nearer 95–100%). This condition can lead to respiratory and renal failure in the elderly. The only treatment is resection of necrotic tissue. Patients who recover may have recurrent attacks. Septic pancreatitis can produce gas formation (seen in 10%) and, at worst, cause death.

Patients present with epigastric pain radiating to the back between the scapulae which can be anything from mild to severe. It is accompanied by nausea and vomiting and frequent retching. Movements cause pain and often patients will exhibit shallow breathing to avoid movement and the accompanying pain. In advanced pancreatitis, tetany (muscle cramp and spasm) is seen, caused by hypocalcaemia which

develops if there is extensive fat necrosis. Pancreatitis is seen equally in males and females and can occur at any age but typically peaks at between 40 and 55. There is usually tenderness, some guarding and rigidity and accompanying shock. Pancreatitis can be mistaken for acute perforated ulcer or leaking aneurysm.

Severe necrotising pancreatitis (>50% involvement) has a very poor prognosis with the following factors:

- patient is aged >55 years old
- raised serum amylase (1000 IU/l) but this can be seen in patients with perforated peptic ulcer or appendicitis. It is more specific if five times more than the normal level, but this test cannot be entirely relied on. The high levels may be transitory and not be noted.
- WBC of >16 000 (16 × 10^9/l)
- blood urea of >16 mmol/l.

ULTRASOUND APPEARANCES

Acute interstitial pancreatitis appears on ultrasound as a swelling of the gland and a reduction in reflectivity. There may be an increase in the calibre of the duct. There may also be a collection of fluid exudate lying within the pancreas or in the lesser sac anteriorly; this secondary infection is a pseudocyst (see page 103) which in turn can cause abscess formation. The appearance may affect the whole of the gland or a part of it (Fig. 5.12).

With pancreatitis, it is essential to detect gallstones if present as 30% of patients will have more severe relapses within six months.

With necrotizing pancreatitis, it is important during the ultrasound examination to concentrate on the biliary tree. If the common bile duct measures more

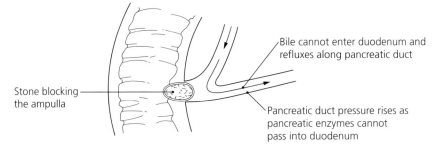

Stone blocking the ampulla

Bile cannot enter duodenum and refluxes along pancreatic duct

Pancreatic duct pressure rises as pancreatic enzymes cannot pass into duodenum

Fig. 5.11 Diagram demonstrating impacted stone in ampulla as reason for onset of pancreatitis.

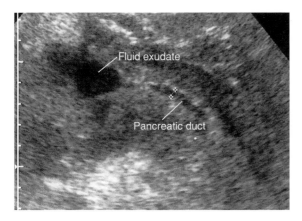

Fig. 5.12 Acute interstitial pancreatitis. Note fluid exudate within head of pancreas and increased duct calibre.

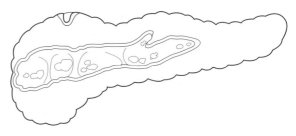

(A)

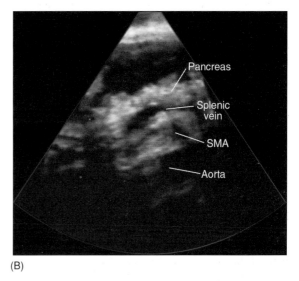

(B)

Fig. 5.13 (A) Chronic pancreatitis showing calculi within dilated ducts. (B) Small, fibrosed pancreas with calcification.

than >6–7 mm, then an urgent sphincterotomy and stone removal must be considered. A scan performed too early can demonstrate a normal pancreas. Later appearances can be patchy from fat necrosis across the surface of the gland; patchy vascular damage can lead to infarction. Patchiness can be confined to one or more lobules and measure 7–8 mm in diameter.

Colour Doppler will show hyperaemia in and around a poorly reflective pancreas with pancreatitis.

Chronic pancreatitis

CLINICAL INFORMATION

Chronic pancreatitis is relatively uncommon, with an incidence of 0.2–3%. It has, however, become more common in the last 20 years, possibly owing to a national increase in alcohol consumption. It causes scarring, stricture of the pancreatic duct and upstream dilatation, calculi in the duct and surrounding inflammation. Protein 'plugs' appear within the pancreatic ducts, leading to dilatation and acinar atrophy. As a result of focal necrosis, fibrous tissue is deposited extensively near the ducts. Eventually, only a few acinar and islet cells remain with a very dilated pancreatic duct. Protein plugs calcify, leading to stone formation.

Chronic pancreatitis is not a reversible condition but can be arrested if alcohol intake is stopped. As this often does not happen, it can then become a progressive disease accompanied by bouts of pain that may be mild and of brief duration or can lead to chronic pain with weight loss from anorexia. Steatorrhoea and diabetes are common with calcified pancreatitis and

30–65% of these patients demonstrate a pancreas speckled with small stones on a plain radiograph.

Serum amylase measurement is of little value in chronic pancreatitis.

ULTRASOUND APPEARANCES

In early chronic pancreatitis, the pancreas is heterogeneous with irregular contours, a dilated pancreatic duct of >2 mm, calculi with associated acoustic shadowing, enlarged and echo poor with patchy inflammatory masses which appear like carcinomas.

In severe chronic pancreatitis, there is often a stricture of the duct with upstream dilatation, the duct measuring more than 4 mm, calculi in the duct, fibrosis of the parenchyma giving a more reflective appearance than usual, cavities of more than 1 cm in diameter and irregular contours (Fig. 5.13).

Pancreatic pseudocysts are a common complication of chronic pancreatitis. Pancreatic ascites can occur in alcoholic pancreatitis with a communication between the pancreatic duct and the peritoneal cavity. There is a high amylase content to the ascites.

Fat infiltration

CLINICAL INFORMATION

With age and in the obese and those with Cushing's syndrome, the pancreas becomes increasingly fatty. Lipomatous pseudohypertrophy of the pancreas is associated with diabetes, alcohol intake and chronic pancreatitis.

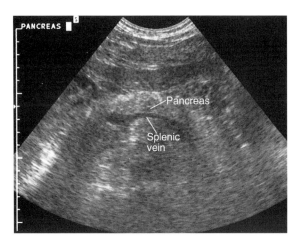

Fig. 5.14   Pancreas with fatty infiltration.

ULTRASOUND APPEARANCES

The pancreas is heterogeneous and is largely replaced with fat. The pancreas appears highly reflective and is generally seen better with a CT scan.

Cystic fibrosis

CLINICAL INFORMATION

Cystic fibrosis is the most common cause of pancreatic disease in childhood. It is an autosomal recessive condition in which a defect in the exocrine glands produces thick viscous secretions. Survival into adulthood has increased owing to better therapy. Patients are treated with a low-fat diet (to reduce steatorrhoea), pancreatic supplements, a high calorie intake and vitamin supplements.

Confirmation of diagnosis is from sweat testing and pancreatic function tests: serum amylase, faecal fat estimation and duodenal enzymes for the exocrine pancreas and serum insulin, glucagon and glucose tolerance tests for the endocrine pancreas.

ULTRASOUND APPEARANCES

The pancreas atrophies and becomes smaller in size. Small cysts can occur, particularly in the tail of the pancreas.

6

THE SPLEEN

Main functions
Anatomy
Scanning
Normal ultrasound appearances
Pathology
Focal disease
Diffuse disease

The spleen is the largest lymphoid organ in the body.

Main functions

- Reticuloendothelial cells take up old fragmented cells, break down haemoglobin and pass constituents to the liver where iron is stored and pigments are excreted in the bile.

- Red blood cells are formed if required in times of disease and especially in 2nd–5th months of intrauterine life.

- The spleen contains masses of lymphatic tissue and forms some of the body's lymphocytes and, together with the other cells of the reticuloendothelial system, forms antibodies and antitoxins.

Anatomy

The spleen measures approximately $12 \times 7 \times 3\text{–}4\,\text{cm}$ and weighs $100\text{–}200\,\text{g}$. It is a lymphoid and a haemopoietic organ, dark purple in colour and approximately the size of a clenched fist. It lies in the posterolateral aspect of the left hypochondrium under the ninth, 10th and 11th ribs with the larger superolateral surface in contact with the left hemidiaphragm. It has a convex diaphragmatic surface and a concave visceral surface and superior, inferior, anterior and posterior borders.

On the visceral surface is the hilum through which vessels and nerves pass. In addition, there are three impressions: the gastric impression formed by the stomach, the colic impression formed by the splenic flexure of the colon and the renal impression formed by the left kidney.

The spleen has a fibrous capsule and is almost entirely covered by peritoneum. On the visceral surface, two ligaments are found, formed from two folds of peritoneum: the gastrosplenic ligament anteriorly which connects the spleen to the fundus and the superior edge of the greater curvature of the stomach, and the lienorenal ligament which runs from the gastric impression anterior to the hilum to the front of the upper pole of the left kidney and attaches the spleen to the posterior abdominal wall. The lienorenal ligament contains the tail of the pancreas, the splenic vessels posteriorly and the portosystemic anastomotic vessels that run from the left renal vein to the splenic vein (Fig. 6.1).

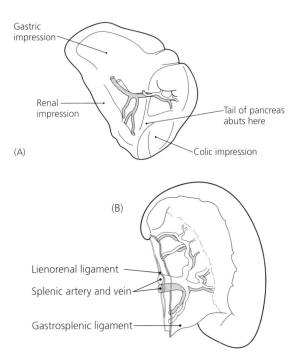

Fig. 6.1 (A) Visceral surface of the spleen. (B) Splenic ligaments.

The ribs protect the spleen to a certain extent but the spleen can be ruptured in traumatic situations, causing severe bleeding, shock and even death (Fig. 6.2).

Blood supply

The splenic artery is a branch of the coeliac axis. It branches into approximately five segments before entering the hilum.

Blood drainage

The splenic vein branches converge outside the spleen to become a single splenic vein which drains into the portal vein, joining the blood from the mesentery.

Lymph drainage

Lymph drainage is via the pancreaticosplenic and coeliac nodes.

Nerve supply

Nerve supply is from the sympathetic nerve chain.

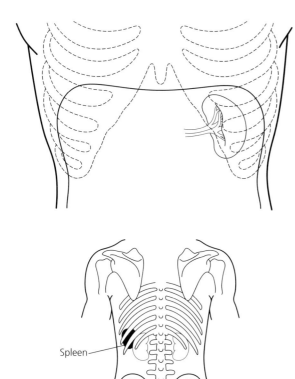

Fig. 6.2 Protection of the spleen by the ribs.

Relations – visceral surface

- Anteriorly – fundus of stomach
- Medially – left kidney
- Anteromedially – tail of pancreas
- Inferiorly – colon
- Superiorly – left hemidiaphragm

Surface markings

The long axis of the spleen corresponds to the 10th rib. The upper pole lies 3–5 cm from the level of the 10th thoracic vertebra. The lower pole can reach the mid-axillary line.

Variations in normal anatomy

- Visceral transposition is seen as the spleen on the right side and the liver on the left (the spleen looks enlarged until you find a portal vein coming from it).

- Accessory spleens (splenunculi) are common, the incidence being 10–31% of the population. Most are found close to the hilum. Sometimes they are found in the left lower abdominal quadrant, usually in the gastrosplenic ligament, and can number up to 20. They are usually about 1–1.5 cm in diameter, are rarely more than 4 cm in diameter and are round or oval in shape. They exhibit a normal splenic texture. In post-splenectomy patients with haematological disease, accessory spleens can occasionally be found.

- Asplenia is a rare anomaly associated with congenital immune deficiency.

- Sometimes the spleen lies posterior to the left kidney.

- There is a phenomenon called the wandering or ectopic spleen. This is a spleen found on a long pedicle which can affect women of childbearing age. It gives no symptoms unless torsion occurs and then appears clinically like a painful digestive condition.

Palpation

To feel for the spleen, stand on the patient's right side. Reach over and place the left hand behind the patient's left ribs. When the patient breathes in deeply, the left hand should push forward to try to push the spleen forward and the right hand push down in the area of the left lower costal margin to try to feel

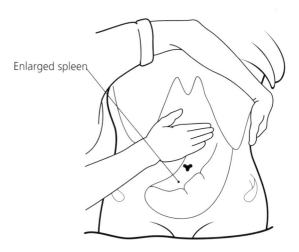

Fig. 6.3 Palpating the spleen.

the spleen with the tips of the fingers. If it is not palpable, try this again with the patient lying on their right side. When the spleen is very enlarged, the lower border can reach as far as the right iliac fossa. As a rule, the spleen can only be felt when it is about three times its normal size (Fig. 6.3).

Relevant tests – normal values

Haemoglobin	130–180 g/l (male), 115–165 g/l (female)
Platelets	$150–400 \times 10^9/l$
White cell count	$4–11 \times 10^9/l$
Neutrophils	$2–7.9 \times 10^9/l$

Scanning

Patient preparation

It is suggested that patients are starved for 4–6 hours prior to the examination. The spleen is affected in cases of portal hypertension when the liver and biliary system is examined, in which case fasting is required. In addition, the portal vessels are enlarged after eating and so fasting is again required in order to measure the vessels accurately. A fluid- and food-filled stomach may also appear similar to splenic pathology (excluded by noting peristalsis or by moving the patient).

Equipment required

A 3.5 or 5 MHz frequency should be used for adults, 7.5 MHz for small children and babies. Sector probes are useful for intercostal scanning but have the disadvantage of missing some information near the skin surface. Curvilinear probes obtain more superficial information but can sometimes be unwieldy for intercostal scanning in the small patient.

Suggested scanning technique

The most comfortable position for the patient is to lie in the supine position. Lying supine allows gas in the stomach to rise away from the spleen. However, it is often difficult to access the spleen like this as it lies in a relatively posterolateral position. The most accessible position may be with the patient in the RLD posture, with the left arm stretched up over the head and the right side draped over pillows in order to open up the

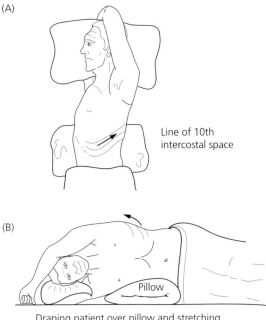

Line of 10th intercostal space

(B)

Pillow

Draping patient over pillow and stretching arm overhead helps to widen intercostal spaces

Fig. 6.4 (A, B) Right lateral decubitus position, one of the positions used when scanning the spleen.

rib spaces. It is important to note, however, that stomach gas will rise towards the greater curvature and consequently nearer to the spleen in this position (Fig. 6.4).

The best compromise is to scan the patient in the RPO position in which the gas rises anteriorly away from the spleen but leaves sufficient room to approach with the transducer. Position according to the patient's condition.

The longest axis of the spleen runs under the 10th rib. Scan along the 10th or 11th interspace; this should give the largest section of spleen. Include from the left hemidiaphragm to the inferior border. Angle the probe mediolaterally to examine the whole spleen. If the spleen is enlarged, it should be possible to scan it subcostally, parallel to the lower costal margin.

Scan on gentle respiration. Deep inspiration draws air into the lungs over the upper portion of the spleen and obscures this area. Also, if air is gulped in, the amount of gas in the stomach bubble increases and prevents good visualization of the spleen.

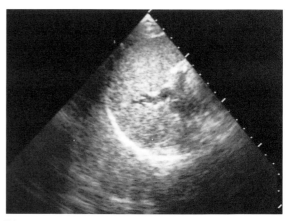

(A)

Suggested minimal sections

- A longitudinal axis of the spleen to include the hemidiaphragm, parenchyma and inferior border with measurement.

- A longitudinal section to include part of the left kidney in order to demonstrate comparative reflectivity.

Normal ultrasound appearances

The spleen is a homogeneous structure, usually either slightly less echogenic than the liver or isoechoic to it. It appears to have similar texture to the liver but without the number of vessels running through it. If the spleen is used to compare reflectivity with the liver, beware as the spleen is often implicated in hepatic disease and vice versa. It is also of higher reflectivity than the normal left kidney. The hilum of the spleen is of higher reflectivity than the parenchyma owing to the interfaces of the vessels entering the hilum and to fat that can accumulate there.

It is often said that the value of imaging the spleen is limited: enlargement is sometimes non-specific and relating echo levels to different pathology is not reliable. Focal lesions, when seen, are a more helpful clinical contribution (Fig. 6.5).

Normal sizes

The size of the spleen is variable and although it is relatively large in relation to the total body size in infants and children, it can reduce in size from middle age onwards.

The normal adult spleen measures about 12 cm from diaphragm to inferior border and is approximately this

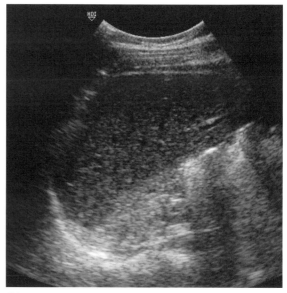

(B)

Fig. 6.5   (A) Normal appearance of vessels entering the spleen. (B) Normal spleen.

size from the early teens onwards. Other sizes (measured from diaphragm to inferior border) related to age are as follows.

Age	Size (cm)
0–3 months	6
3–6 months	6.5
6–12 months	7
1–2 years+	8
12–14 years+	10–12

The spleen is considered enlarged when:

- the anterior border lies anterior to the aorta and the IVC and is as thick as a normal kidney

- in the RLD position, the spleen is twice the kidney size

- the diaphragm–inferior border measures >14 cm.

With splenomegaly, the spleen grows inferiorly and medially. The larger it gets, the more superficial it lies. In extreme cases, it can cross to the midline and lie anterior to the stomach and colon – an excellent acoustic window.

Box 6.2　Advice

If the spleen is not seen, look for a fine scar and read the patient's notes (the patient has probably had a splenectomy). The left kidney and the splenic flexure of the large bowel tend to move upwards and to occupy space vacated by the spleen.

Pathology

Focal disease:

- lymphoma

- abscess

- metastases

- cyst

- hydatid cyst

- haemangioma

- lymphangioma

- infarcts

- trauma

Diffuse disease:

- lymphoma

- leukaemia – acute and chronic

- tuberculosis

- others

- congestive disorders

Focal disease

Focal lymphoma

CLINICAL INFORMATION

Lymphoma is a malignant tumour of the reticulo-endothelial system, divided into Hodgkin's and non-Hodgkin's lymphomas. It is rare in children, affecting boys twice as often as girls. As age increases, males and females are equally affected. The condition peaks twice, once in the 20s and then later in middle age. Patients present with cervical and possibly axillary and inguinal lymphadenopathy. The enlarged glands are painless and rubbery to feel. Patients may be tired, weak and anorexic and have fever, night sweats, weight loss and pruritus. Diagnosis is from biopsy of a whole node and treatment is usually by radiation therapy or combination chemotherapy.

Lymphoma can appear in the spleen as a single, relatively large lesion or as multiple lesions (rare) or as a diffuse appearance, which is more common. The incidence of focal lesions in the spleen is 0.1%.

ULTRASOUND APPEARANCES

With focal lymphoma the spleen is not usually enlarged. The lesions are usually echo poor and have boundaries which are not clearly defined. Occasionally they are more highly reflective than the normal splenic tissue. If the lesions are large, they are seen to be heterogeneous and sometimes to 'bulge'. Appearances are non-specific and they are often difficult to differentiate from other splenic focal pathologies. As the incidence of splenic focal lesions is so low, it can be assumed that focal lesions in a patient with lymphoma is lymphomatous involvement. This can be confirmed by ultrasound-guided biopsy of the lesion using 21 or 22 gauge needles (see also section on Diffuse lymphoma below) (Fig. 6.6).

Abscess

CLINICAL INFORMATION

Splenic abscesses are uncommon. They can be caused by spread of infection in the blood system or after trauma or infarction.

ULTRASOUND APPEARANCES

The general appearance of abscesses varies according to the number, size, texture, shape and position. They can be echo free or of mixed echogenicity with solid and cystic components, thick walled and irregular and

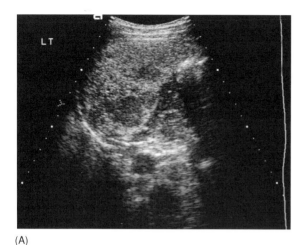

(A)

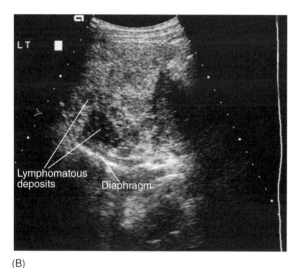

(B)

Fig. 6.6 (A, B) Lymphomatous deposits in the spleen.

may contain septations, gas and/or debris. They can be mistaken for focal malignant change.

Metastases

CLINICAL INFORMATION

Metastases are rare in the spleen except from lymphoma but they can be spread from the ovary, melanoma and occasionally from breast or lung.

ULTRASOUND APPEARANCES

The appearance of splenic metastases can be as varied as metastases in the liver (see pp. 46–48). Metastatic

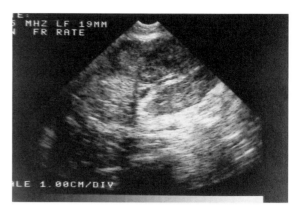

Fig. 6.7 Splenic metastases.

involvement of the spleen in carcinomatosis can often be seen (Fig. 6.7).

Cysts

CLINICAL INFORMATION

Cysts can be congenital or acquired from infection or trauma. Simple cysts are less common than renal or hepatic cysts. Splenic epidermoid cysts are rare congenital lesions which, if infected, can lead to septicaemia.[1]

ULTRASOUND APPEARANCES

Cysts are seen as echo-free spherical lesions with posterior acoustic enhancement. They can calcify and sometimes contain cholesterol crystals, giving the cyst a

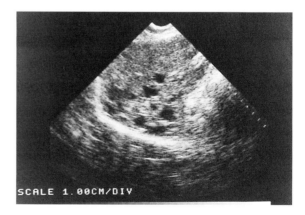

Fig. 6.8 Splenic involvement in adult polycystic kidney disease.

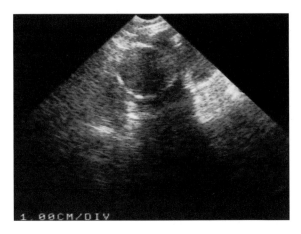

Fig. 6.9 Calcified cyst.

solid appearance. When the cyst is haemorrhagic, gravity causes the clot to layer within the cystic fluid. Cysts are seen in 5% of patients with polycystic renal disease (Figs 6.8, 6.9).

Box 6.3 Advice

Sometimes the appearance of fluid in the stomach can be mistaken for a cyst or cysts in the spleen. Ensure it is not fluid in the stomach by giving water to outline the stomach. A splenic cyst is sometimes difficult to differentiate from a retroperitoneal cyst, a pseudocyst at the tail of the pancreas, a renal cyst, blood from a leaking aortic aneurysm or a haematoma in childhood trauma.

Hydatid cyst

ULTRASOUND APPEARANCES

Hydatid cysts of the spleen are rare. Their appearance is similar to that of hydatid cysts in the liver (see p. 50). They appear as multiple cysts within a cyst (daughter cysts). Often these hydatid cysts will present as a normal echo-free cyst although the wall can be thick and highly reflective. The cyst content can occasionally be highly reflective owing to several membranes and hydatid sand being present.

Haemangioma

ULTRASOUND APPEARANCES

Haemangiomas are rare in the spleen. They can be seen in childhood as a solid mass. They range in appearance from being reflective with some posterior acoustic shadowing to echo-poor lesions with posterior acoustic enhancement to both types being present at the same time.

Lymphangioma

ULTRASOUND APPEARANCES

Lymphangiomas (benign congenital malformations of the lymphatic system) are rarely seen in the spleen. The spleen is often enlarged and contains multiple lesions of low reflectivity.

Infarction

CLINICAL INFORMATION

Infarction can occur with splenomegaly and sickle cell anaemia and also with intravenous drug abuse, atrial fibrillation, leukaemia, pancreatitis and subacute bacterial endocarditis. With sickle cell disease (occurring mainly in Africans, Caribbeans and Mediterraneans) the sickle shape of the red cells makes passage through the small vessels difficult and leads to their obstruction, reducing oxygen supply to the relevant tissues. A typical sickle cell crisis can include bone pain, pleuritic chest pain and painful splenic infarcts. The haemoglobin level usually falls drastically.

ULTRASOUND APPEARANCES

The infarct appears usually as an echo-poor wedge shape with the apex pointing to the splenic hilum and the base to the periphery. The infarct can sometimes be smooth and rounded. As the infarct heals, the scar becomes highly reflective. Recurrent splenic infarctions can lead to fibrosis and shrinking of the spleen and it can eventually be almost impossible to detect.

Box 6.4 Advice

Splenic infarction can be very painful: be gentle when scanning.

Trauma

CLINICAL INFORMATION

After blunt abdominal trauma, the spleen often enlarges owing to changed blood volume and adrenaline stimulation. This increase in size does not necessarily signal deterioration. Fractured ribs on the lower left and injury to left upper lumbar transverse processes can often cause a ruptured spleen. Ultrasound has been considered 94.6% sensitive, 95.1% specific and 94.9% accurate in detecting injuries in general after trauma and is 90% sensitive in identifying injury to the spleen.[2] The modern trend after splenic trauma is to conserve the spleen whenever possible rather than to remove it.[3] If a spleen is removed, susceptibility to pneumococcal infection increases, necessitating long-term penicillin treatment.

Disruption of the spleen can cause seeding of splenic tissue to such places as the liver, stomach and pleura.

ULTRASOUND APPEARANCES

- Subcapsular haematoma – shows as an echo-free or echo-poor area outside the splenic body but within the splenic capsule. Sometimes the left lobe of the liver can lie between the spleen and the left hemi-diaphragm and, if of low echogenicity, can appear like a haematoma.

- Extracapsular haematoma – shows as an area of low reflectivity that has breached the splenic capsule. As clot forms, the echogenicity increases. The area may increase in size then resolve in time (Fig. 6.10).

- Splenic rupture – shows as an irregular area of decreased reflectivity from haemorrhage. A focal pattern of blood pooling seen as local areas of reduced reflectivity is rare. Lacerations are often difficult to see as the appearance is similar to normal splenic tissue.

- Acute haematomas – are seen as well or poorly defined crescentic shapes of increased reflectivity. They enlarge in time then reduce in reflectivity and can appear similar to a cyst. Blood in the lesser or greater sac suggests much blood loss from the spleen.

After healing, the damaged part of the spleen fibroses and can appear on ultrasound as an area of increased reflectivity compared with the surrounding tissue.

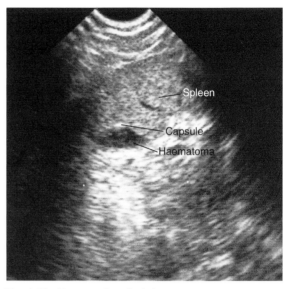

Fig. 6.10 Extracapsular splenic haematoma.

Box 6.5   Advice

It is essential to scan the pelvis in patients in whom a ruptured spleen is thought to have occurred. Not all ruptures are easily seen on ultrasound and the pelvis may be the only area in which fluid can be seen to collect.

Diffuse disease

Diffuse lymphoma

ULTRASOUND APPEARANCES

Focal lesions accompanying lymphoma have been described above. However, it is far more common to see a diffuse appearance than focal lesions with this disease.

The spleen can be enlarged, homogeneous in texture with reduced reflectivity although it is often of normal size and echogenicity. Splenomegaly has a 36% sensitivity and 61% specificity in diagnosing lymphoma. The spleen can be enlarged without involvement or can be of normal size when involved in the disease (Fig. 6.11).

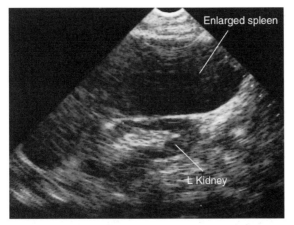

(A)

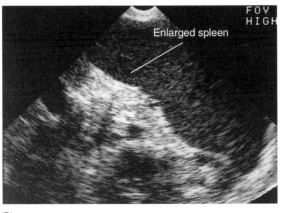

(B)

Fig. 6.11 (A) Diffuse lymphoma (compare size of spleen with left kidney). (B) Transverse section of enlarged spleen (different patient).

Acute leukaemia

CLINICAL INFORMATION

Leukaemia is the term given to an increase in malignant white cells within the circulatory system. Features of acute leukaemia are anaemia and malaise, repeated infections, bruising and painful and enlarged lymph nodes. The spleen and/or liver may be enlarged.

The white cell count is raised and the platelet count reduced.

ULTRASOUND APPEARANCES

The spleen is often of normal size or slightly enlarged although hepatomegaly may occur. It will often be of reduced echogenicity.

Chronic leukaemia

CLINICAL INFORMATION

Patients present with anaemia, sweating, fever, loss of weight owing to high metabolic rate and pain and perhaps gastrointestinal disorders resulting from splenomegaly. They may have gout from a raised serum uric acid.

ULTRASOUND APPEARANCES

The spleen may be grossly enlarged with reduced reflectivity. However, it may be normal or even increased in reflectivity and homogeneous in texture. It is thought that chemotherapy can cause the reflectivity of the spleen to be increased.

Tuberculosis

CLINICAL INFORMATION

Active tuberculosis is usually miliary.

ULTRASOUND APPEARANCES

The spleen has a diffuse, uniform, highly reflective appearance. Old tuberculosis can appear as a number of small, highly reflective focal areas throughout the spleen.

Others

POLYCYTHAEMIA RUBRA VERA

The spleen is often enlarged with a uniform texture.

ACUTE INFECTION

A normal-sized spleen often shows with low reflectivity.

CHRONIC INFECTIONS

Chronic infections can show moderate to gross splenomegaly usually with higher level echoes and sometimes with calcification.

Congestive disorders

ULTRASOUND APPEARANCES

A congestive spleen can be seen in portal hypertension and portal vein thrombosis as a complication of cirrhosis, splenic vein thrombosis and congestive cardiac failure (CCF). The spleen can be moderately to

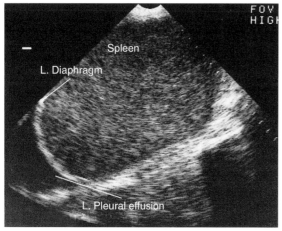

(A)

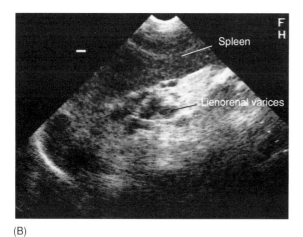

(B)

Fig. 6.12. (A) A large congested spleen with accompanying left pleural effusion. (B) Lienorenal varices.

severely enlarged with the reflectivity normal. The portal system (portal vein, superior mesenteric vein and splenic vein) is usually enlarged. The branches are obvious when viewing the splenic hilum. At the same time there may be varices in the lienorenal ligament which are seen as echo-poor irregular and tortuous areas around the hilum (Fig. 6.12). If the portal hypertension is severe, the paraumbilical vein within the ligamentum teres in the liver may recanalize (see p. 56).

References

1. Morris-Stiff G, Foster M 1998 Chicken fancier's spleen. Int J Clin Pract 52(4): 272–273

2. Yoshii H, Sato M, Yamamoto S *et al* 1998 Usefulness and limitations of ultrasonography in the initial evaluation of blunt abdominal trauma. J Trauma 45(1): 45–50

3. Bain IM, Kirby RM 1998 10 year experience of splenic injury: an increasing place for conservative management after blunt trauma. Injury 29(3): 177–182

Further reading

Venkataramu NK, Gupta S, Sood BP *et al* 1999 Ultrasound guided fine needle aspiration biopsy of splenic lesions. Br J Radiol 72: 953–956

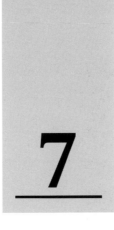

7

LYMPH NODES

Main functions
Anatomy
Position of relevant lymph node groups
Ultrasound appearances

Main functions

Lymph nodes act as a filter for lymph, preventing foreign particles and bacteria from entering the bloodstream, and produce lymphocytes.

Anatomy

Lymph nodes are small round or bean-shaped structures. Normal nodes measure between 1 and 15 mm in diameter and are distributed along the lymph vessel chains. Lymph passes through at least one node on its way into the bloodstream.

Lymph from the abdomen, left side of the thorax, head, neck, arm and both legs drains into the thoracic duct and subsequently into the left subclavian vein. Lymph from the right side of the thorax, head, neck and right arm drains into the shorter right lymphatic duct and eventually into the right subclavian vein. An expanded part of the thoracic duct, the cisterna chyli, receives several lymph vessels from the lower limbs and the abdomen, especially from the digestive tract. It is about 5–7 cm long and lies behind and to the right of the abdominal aorta at the level of the first and second lumbar vertebra.

Position of relevant lymph node groups

Preaortic (coeliac, superior mesenteric and inferior mesenteric)

These lie on the anterior surface of the abdominal aorta. The coeliac group lies near the coeliac axis of the aorta and drains lymph from secondary lymph nodes (gastric nodes draining lymph from the stomach, hepatic nodes draining lymph from the stomach, duodenum, gallbladder, liver and pancreas and pancreatico-splenic nodes draining lymph from the stomach, pancreas and spleen).

The superior and inferior mesenteric groups lie near the origins of the superior mesenteric and inferior mesenteric arteries on the anterior aspect of the aorta. These drain lymph from the intestinal tract, the efferent vessels from these nodes passing to the cisterna chyli.

Lateral aortic (paraaortic)

These lie on either side of the abdominal aorta anterior to the lumbar spine. They receive lymph from the

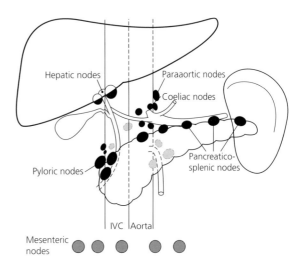

Fig. 7.1 Main lymph node groups.

kidneys, ureters, gonads, pelvic viscera and abdominal walls. Common iliac lymph nodes also drain into the lateral aortic group. The first nodes from the testes lie at the renal level as the testes first descend from the abdomen (Fig. 7.1).

Ultrasound appearances

Normal lymph nodes

Normal lymph nodes are rarely seen on ultrasound with 3.5–5 MHz transducers but normal fleshy nodes in children can be seen with high-resolution 7.5–10 MHz probes.

They can be calcified and appear as highly echogenic round structures with characteristic acoustic shadowing posteriorly or can rarely be infiltrated with fat and again appear highly reflective but without the shadowing.

Abnormal lymph nodes

In illness causing enlarged lymph nodes such as tumour infiltration or inflammatory disease, clumps of enlarged nodes can be seen at the porta hepatis, the renal and splenic hila, and close to the pancreas, as well as around the aorta.

Enlarged lymph nodes, seen when 1.5–2 cm diameter and considered to be pathological at this size, are uniformly low in echogenicity and can be almost anechoic when very large. Large nodes can display colour Doppler flow through them. The appearance of the enlarged nodes does not give any clue as to the reason for the lymphadenopathy. Care has to be taken when scanning to ensure that incorrect gain settings do not make the enlarged lymph nodes appear like cysts.

Enlarged lymph nodes can cause extrinsic pressure, leading to obstruction and dilatation of some vessels, and can distort and change the normal direction of others. Obstruction of the biliary or renal systems from enlarged lymph nodes is not unknown. Lymphoma can give rise to large anechoic nodes. If enlarged lymph nodes are seen by chance on scanning, all abdominal organs should be scanned for evidence of a primary tumour. If not found, an examination of the testes and thyroid must also be undertaken.

Paraaortic lymph node enlargement can elevate the aorta and the superior mesenteric artery. These nodes also frequently push the IVC forwards. The enlarged nodes can be lobulated or smooth bordered and may surround the aorta so closely that the aortic boundaries are lost (Figs 7.2, 7.3).

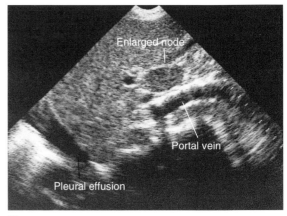

(A)

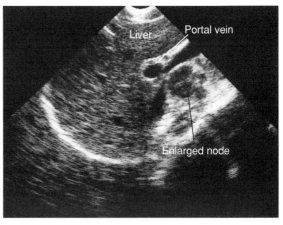

(B)

Fig. 7.3 (A, B) Enlarged lymph nodes at the porta hepatis.

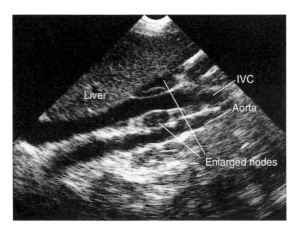

Fig. 7.2 Paraaortic lymph nodes.

Enlarged coeliac axis nodes can extend into the porta hepatis and can cause obstruction to the biliary system. They can push the pancreas forwards and surround and straighten the coeliac axis. Enlarged paraaortic lymph nodes are involved in 25% of Hodgkin's disease and 40% of non-Hodgkin's disease. Enlarged lymph nodes are also frequently seen in patients with AIDS. In patients with tuberculosis, enlarged lymph nodes can liquefy, giving a characteristic appearance of fluid areas within the node.

Enlarged mesenteric nodes can be seen anterior and posterior to the superior mesenteric vein, forming a 'sandwich' sign. It must be noted that occasionally, large amounts of fat in the mesentery can imitate this sign although fat is usually more highly reflective: take into consideration the size of the patient and the gain settings being used (Fig. 7.4).

Enlarged lymph nodes appear in patients with lymphoma, metastases and inflammatory reactions. Non-Hodgkin's lymphoma appears to produce the most numerous and enlarged nodes but this pathology is rare in Hodgkin's lymphoma. The size of the nodes is not related to the severity of the disease process and so measurements of the nodes need not be taken when monitoring progress.

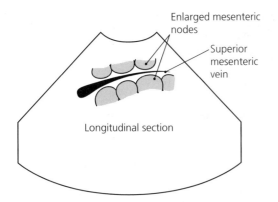

Fig. 7.4 The mesenteric node 'sandwich' sign.

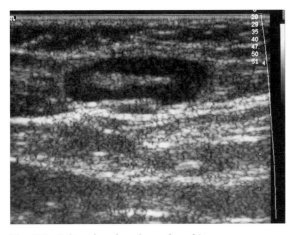

Fig. 7.5 Solitary lymph node – enlarged image.

Box 7.1   Advice

Multiple enlarged lymph nodes closely surrounding the abdominal aorta can appear similar to an aortic aneurysm, more on longitudinal sections than transverse sections. Echo-poor areas produced by spinal bodies seen posterior to the aorta may be mistaken for the aorta itself.

Lower than normal gain settings give enlarged nodes a cystic appearance.

Accessory spleens are sometimes solitary and although they are of the same echogenicity as the spleen, an enlarged node is hard to exclude especially as splenunculi and enlarged nodes are often found in similar positions. Enlarged nodes in the region of the pancreas can appear similar to pancreatic masses.

Enlarged mesenteric nodes can appear like loops of bowel, but without the peristalsis.

Further reading

Watanabe M, Yoshi H, Ishi E *et al* 1997 Evaluation of abdominal lymphadenopathy in children by ultrasonography. Pediatr Radiol 27(11): 860–864

8

ABDOMINAL AORTA AND INFERIOR VENA CAVA

Main functions
Anatomy
Scanning
Normal ultrasound appearances
Pathology:
  Abdominal aorta
  IVC

The abdominal aorta and the inferior vena cava (IVC) are major retroperitoneal blood vessels.

Main functions

The abdominal aorta is the part of the main artery in the body that runs from the diaphragm and supplies blood to all parts of the body from the diaphragm inferiorly.

The IVC returns blood to the right atrium of the heart from those parts of the body distal to the diaphragm.

Anatomy

Abdominal aorta

The abdominal aorta penetrates through the diaphragm at the level of the 12th thoracic vertebra (T12) and bifurcates at the level of the fourth lumbar vertebra (L4) where it continues as the right and left common iliac arteries. It lies to the left of the anterior part of the lumbar bodies just posterior to the centre of the abdomen in cross-section.

Inferior vena cava

The IVC begins at the junction of the left and right common iliac veins a little to the right of the fifth lumbar vertebra (L5), widening at the level of the renal veins and coursing slightly anteriorly at L2 where it passes through the liver. Here it runs through a groove in the posterior part of the liver, receiving the hepatic veins before leaving the abdomen through the right leaf of the central tendon of the diaphragm at the level of T8. It lies to the right of the anterior part of the lumbar bodies.

Branches of the aorta seen on ultrasound

- Coeliac axis, which is 2–3 cm in length, arises from the anterior part of the aorta just below the liver. It branches into the splenic artery on the left and the common hepatic artery on the right. The left gastric artery also originates from the coeliac axis but is not often seen on ultrasound. The gastro-duodenal artery branches from the common hepatic artery and supplies the stomach and duodenum. The hepatic artery continues from the common hepatic artery and courses to the liver via the porta hepatis.

- Superior mesenteric artery originates just below the coeliac axis from the anterior or antero-lateral part of the abdominal aorta and runs parallel to it, supplying the small bowel, caecum, ascending colon and the proximal third of the transverse colon.

- Renal arteries originate from the lateral aspects of the abdominal aorta at a more inferior level than the superior mesenteric artery. They supply the kidneys, provide branches for adrenal glands and ureters and lie posterior to the renal veins. A double renal artery is sometimes seen.

- Inferior mesenteric artery is sometimes seen at its origin close to the bifurcation of the aorta. It supplies the rest of the large bowel not supplied by the superior mesenteric artery down to and including part of the rectum.

- Right and left common iliac arteries are the continuation from the bifurcation of the abdominal aorta at L4 towards each leg (Fig. 8.1).

Tributaries of the IVC seen on ultrasound

- Left and right common iliac veins which join the IVC at the level of L5.

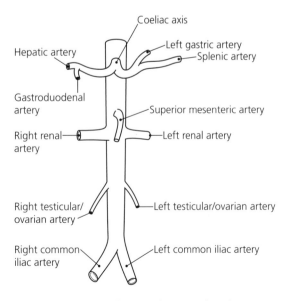

Fig. 8.1 The abdominal aorta and its major branches.

- Left and right renal veins which drain into the lateral aspect of the IVC. The left renal vein is longer than the right as it lies anterior to the aorta in order to receive blood from the left kidney. It receives blood from the left testicular/ovarian vein and the left suprarenal vein. The right suprarenal vein and testicular/ovarian vein drain directly into the IVC.

- Hepatic veins drain blood from the liver into the anterior part of the IVC, the right draining into the IVC separate to the middle and left hepatic veins which join to form a short trunk which then drains into the anterior part of the IVC (Fig. 8.2).

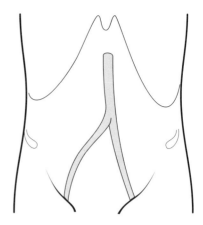

Fig. 8.3 Surface markings of the aorta.

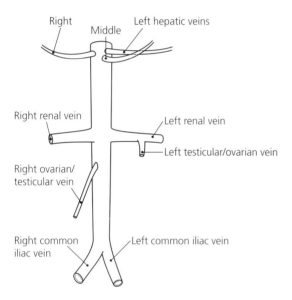

Fig. 8.2 The inferior vena cava and its major tributaries.

Relations: abdominal aorta and IVC

- Posteriorly – thoracic and lumbar spines.
- Anteriorly – mesentery, small intestine, transverse colon, stomach, duodenum, pancreas.
- Laterally – left and right kidneys, spleen.

Surface markings

The abdominal aorta lies under a line drawn 2.5 cm above the transpyloric plane (the line bisecting a point between umbilicus and xiphisternal joint) and slightly to the left of midline to 1.5 cm below and to the left of the umbilicus (Fig. 8.3).

The IVC starts about 2.5 cm below and 1.5 cm to the right of the umbilicus and runs to a point between the fifth right interspace and the right border of the sternum.

Variations in normal anatomy

- Transposition of the great vessels – situs inversus (aorta lies on the right). The IVC can appear completely on the left (0.2%), the more common variant being one where a large left renal vein crosses the aorta and drains into a normally sited upper part of the vena cava.

- The abdominal aorta is often tortuous in the elderly (Fig. 8.4)).

- The amount of distension in the IVC varies with posture, respiration and dehydration.

Palpation

The abdominal aorta can be palpated in cases where there is a large aneurysm or when the patient is thin and a haemodynamic aortic can be felt (see Abdominal aortic aneurysm, below).

Relevant tests – normal values

Normal blood pressure	120/80
Normal pulse rate	60–80 beats per minute in the resting adult

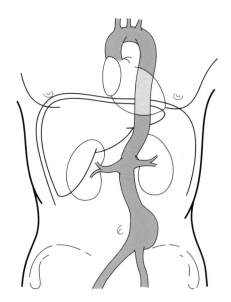

Fig. 8.4 The tortuous aorta.

Scanning

Patient preparation

Clear, still fluid only to be taken for 4–6 hours prior to the examination. This may help reduce gas but is not always strictly necessary.

Equipment required

3.5–5 MHz in the adult and child, 7.5 MHz in the infant and neonate, all dependent on patient size. Curved linear and linear array transducers offer a wider field of view than a sector transducer.

Use must be made of appropriate focusing bearing in mind that the abdominal aorta can be quite superficial in some subjects and quite deep in others.

Suggested scanning technique – aorta

SUPINE POSITION

When scanning the aorta, it is essential to first exclude an abdominal aortic aneurysm before applying any form of pressure to the abdomen, especially in the elderly. Scan longitudinally from the xiphisternum towards the left, using the small amount of the liver as an acoustic window for the proximal part. Set the gain and the focusing zones appropriately so that the near

wall of the aorta is seen as clearly as possible. In the longitudinal position, scan from as superior a position as possible and try to scan down the length of the aorta. When at the level of the bifurcation, angle the probe first to the right then to the left in order to survey the common iliac arteries. While scanning longitudinally, find the angle and the lie of the aorta to the horizontal.

Turn the probe at right angles and scan transversely from the upper aorta to the bifurcation and just below. When scanning transversely, it will be necessary to scan with the probe angled at 90° to the long axis of the aorta in order to avoid elongation and to obtain an accurate measurement.

Lower the sensitivity to obtain a better wall outline. Note the measurement of the aorta and the position and relative size of the vessels originating from it.

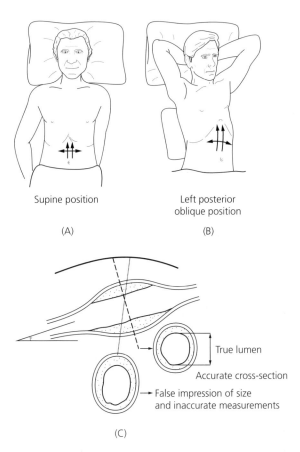

Fig. 8.5 (A) Supine position for scanning the aorta and IVC. (B) Left posterior oblique position for scanning the aorta and IVC. (C) Measuring the cross-section of an aortic aneurysm.

The aorta can sometimes be seen for most of its length in a slim, gas-free subject but this is unusual and owing to the overlying gas-filled bowel, other positions are often required to visualize the length of the aorta clearly, such as the oblique coronal view taken in the LPO position. (In the obese patient, it may be helpful to scan through the left posterolateral area with the patient in the RLD position using the left kidney as an acoustic window.) (Fig. 8.5.)

RIGHT CORONAL OBLIQUE VIEW

In this position, described by Creagh-Barry *et al* in 1986, the right lobe of liver and right kidney move anteriorly and inferiorly to act as acoustic windows and fat and gas-filled bowel move to the left which allows slightly more access to the retroperitoneum when scanning in the right oblique coronal plane.[1]

The patient is turned 45° with the left side down (LPO position) and scanned longitudinally from the right side in a plane oblique to the coronal plane. This plane can vary in obliquity from 0° to 30°. The patient can be scanned from the left side while in the RPO position (the left coronal oblique view) (Fig. 8.6).

This is sometimes called the 'rosethorn view' owing to the appearance of the renal arteries (the thorns) and the aorta (the stem) (Fig. 8.9).

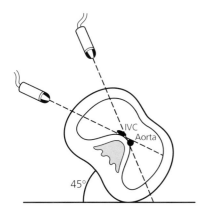

Left side down

Fig. 8.6   The right oblique coronal view.

Suggested scanning technique – IVC

SUPINE POSITION

The IVC may be scanned in a similar way to the aorta in either supine, LPO or LLD positions. When scan-

ning the upper part of the IVC, it is important to scan transversely and angle towards the head in order to visualize the confluence of the hepatic veins into the IVC. It may be necessary to scan during the Valsalva manoeuvre in order to fill the IVC and see it clearly. At the level of the renal veins, the transverse section demonstrates the left renal vein passing anterior to the aorta and the right renal vein entering the right kidney anterior to the right renal artery.

Suggested minimal sections

AORTA

- A longitudinal section showing the coeliac axis and superior mesenteric artery.

- A longitudinal section showing lower aorta and bifurcation.

- A longitudinal oblique section demonstrating the length of the aorta, the proximal renal arteries and the bifurcation.

- Transverse sections at the levels of coeliac axis, superior mesenteric artery, renal arteries and bifurcation (Fig. 8.7A).

IVC

- Longitudinal section through the liver.

- Transverse sections at level of portosplenic junction and renal veins.

Normal ultrasound appearances

Aorta

LONGITUDINAL SECTION

The aorta appears as an anechoic tubular structure, gently tapering inferiorly and following the direction of the lumbar curve so that the inferior end is more anterior than the superior end. It is bordered by characteristic highly reflective walls. On longitudinal section the coeliac axis can be seen protruding from the anterior superior part of the abdominal aorta. Just below the coeliac axis, the superior mesenteric artery (SMA) protrudes out and follows the aorta anteriorly or antero-laterally. The SMA is recognized by its highly reflective walls (Fig. 8.8A).

TRANSVERSE SECTION

Providing it is scanned at right angles to its long axis, the aorta is circular in shape in transverse section.

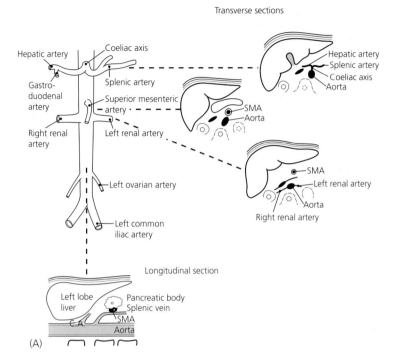

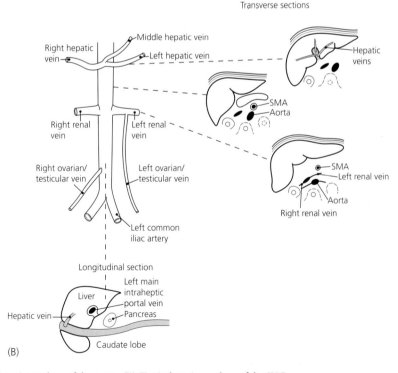

Fig. 8.7 (A) Typical sections taken of the aorta. (B) Typical sections taken of the IVC.

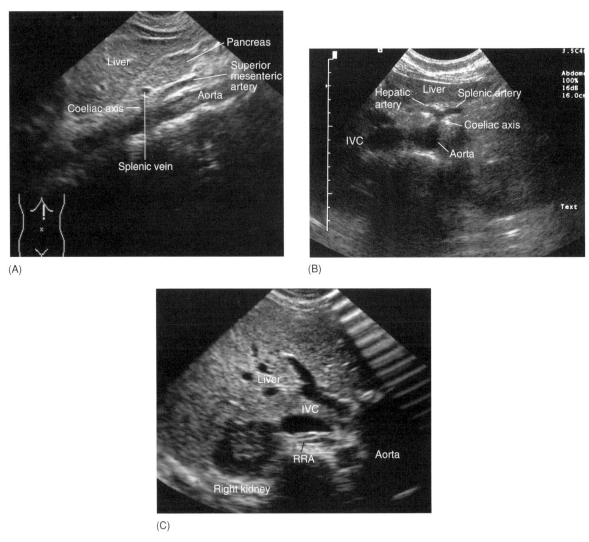

Fig. 8.8 (A) Longitudinal section through the abdominal aorta showing coeliac axis and SMA. (B) Transverse section through the abdominal aorta showing coeliac axis, hepatic artery and splenic artery. (C) Transverse abdominal section showing the right renal artery lying posterior to the IVC.

The coeliac axis and branches appear like a gull's wings. Further inferiorly, the SMA appears as a round, anechoic vessel surrounded by a highly reflective ring. Just below this level, the renal arteries can sometimes be seen from the side of the aorta. On some thin patients without the use of Doppler, the renal arteries appear quite clearly in the supine position. On scanning inferiorly in the transverse plane, the aorta eventually divides into the left and right iliac arteries. On transverse sections, the aorta is seen as lying more posterior than the IVC superiorly, at about the same level as the IVC at the level of the

renal vessels and more anterior inferiorly (Figs 8.8B, C).

In the right oblique coronal view, the scanning plane often passes through the IVC before passing through the aorta. In the right subject, this position is helpful in showing both renal artery origins in 79% and right renal artery origin in 92%. In this position, the renal arteries appear as two hooks or rosethorns on each side of the aorta. The entire length of the aorta can often be seen in this view. The proximal common iliac arteries can be seen in 80% of patients (Fig. 8.9).

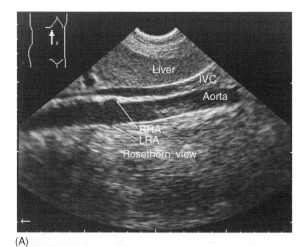

(A)

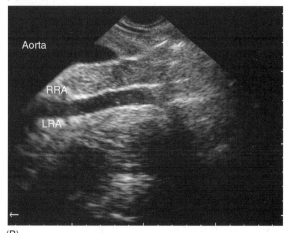

(B)

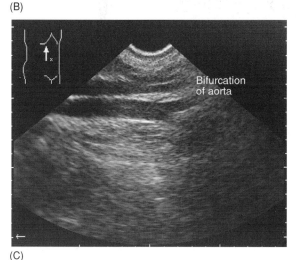

(C)

Fig. 8.9 (A) The right oblique coronal or 'rosethorn' views of the aorta.

Normal ultrasound appearances – IVC

LONGITUDINAL SECTION

The IVC is seen on longitudinal section as a gently curving, tapering anechoic structure surrounded by a reflective wall. The wall is, however, not as highly reflective as that of the aorta. It is usually well seen as it passes posterior to the liver but, as with the aorta, is not often seen behind mid-abdominal gas. The distinct appearance of the right renal artery in cross-section can often be seen posterior to the IVC in this section (Fig. 8.10A). (There may be two renal arteries seen in this section which is a normal variation see Fig. 9.8B.)

The hepatic veins can be seen anterior to the upper part of the IVC within the liver, curving towards it before entering the right atrium of the heart. The hepatic veins appear different to the other vessels on ultrasound as they have no distinct white vessel walls.

TRANSVERSE SECTION

In transverse section, the IVC is sometimes barely visible. It can be oval or slit-like and the calibre varies depending on the patient position or phase of respiration. It distends with the Valsalva manoeuvre in normal subjects. At the level of the renal vessels, a transverse scan will show the left renal vein stretching between the aorta and the SMA (Figs 8.10B, C).

Normal sizes

AORTA

Maximum diameter:

- at the level of the diaphragm – 2.5 cm
- at the level of the renal arteries – 2 cm
- at the level of the bifurcation – 1.5–1 cm
- iliac arteries just distal to the bifurcation – 1.0 cm.

Box 8.1 Advice

Research from Germany has shown that the great abdominal arteries of endurance athletes undergo morphologically adaptive processes and enlarge, compared to athletes undergoing relatively moderate training and to sedentary males. Bear this in mind when measuring the arteries of German endurance athletes.[2]

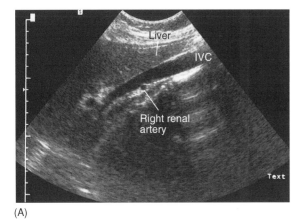

(A)

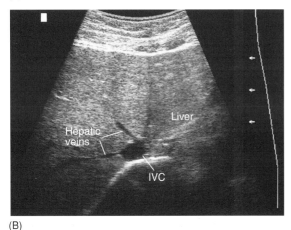

(B)

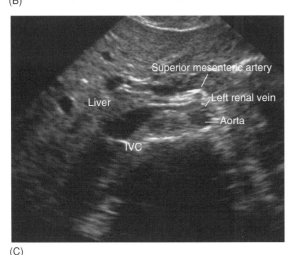

(C)

Fig. 8.10 (A) Longitudinal section of the IVC with right renal artery passing posteriorly towards the right kidney. (B) Transverse section of the IVC showing confluence of the hepatic veins. (C) The left renal vein passing between the SMA and the aorta.

IVC

The calibre varies depending on the phase of respiration and position of the patient; as mentioned, it often appears slit-like and thin but distends with the Valsalva manoeuvre.

Measuring

When measuring the abdominal aorta, the measurement should be taken from outer wall to outer wall, at the level just inferior to the renal arteries. Some centres use the mean of the anteroposterior and lateral measurements. Most of the literature concerning accuracy of measurements fails to state whether an anteroposterior measurement, lateral diameter measurement or the mean of both measurements should be taken although axial resolution is known to be better than lateral resolution. Anteroposterior measurements can be inaccurate owing to oblique measurements being made when the incident sound beam is not at right angles to the long axis of the aorta.

Normal pulsed wave Doppler

Pulsed wave Doppler of the aorta demonstrates more decreased flow during diastole the nearer the sample is to the lower end of the aorta. This is due to the high resistance in the lower limbs. Some reversal of flow is seen near to the bifurcation of the aorta and a greater degree of flow reversal is seen in the common iliac arteries (Fig. 8.11).

Pathology

Aorta:

- abdominal aortic aneurysm (AAA) with atheroma
- aortic dissection
- dissecting aneurysm
- graft monitoring
- ectatic aorta

IVC:

- distension
- intraluminal mass
  - tumour thrombus
  - non-tumour thrombus

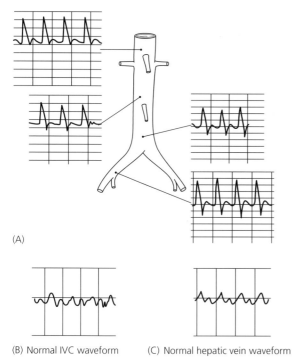

(A)

(B) Normal IVC waveform   (C) Normal hepatic vein waveform

Fig. 8.11 (A) Examples of pulsed wave Doppler signals from the normal upper aorta to the common iliac artery. (B) Pulsed wave Doppler signals of the normal IVC. (C) Hepatic veins.

- IVC filter
- primary IVC tumour

Abdominal aorta

Abdominal aortic aneurysm (AAA) with atheroma

CLINICAL INFORMATION

An aneurysm is an abnormal focal dilatation of an artery. The dilatation occurs when arterial disease causes the tunica media in the arterial wall to become weak and thin, the smooth muscle cells and elastic fibres are lost and the tunica media is replaced by non-contractile inelastic collagen. The tunica media becomes incompetent and the artery gradually dilates over a number of years. Two types of aneurysm are usually seen: the fusiform or wedge-shaped type which tapers to a maximum diameter and the saccular type (not often seen in the abdominal aorta) which is rounded and enlarges within a relatively short distance (Fig. 8.12).

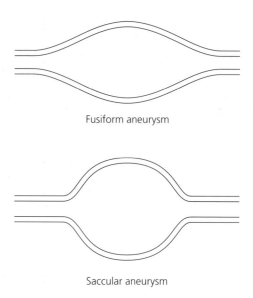

Fusiform aneurysm

Saccular aneurysm

Fig. 8.12 Types of aneurysm.

By far the most common disease to cause weakening of the abdominal aorta is atheroma (from the Greek for gruel, a porridge-like substance composed of muscle cells, macrophages, cholesterol-rich lipids and collagen) forming on the tunica intima. Atheroma leads to 97% of AAAs. Apart from atherosclerosis, other causes of intimal weakening are trauma, bacterial infection and syphilitic aortitis, but this is now rare.

An AAA is considered to be present when the aorta just below the level of the renal arteries measures >3 cm in diameter or where the diameter is 1.5 times the normal size for that person.

The main factors in atheroma and subsequent AAA formation are:

- smoking
- a cholesterol-rich diet
- diabetes mellitus
- hypertension.

The incidence of AAAs is increasing with the general ageing of the population and the increase in diagnostic and clinical testing. Seven percent of men and 1% of women aged 65–80 are reported to have an AAA >3 cm in diameter but only 0.6% have AAAs >5 cm and 0.3% have AAAs >6 cm.

Rapid death from rupture of an AAA and the subsequent massive intraabdominal haemorrhage accounts for about 6000 deaths in the United Kingdom each year. One in 90 people between the ages of 60 and 84 dies from a ruptured AAA. Less than 20% of those with a ruptured AAA will survive if they have not reached a hospital; in those who survive to hospital and are operated on, the operative mortality is reported to be between 27% and 50%.

Although recommendations for surgery have been made if the AAA is more than 4–5 cm in diameter, the usual criterion for elective surgery on previously diagnosed AAAs is where the diameter is >6 cm, where it grows at more than 1 cm/year or where it causes symptoms.[3] The mortality rate from elective surgery is, according to various reports, 1–8% and surgical repair is said to restore life expectancy to normal. The traditional method of repair by graft and its associated mortality rate is being improved by the insertion of a graft–stent combination via a peripheral artery as outlined by Nasim et al.[4]

The size of the AAA is an important factor. The risk of fatal rupture with AAAs over 7 cm in diameter is 75% and less than 5 cm in diameter is 1%. The mean survival rate of one year for those with an AAA of <6 cm diameter is said to be 75% and for those of >6 cm diameter is 50%. If untreated, 42% of patients with AAAs >6 cm diameter die within two years.

The rapidity of growth is also important. An estimation for the rate of growth is, on average, 2 mm per year for AAAs under 4 cm diameter and 5 mm per year for those over 6 cm in diameter. Research has shown that the growth of an AAA is exponential, i.e. the larger the AAA, the greater the rate of growth, but also that large and small AAAs grow linearly and other research shows that the growth rate of aneurysms is unpredictable and varies between patients.

AAAs usually affect men >60 years of age. More men than women are affected in a ratio of 5:1 although with the increase in smoking amongst young females, this ratio may reduce in the next three to four decades. It has been called 'the silent killer' as it may be symptomless and, as such, unnoticed until it ruptures. Screening on a national scale based on local studies has been advocated, producing arguments for and against but also unearthing concerns such as finding other pathologies which will cause further anxiety, whether to operate on smaller AAAs with the resultant better mortality rate, the increase in mortality rates at operation with larger AAAs and cost and life expectancy.[5-9]

A table of intervals between scans for monitoring aortic growth has been produced to try to rationalize the monitoring process (see Appendix 3) but it would seem that it does not take into account the unpredictability of growth of the aneurysm. Research is, at present, taking place on aortic wall compliance or distensibility where the maximum change in aneurysmal diameter with the cardiac cycle is measured. The research aims to see if compliance is related to rupture.[10]

The patient with an AAA commonly presents with a persistent, aching pain in the epigastrium and central abdomen, not relieved by antacids and not related to eating. It can be related to backache and mistaken for sciatica as pain can radiate down one buttock or leg. With a large, leaking or ruptured AAA, a severe pain is often felt, radiating to the back. The patient may feel a pulsatile mass in the abdomen. There may be a family history of arterial disease and a pulsatile mass may or may not be visible. The only palpation undertaken by the sonographer should be very lightly with the fingers of one hand to confirm the position of the AAA prior to scanning.

With a leak or rupture of an AAA, the patient shows signs of massive blood loss: tachycardia and hypotension, pallor, sweating, laboured and heavy breathing. The patient has abdominal tenderness and guarding and the femoral pulses are usually present but weak. There can be gastrointestinal bleeding and haematemesis from an aortoduodenal fistula. Clinical signs are sufficient to diagnose an AAA in 75% of patients. AAAs can only be seen on about two-thirds of all radiographs as not all contain enough calcification to be seen clearly.

ULTRASOUND APPEARANCES

An AAA is seen on longitudinal section as a swelling of the aorta, making it lose its smooth, tapering shape. It usually has a central, anechoic, true lumen and often thrombus or plaque surrounding the true lumen which is of higher reflectivity. The thrombus can be calcified in places which can produce posterior acoustic shadowing. In transverse section, the AAA is seen as a large, roundish, mass with a central anechoic true lumen and thrombus of relatively higher reflectivity often surrounding it. The thrombus is thickened and irregular and the length of the AAA can be difficult to trace (Fig. 8.13).

A false aneurysm is sometimes seen, usually to the left of the aorta. This is where the wall of the aneurysm has leaked and has been replaced by clot. It may suddenly give way and is considered to be a surgical emergency. In transverse section, it appears as a mass with echogenic material inside, the true lumen being relatively small. Ultrasound has been considered to be relatively poor at demonstrating acute paraaortic fluid collections, with a sensitivity of 4%, and CT is considered to be more accurate at identifying the precise site of split or rupture in the stable patient.

Box 8.2   Advice

When scanning the AAA, it is essential not to have the gain setting too low or too high as anterior wall thrombus may be missed or reverberation artefacts may mimic anterior thrombus respectively. Any loose thrombus seen must be reported as it can break away and cause an embolus in the leg.

The following can be mistaken for an AAA:

- paraaortic lymph nodes
- retroperitoneal haematoma around the midline
- an overlarge oblique section through an ectatic aorta (page 139).

Aneurysms of the abdominal aorta are mostly always of the fusiform (or wedge-like) variety and 90–95% begin below the renal arteries. AAAs often extend to and involve the common iliac arteries (66% of cases). If there is an aneurysm in the common iliac artery, scan the popliteal arteries (popliteal aneurysms are often bilateral).

Box 8.3   Advice

It is essential to scan and measure the kidneys when examining the aorta. Atheromatous disease involving the aorta can involve the renal arteries, causing renal artery stenosis. This will frequently cause hypertension and lead to renal failure. Renal artery occlusion can lead to reduced arterial perfusion and subsequent small kidneys. Doppler is often not able to confidently confirm stenosis, although reduction of renal cortex can suggest a stenosis of >60%.

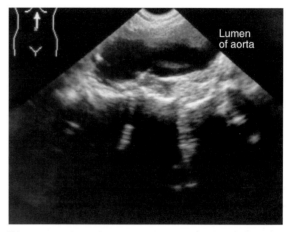

(A)

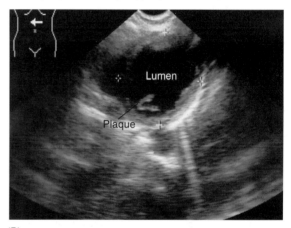

(B)

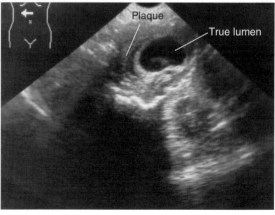

(C)

Fig. 8.13 (A) The abdominal aortic aneurysm – longitudinal section. (B, C) Transverse sections.

The role of ultrasound is to:

- confirm or exclude the presence of AAA or other abdominal masses mimicking an AAA. The accuracy in detecting AAAs by ultrasound is near to 100%

- measure the aneurysm (ultrasound could assess the size to within ±3 mm in 1980 and to ±1.3 mm in 1992). This is useful for serial monitoring and prior to surgery

- demonstrate the site of the AAA and its relationship to the coeliac axis, superior mesenteric and renal arteries as surgical treatment depends on this (demonstrating the renal arteries in the presence of an AAA is often better using the oblique coronal view) (Fig. 8.14)

- demonstrate the extension of the AAA into the common iliac arteries, if present

- measure renal size in order to confirm normality or infer renal artery involvement.

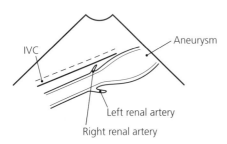

Fig. 8.14 Typical position of abdominal aortic aneurysm below renal arteries as shown using the oblique coronal plane.

THE EMERGENCY SITUATION

A ruptured AAA is a surgical emergency and as such, there is little time available and an ultrasound scan would be inappropriate. However, there can be a place for a quick scan in patients suspected to have a ruptured AAA as long as the equipment is in the emergency room, is part of the initial clinical evaluation and is quick. Demonstrating an AAA on ultrasound must be seen as a back-up to a strong clinical suspicion to confirm the decision to operate.

Aortic dissection

CLINICAL INFORMATION

Dissection of the aorta is usually caused by hypertension (70%) and degenerative changes in the tunica media. The tunica intima tears and blood tracks down inside the tunica media which splits and forms a channel. The blood often reemerges into the true lumen lower down. Dissection can occur in those with Marfan's syndrome where there is defective fibrillin or iatrogenically after arterial puncture or cannulation, although this area usually heals itself relatively quickly as the puncture should take place at a healthy site rather than a site where the wall is weakened by disease. In conjunction with an AAA, dissections can occur at the edge of an atheromatous plaque, forming a dissecting aneurysm. Dissection of the abdominal aorta alone is rare, accounting for 2–3% of aortic dissections. Dissections tend to start in the thoracic aorta and extend into the abdominal portion.

ULTRASOUND APPEARANCES

In the transverse section of the aorta, the diameter is often within normal limits. The inner wall can be seen

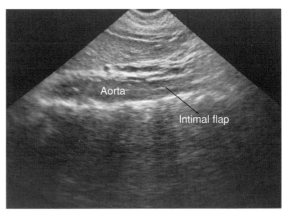

(A)

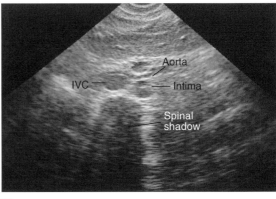

(B)

Fig. 8.15 (A) Longitudinal and (B) transverse sections demonstrating an aortic dissection.

as a thin echogenic septum dividing the lumen. On longitudinal section, it shows as a vessel with a loose or flapping inner wall. Colour Doppler can show the separate vascular channels and their respective differing velocities (Fig. 8.15).

Dissecting aneurysm

ULTRASOUND APPEARANCES

In the transverse section, the aneurysm appears as described before with an echo-poor false channel of blood obliquely positioned to one side of the true lumen within the mass of the aneurysm, this channel rejoining the true lumen at some distal point.

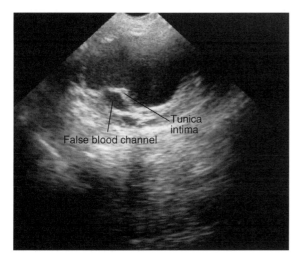

Fig. 8.16 Transverse section through a dissecting aneurysm.

Graft monitoring

ULTRASOUND APPEARANCES

Grafts are seen by their well-defined, reflective, parallel walls. Bleeding after the operation can show echo-poor blood tracking between the graft and the sac of the aneurysm that has been wrapped around it, appearing as a lumen inside a lumen. False aneurysms can appear at the sites of the anastomoses and can be due to infection or stitch breakdown. Any fluid seen around the graft could mean an abscess, haematoma or lymphocoele. Small fluid collections which would be difficult to see often resorb in time but larger collections suggest abscess, false aneurysm or aorto-duodenal fistula. A Doppler examination is required to exclude occlusion of the graft.

Ectatic aorta

ULTRASOUND APPEARANCES

Aortas that contain an aneurysm lose their characteristic shape and often become very tortuous and therefore it is difficult to obtain a clear longitudinal section. Attempts must be made to obtain a true transverse section by following the line of the aorta and scanning at right angles to the line in order to avoid giving over-sized measurements. Tortuous aortas do not have to have aneurysms; they are sometimes just large.

IVC

Distension

CLINICAL INFORMATION

The IVC can distend in patients with raised central venous pressure such as right heart failure and fluid overload.

ULTRASOUND APPEARANCES

The normal difference in appearance and dimension seen with respiration becomes less marked and eventually ceases. If the obstruction occurs above the level of the hepatic veins, these are also distended.

Tumour thrombus

CLINICAL INFORMATION

Tumour thrombus from renal tumours breaks away and enters the IVC by means of the renal veins in about 10% of cases.

ULTRASOUND APPEARANCES

The thrombus shows as an irregular area of high reflectivity compared to the blood in the vessel. Depending on the amount of obstruction the thrombus is causing, Doppler ultrasound will show a decreased or absent signal or an area of turbulence (Fig. 8.17).

Non-tumour thrombus

Non-tumour thrombus, such as extension of deep vein thrombosis, may extend to the IVC and not be suspected clinically. The clot appears similar to that from tumour thrombus.

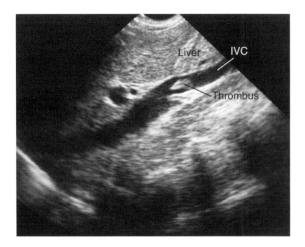

Fig. 8.17 Longitudinal section of an IVC containing thrombus or tumour.

IVC filter

Metallic or plastic filters can be inserted into the IVC to prevent a pulmonary embolus. Doppler ultrasound is a useful and accurate method of assessment of the IVC for patency and presence of clot before the insertion of a caval filter as it may be difficult to see owing to overlying bowel gas on B-mode scanning. Ultrasound can also be used to position the filter and check it after positioning. Ultrasound is accurate if the filter is clearly seen and the IVC is seen above and below the filter site, although MRI is more accurate. The filter is seen as an area of high-level echoes within the lumen of the IVC with reverberation posteriorly.

Primary IVC tumours

Leiomyosarcomas and liposarcomas are two of the most common retroperitoneal tumours. Most arise from the kidneys and approximately 80% are malignant. Invasion of the IVC can obstruct the flow of returning blood (best seen with Doppler) and make the vessel difficult to see distal to the obstruction. Oedema of the lower limbs often occurs. The vessel can also become encased with tumour.

The IVC can also be elevated by several causes, losing its characteristic shape, such as:

- right adrenal tumour
- renal tumour
- right renal artery aneurysm
- enlarged paraaortic lymph nodes
- retroperitoneal tumour
- abscess

and be pushed posteriorly by anterior masses such as:

- lymph nodes
- pancreatic head masses
- liver tumours.

References

1. Creagh-Barry M, Adam EJ, Joseph AEA 1986 The value of oblique scans in the ultrasonic examination of the abdominal aorta. Clin Radiol 37: 239–241

2. Gabriel H, Kindermann W 1996 Ultrasound of the abdomen in endurance athletes. Eur J Appl Physiol Occup Physiol 73(1–2): 191–193

3. Scott RAP, Wilson NM, Ashton HA, Kay DN 1993 Is surgery necessary for abdominal aortic aneurysm less than 6 cm in diameter? Lancet 342: 1395–1396

4. Nasim A, Thompson MM, Sayers RD et al 1996 Endovascular repair of abdominal aortic aneurysm: an initial experience. Br J Surg 83: 516–519

5. Cheatle TR 1997 The case against a national screening programme for aortic aneurysms. Ann Roy Coll Surg Engl 79: 90–95

6. Mason JM, Wakeman AP, Drummond MF, Crump BJ 1993 Population screening for abdominal aortic aneurysm: do the benefits outweigh the costs? J Publ Health Med 15: 154–160

7. Emerton ME, Shaw E, Poskitt K, Heather BP 1994 Screening for abdominal aortic aneurysm: a single scan is enough. Br J Surg 81: 1112–1113

8. Frame PS, Fryback DG, Patterson C 1993 Screening for abdominal aortic aneurysms in men aged 60 to 80 years. Ann Intern Med 119: 411–416

9. Smith FCT, Grimshaw G, Paterson I et al 1993 Ultrasonographic screening for abdominal aortic aneurysm in an urban community. Br J Surg 80: 1406–1409

10. Wilson K, Bradbury A 1997 Aortic compliance and the risk of aneurysm rupture. Reflections 3: 5–7

9

KIDNEYS AND URETERS

Main functions
Anatomy
Scanning
Pathology
Cystic disease
Benign tumours
Malignant tumours
Urinary tract infections and
    inflammatory conditions
Diffuse renal disease
Vascular pathology
Obstruction
Calculi
Renal trauma
Renal transplant
Normal ultrasound appearances
Post transplant complications
Interventional procedures

The kidneys excrete urine which is then conveyed to the urinary bladder via the ureters before micturition.

Main functions

- Removing waste products such as urea and creatinine through a process of filtration, secretion and reabsorption.

- Helping to regulate normal blood pressure. When the flow of blood to the kidneys falls, renin is released, which raises the blood pressure.

- Involvement in the regulation of red blood corpuscle production. Patients with renal failure are very often anaemic and those with a renal tumour often have an increased red blood cell count.

- Regulating the volume and composition of the extracellular fluid.

Anatomy

Kidneys

The two kidneys are bean shaped and weigh about 150 g in adult males and 135 g in adult females. In the infant, the kidney is larger in proportion to the total body mass than in the adult, being proportionally three times as large. The volume of urine passed by an adult in a temperate climate is between 800 and 2500 ml per day.

The kidneys have a curved, sometimes mildly lobulated but smooth lateral border, an upper and a lower pole, a concave medial border and a hilum. The hilum allows the renal arteries and nerves to enter the kidney and the veins and ureters to leave. It expands into the renal sinus, a space inside the kidney that contains the superior ureteral segment and renal calyces. They lie in the retroperitoneum on either side of the upper lumbar vertebrae. They are surrounded by three layers of fat and fascia, an outer perirenal capsule, a middle adipose capsule and an inner fibrous capsule. Generally, they lie with the upper poles at approximately the level of T12 and the lower poles at the level of L2–3. They move superiorly and inferiorly during respiration. The right kidney lies slightly lower than the left owing to the position of the liver. The kidneys lie in three angled planes. The lower poles lie more laterally and more anteriorly than the upper poles and the hila are more anterior than the lateral borders.

Each kidney consists of an outer cortex, containing many of the glomeruli and convoluted tubules, and an inner medulla, containing many tubules and collecting ducts. The renal cortex can extend to the renal sinus and appear as thin strips or columns of Bertin which lie between the medullary pyramids. The

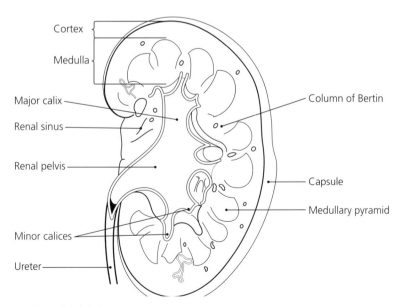

Fig. 9.1 Coronal section through left kidney.

medullary pyramids consist of straight tubules and collecting ducts and are situated so that the bases face laterally and the apices face towards the renal sinus. At this point, they end in a papilla which projects into the minor calyces (Fig. 9.1).

Ureters

The ureters are muscular tubes situated on either side of the major vessels which convey urine to the bladder using a peristaltic action. They consist of three layers: the outer, fibrous layer continuous with the renal capsule, an outer circular and inner longitudinal layer of smooth muscle fibres and an inner layer of mucous membrane lined with transitional epithelium which lies in folds when the ureter is empty but is smooth when full. The ureters are also described in three parts. The pelvic portion is described above. The abdominal portion runs downwards, forwards and slightly medially behind the peritoneum on the anterior part of the psoas muscle and the pelvic portion, which starts at the pelvic brim, crosses the common iliac vessels, runs downwards and backwards beneath the peritoneum to the ischial spine where it turns medially and forwards and enters the base of the bladder at the trigone.

Blood supply

The kidneys are supplied with blood from the left and right renal arteries which arise from the lateral aspect of the abdominal aorta at approximately the level of L1–2. The right renal artery is longer and slightly inferior to the left and passes behind the IVC and the left renal vein towards the hilum of the right kidney. The left renal artery lies posterior to the left renal vein as it passes towards the hilum of the left kidney. The renal arteries branch and each branch runs along each column of Bertin. At the border of cortex and medulla, they become arcuate arteries which in turn become the afferent arterioles of the glomeruli. The efferent arterioles branch into capillary networks surrounding the renal tubules. Each artery gives rise to the inferior suprarenal artery before entering the hilum. Accessory renal arteries can be seen arising from the aorta or common iliac arteries, more common on the left. Sometimes the renal artery branches before entering the kidney; sometimes a double renal artery is seen.

Blood drainage

The blood leaving the kidneys drains into the IVC via the left and right renal veins. They are larger than the renal arteries and lie anterior to them. Accessory renal veins are rare. The left renal vein is longer than the right and lies about 1 cm superior to the level of the right renal vein. It passes anterior to the abdominal aorta just below the origin of the superior mesenteric artery. It receives, in addition, blood from the left testicular or ovarian vein, left suprarenal vein and left inferior phrenic vein. The right renal vein is short and runs anterior to the right renal artery. Blood from the right ovarian or testicular vein does not pass into the right renal vein but drains directly into the IVC (Fig. 9.2).

Lymph drainage

From the renal hilum, along the path of the renal vein to the lumbar lymph nodes.

Nerve supply

From the renal plexus in turn from the lowest splanchnic nerves. The efferent nerve supply to the kidneys is autonomic with vasomotor fibres to both afferent and efferent renal arterioles. Renal nerves connect with testicular nerves, accounting for testicular pain in some renal diseases.

Relations

RIGHT KIDNEY

- Superiorly – the right adrenal gland.

- Laterally – the liver.

- Medially – the duodenum, renal arteries, veins and nerves entering and leaving the renal hilum, the ureters, the IVC.

- Inferiorly – the hepatic flexure of the colon.

- Anteriorly – the right lobe of the liver.

LEFT KIDNEY

- Superiorly – the left adrenal gland.

- Laterally – the spleen for the upper two-thirds, the splenic flexure of the colon.

- Medially – renal arteries, veins and nerves entering and leaving the renal hilum, the ureters, the stomach (variable), the pancreas, the abdominal aorta.

- Inferiorly – jejunum.

- Anteriorly – stomach, small intestine.

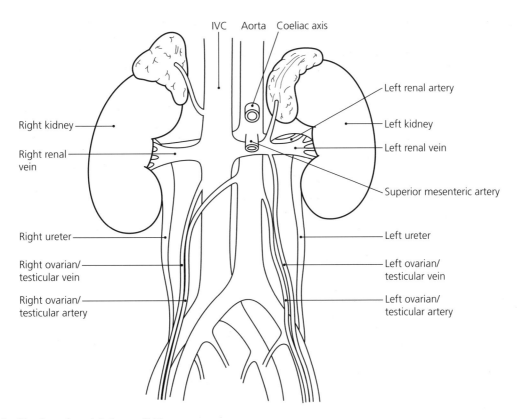

Fig. 9.2 Blood supply and drainage of kidneys.

BOTH KIDNEYS

● Posteriorly – the diaphragm, muscles (from lateral to medial: the tendon of the transversus abdominis, quadratus lumborum and psoas major). This surface is not covered by peritoneum and adheres to fatty areolar tissue.

Surface markings

RIGHT KIDNEY

The right kidney lies lower than the left kidney and the lower pole lies opposite the umbilical plane.

LEFT KIDNEY

The hilum lies just medial to the anterior extremity of the ninth costal cartilage. The upper pole lies half way between the xiphisternum and the transpyloric planes; the lower pole lies on the subcostal plane.

Variations in normal anatomy

● The kidney may be tilted forward inferior to the liver and the lower pole of the kidney palpated anteriorly.

● Lobulation from the developing kidney in utero can sometimes be seen on the lateral border, especially on the left side (Fig. 9.3A).

● The lateral border can also show a single, larger lobule which is known as a dromedary hump. This may be a result of the kidney developing in a certain shape to fit the contour of the spleen (Fig. 9.3B).

● Thickened septa or columns of Bertin can be seen as thickened areas between the medullary pyramids. Sometimes these are mistaken for masses although they do not cause the renal outline to bulge outward and the parenchymal appearance is not changed from the normal (Fig. 9.3C).

- Unilateral renal agenesis (absent kidney) is found in one in 1000 people. The contralateral kidney will often be larger than usual (compensatory hypertrophy) and can grow up to 20 cm long. It is often associated with other anomalies (58%), especially in women, and of these 48% are genital tract anomalies such as bicornuate uterus. It is more common on the left side. Bilateral renal agenesis (known as Potter's syndrome and occurring in three in 10000 of the population) is fatal after birth.

- Kidneys may be hypoplastic and fibrosed and can be small or barely visible. Sometimes a single kidney is a result of developmental fusion of both kidneys into one, with two ureters (Fig. 9.3D)

- Horseshoe kidneys (found in one in 400–600 of the population) have an abnormal lie, being more anterior and medial. The kidneys are usually fused at the lower pole (90%) by renal tissue or a fibrous band. Horseshoe kidneys are prone to infection, obstruction and stones and have been associated with Wilms' tumours (Fig. 9.3E).

- Ectopic kidneys are rare, usually found low in the pelvis. They sometimes cross to the other kidney and fuse to its inferior part(Fig. 9.3F).

- There can be multiple renal vessels, a bifid ureter or a double ureter.

- Duplitized collecting system and ureters are seen in about one in 70 of the population and range from two completely separate ureters to a double collecting system draining into a single ureter.

- Extrarenal pelvis is seen when the renal pelvis lies outside the kidney. It usually contains urine and can be mistaken for pathology.

Palpation

The kidneys should be palpated with both hands. For the right kidney, with the patient supine, the left hand should be placed behind the kidney underneath the patient and pushed anteriorly. The right hand should push the anterior abdominal wall upwards and posteriorly. An enlarged kidney can be felt between the two hands. The lower pole can be felt relatively easily in thin subjects but the left kidney is rarely felt unless abnormal (Fig. 9.4).

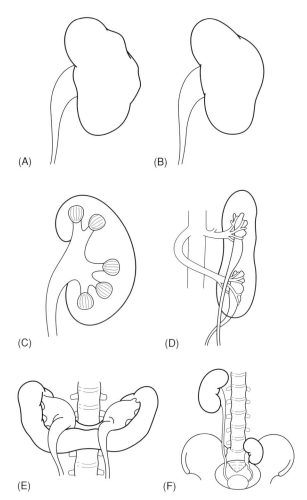

Fig. 9.3 Normal variations. (A) Lobulation. (B) Dromedary hump. (C) Enlarged column of Bertin. (D) Single kidney. (E) Horseshoe kidney. (F) Ectopic kidney.

Relevant tests – normal values

BLOOD TESTS

Haemoglobin	130–180 g/l (male)
Creatinine	62–132 μmol/l
Urea	2.5–7.0 mmol/l

URINE TESTS

Creatinine	0.13–0.22 mmol/kg/24 h
Creatinine clearance	1.7–2.1 ml/s
Glucose	Nil
Protein	<0.15 g/24 h

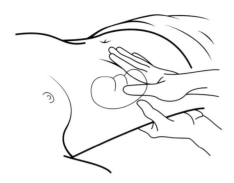

Fig. 9.4 Palpating a kidney.

Scanning

Patient preparation

The practice of preparation for kidney scanning varies from department to department. If the kidneys are to be scanned in isolation for serial measurements, for example, no preparation is usually necessary. However, if solving a problem such as a cause for haematuria or whether there is residual urine in the bladder after micturition, then it is necessary to fill the patient's bladder by asking them to drink a litre or so of still, clear fluid one hour before arrival as an investigation of the bladder is an essential part of the examination.

Children should have this amount reduced according to age and size; for example, a five year old may require a glass or two of squash half an hour before the scan. There is no preparation required for the scanning of babies' kidneys except to note that scans should not be performed during the first 72 hours after birth owing to the natural process of dehydration that occurs at that time which can mask a small renal pelvic dilatation if present.

Equipment required

For adults, the transducer of choice is often a 3.5 MHz sector or curved linear transducer if examining the right kidney from the front through the liver. If the patient is thin or if scanning a child, 5 MHz can be used and babies can be scanned using a 7.5–10.0 MHz transducer.

The difficulty in scanning the left kidney through the spleen in the left posterolateral position is that it is relatively superficial and if using a sector transducer, information in the near-field can be lost (see Chapter

1). This can happen to a certain extent with curved linear transducers and makes measuring the long axis rather difficult.

The appropriate focusing zone should be selected and use of the cine-loop facility, if available, is essential when scanning infants in order to obtain the best image.

Warm acoustic coupling gel should be used, in particular for infants and babies.

Suggested scanning technique – adults

RIGHT KIDNEY

This side is usually easier to image than the left side. Use the liver as an acoustic window. With the patient supine, place the transducer in the subcostal position in approximately the mid-clavicular line and angle up until the kidney is seen. Alter the longitudinal axis until the longest measurement is found, bearing in mind the angle at which the kidney lies. The position of the kidney can be lowered by scanning on inspiration in order to make subcostal scanning easier, but this may add to the amount of gas present. An intercostal approach can similarly be made. Often, gas present in the region of the hepatic flexure can lie between the probe and the kidney and does not allow visualization of at least the lower half of the kidney.

If gas is too much of a problem, raise the right side and turn the patient into the left posterior oblique or left lateral decubitus position and scan from the right lateral or posterolateral aspect. Once the longitudinal axis of the kidney has been established, it should be scanned from medial to lateral border then from upper to lower pole in transverse section by turning the transducer 90° to the long axis.

LEFT KIDNEY

The left kidney is more difficult to scan than the right owing to the amount of gas in the stomach, jejunum and splenic flexure. The smaller acoustic window, the spleen, is also less convenient, giving access to only the upper half of the kidney at most unless the spleen is enlarged.

With the patient rolled slightly to the right in the RPO position, the transducer should be positioned on the left posterolateral aspect just below the ribs and then intercostally in search for the kidney. In this position, the gas rises anteriorly away from the kidney. Full inspiration can be used in order to lower the kidney so that scanning from below the ribs gives better results. Scanning posterolaterally allows the transducer to be positioned higher than scanning from the front, owing to the position of the ribs at the back. Again, the longest section must be sought by rotating the transducer to find the longest axis. When this is found, scan from medial to lateral border then scan transversely at 90° to this axis from the upper to the lower pole.

Alternatively if visualization is difficult, turn the patient into the RLD position. Although gas should rise towards the kidney, the bowel should move away from that area. In order to obtain clear access to the kidney,

a pillow should be placed under the right side and the patient should stretch the left arm up over the head. In addition, the examination can be performed under inspiration (Fig. 9.5).

The prone position is rarely used for adults except for renal biopsies as the ribs and paraspinal muscles interfere with the image. If this position has to be used, drape the patient over two pillows in order to thin out the paraspinal muscle thickness. Quite often, separate views of the left kidney are required as the organ is close to the skin surface and the full picture of the lateral border cannot always be seen. Similarly, rib shadows can interfere with the image.

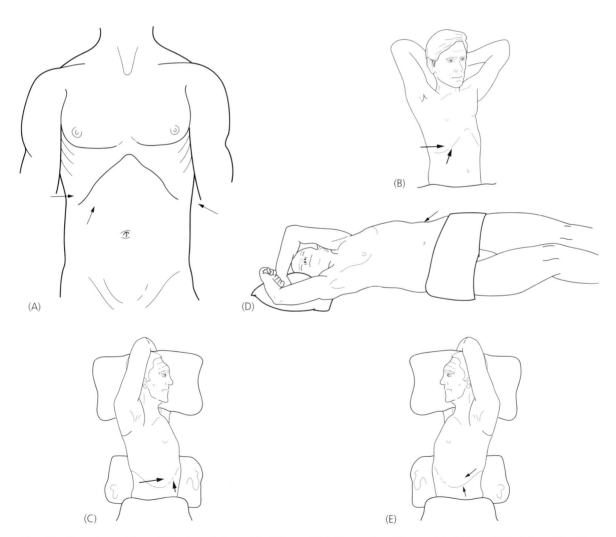

Fig. 9.5 Scanning positions. (A) Supine – left and right kidneys. (B) Left posterior oblique – right kidney. (C) Left lateral decubitus – right kidney. (D) Right posterior oblique – left kidney. (E) Right lateral decubitus – left kidney.

The kidneys should be measured, assessment of renal pelvis dilatation made if present and an assessment made of the size of the cortex, the echo pattern of the parenchyma, renal vessels and contour.

Note that when scanning the kidneys, as with any structure, the incident sound should be directed whenever possible at right angles to the organs' interfaces in their long axis. It is often necessary to approach the kidney from a higher intercostal space and angle down to the feet to obtain this view owing to the angle at which the kidney lies. This helps to produce a clearer outline and reduce upper pole artefact.

Suggested scanning technique – children and babies

With toddlers, it is probably better to let them see and get used to what is happening by lying them supine first and turning them prone if necessary afterwards. Young children have much thinner paraspinal muscles than adults. Usually, however, young children can be scanned in a similar way to adults. Longitudinal and transverse sections of the kidneys should be taken and their reflectivity compared with the liver and kidney.

Babies can be easily scanned when cuddled by their mother, either with the mother lying supine with the baby lying on top of them or sitting upright. A vest can be left on them and just lifted to reveal sufficient skin at the back for the scan. If soothed in this way, the baby is more likely to move less than when lying supine or prone in the middle of a couch. The majority of scans of babies' kidneys are to assess the prenatal findings of dilated renal pelvices. An assessment of the bladder and as much of the ureters as can be seen must be made so at some time, the baby will have to be laid in the supine position.

When scanning neonates 72 hours after birth, ensure the use of warm gel; use a heat lamp to keep the baby warm if not in an incubator. Be extremely careful of catheters and lines being caught up with the probe and cable (Fig. 9.6).

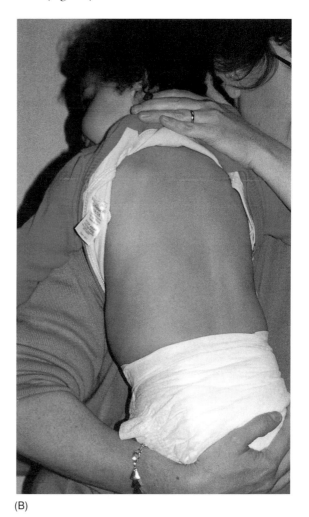

(A)

(B)

Fig. 9.6 Scanning positions for babies and toddlers. (A) The 'cuddle' position for babies. (B) The same position can be tried for toddlers but they will usually want to see what is behind them.

Suggested minimal sections

- Longitudinal section of kidneys with liver and spleen tissue to compare reflectivity.

- Transverse sections at the hila to show renal vessels and ureters. Measurements taken of both kidneys in longitudinal and transverse sections (either length or length, width and breadth according to departmental protocols).

Normal ultrasound appearances

In neonates, kidneys often have foetal lobulations (scalloped edges). The cortex is hyperechoic and thinner than the equivalent adult kidney and the medulla darker, with pronounced medullary pyramids. The cortex should be of an even size around the pyramids. Where the cortex is thinned focally in children, scarring is suggested. The medullary pyramids are triangular in shape with the base on the cortex and the apex pointing towards the hilum. The capsule is hardly noticeable in babies and very thin in young children. The renal sinus is less noticeable as the cortex is of greater reflectivity than in the adult and older children, therefore the contrast between cortex and sinus is less. There may be a small amount of urine seen in the renal sinuses in a hydrated baby. This appearance can last for anything between two and six months after birth.

Size is important in neonates; the kidney should be 4.5–5 cm in length or 1 mm for every gestational week. With paediatrics, the comparison between the two kidneys is more important than the individual size as a difference of more than 15% may be an indication of renal scarring.

In adults, the normal kidneys have an echogenicity that is of lower reflectivity than that of the normal liver and spleen. The medullary pyramids are less obvious than those of the infant but are still recognizable as being areas of lower reflectivity than the cortex. Arcuate and interlobar arteries are seen as highly reflective foci at the corticomedullary junction or the base of the pyramids which can be identified by colour Doppler. The collecting or calyceal system should be symmetrical and is of higher reflectivity than the cortex. It becomes even more so with age as the amount of fat in the sinus increases (sinus lipomatosis). The collecting system should not demonstrate fluid in a dehydrated patient but some fluid can be seen in patients that are hydrated or who have a full bladder.

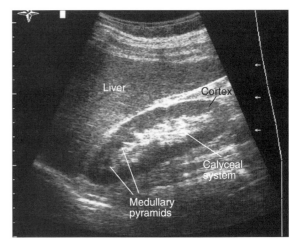

(A)

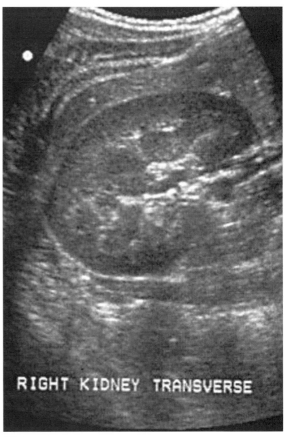

(B)

Fig. 9.7 (A) Normal adult right kidney in longitudinal section. (B) Transverse section through right kidney. (Image courtesy of Acuson, a Siemens Company.)

To see if the fluid is persistent, the patient should be asked to void their bladder and then rescanned in order to exclude a renal obstruction. The renal pelvis can also appear relatively full in pregnancy. It can lie partially or completely outside the sinus and can be mistaken for a cyst.

The cortex also reduces in size with age but the kidney remains more or less the same size as the increasing size of the sinus compensates for this. The sinus fat reduces in echogenicity when the patient starves and loses body fat. The contour should be smooth and evenly circumscribed.

When scanned in the transverse section, the small tubular right renal artery (RRA) runs from the aorta behind the IVC to the right kidney. It is a relatively long vessel owing to the distance from the aorta to the right kidney. The left renal artery (LRA) is shorter and exits the aorta from a more posterolateral position. The renal veins lie anterior to the arteries. The right renal vein drains into the IVC and can be large in patients with congestive heart failure. The left renal vein runs from the left kidney anterior to the aorta and posterior to the superior mesenteric artery.

In longitudinal section, the RRA can frequently be seen as a highly reflective circle lying posterior to the IVC. There may be two or even three renal arteries seen (Fig. 9.8).

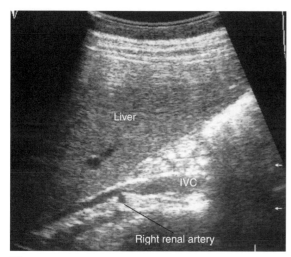

(A)

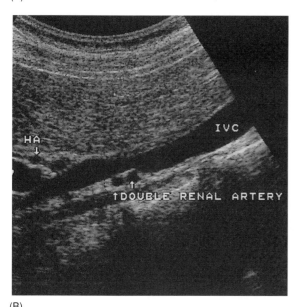

(B)

Fig. 9.8 (A, B) The position of the right renal artery relative to the IVC.

Normal sizes

It must be noted that, when measuring the long axis of the kidney, scanning in any oblique plane will result in a smaller measurement. Two or three measurements should be taken to obtain the longest one for the sake of accuracy (Fig. 9.9).

● At birth, the kidneys can measure 4–5 cm long.

● Up to one year old, they measure 5½–6½ cm long.

● Five years old, they measure 7½–8½ cm long.

● Ten years old, they measure 8½–10 cm long.

● The normal adult kidney size is 9.5–12.5 cm long; average 11 cm long. They measure 5 cm wide and 3 cm thick, although this depends on the size of the patient.

Renal volume has been calculated as width × length × thickness × 0.5233 cm³. At birth, the renal volume has been calculated as 20 cm³; at one year, 30 cm³ and 155 cm³ at 18 years.

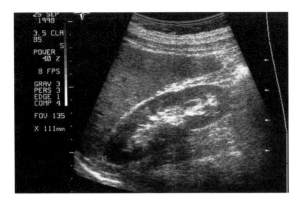

(A)

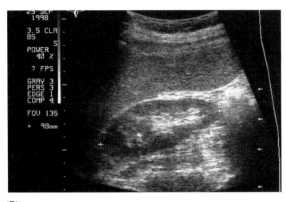

(B)

Fig. 9.9 (A) Largest measurement. (B) Foreshortened view of the same kidney reduces its length by over 1 cm.

Box 9.1 Advice

Understanding the variations in normal anatomy can help to avoid mistakes in identity. Bowel loops can imitate a kidney if the kidney is ectopic and the bowel occupies the kidney's normal place. Observe peristalsis in order to differentiate between bowel and kidney.

Medullary pyramids can be mistaken for cysts. Observe them for triangularity and regular positioning compared to spherical and irregularly placed cysts.

A dromedary hump caused by splenic indentation of the lateral border of the left kidney, or foetal lobulations, can be mistaken for tumours.

Thickened columns of Bertin can also be mistaken for tumours. These are rarely more than 3 cm in size and do not distort the renal architecture.

If the kidneys, especially the right kidney, are scanned with the probe angled towards the head, the upper pole is hard to visualize and can appear, through lack of information, to be cystic.

Renal measurements in all dimensions can be inaccurate owing to foreshortening of the image.

Inappropriate gain control settings can mask pathology (Fig. 9.11).

An extrarenal pelvis can be mistaken for a dilated pelvicalyceal system.

Normal pulsed wave Doppler

As the vascularity of the kidneys offers a low resistance, the arterial signal shows as having a high diastolic flow, seen in the main renal, interlobar and arcuate arteries.

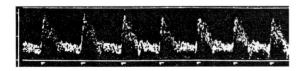

Fig. 9.10 Normal pulsed wave Doppler signal of the right renal artery.

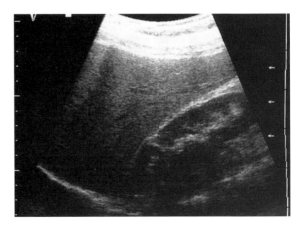

Fig. 9.11 Example of poor gain setting. This could mask a cystic lesion in the upper pole of the kidney.

Pathology

CYSTIC DISEASE

- Simple cyst
- Adult polycystic disease
- Infantile polycystic disease
- Multicystic dysplastic kidneys
- Medullary cystic disease
- Juvenile nephronophthosis
- Medullary sponge kidney
- Renal cysts in dialysis

BENIGN TUMOURS (ADULT)

- Adenoma
- Oncocytoma
- Angiomyolipoma
- Urinoma

BENIGN TUMOURS (PAEDIATRIC)

- Mesoblastic nephroma

MALIGNANT TUMOURS (ADULT)

- Renal cell carcinoma
- Transitional cell carcinoma
- Metastases

MALIGNANT TUMOURS (PAEDIATRIC)

- Wilms' tumour
- Lymphoma

URINARY TRACT INFECTIONS AND INFLAMMATORY CONDITIONS

- Acute pyelonephritis
- Chronic pyelonephritis
- Renal abscess
- Pyonephrosis
- Xanthogranulomatous pyelonephritis
- Fungal infection

DIFFUSE RENAL DISEASE

- Acute tubular necrosis
- Interstitial nephritis
- Glomerulonephritis
- Diabetes mellitus
- AIDS

VASCULAR PATHOLOGY

- Renal vein thrombosis
- Renal artery occlusion
- Renal artery stenosis

OBSTRUCTION

- Obstruction in pregnancy
- Obstructed moiety in duplex kidney
- Reflux in children
- Obstruction by posterior urethral valves

CALCULI

- Staghorn calculus
- Nephrocalcinosis or medullary calcinosis

RENAL TRAUMA

RENAL TRANSPLANT

- Normal appearances
- Post transplant complications

INTERVENTIONAL PROCEDURES

Cystic disease

Simple cyst

CLINICAL INFORMATION

Simple renal cysts are common incidental findings found with advancing age (seen in 50% of over-50s) but are uncommon in children. They have a smooth lining and contain clear watery fluid. They may be single or multiple and are variable in size up to 5 or 6 cm in diameter. Simple renal cysts can haemorrhage or become infected but have no effect on renal function. They are usually asymptomatic unless they cause obstruction through their size or become infected or haemorrhage.

ULTRASOUND APPEARANCES

Most renal cysts are found in the cortex and sometimes in the medulla. They are more commonly seen within the renal parenchyma but can be found as tangential cysts projecting outwards from the kidney. The classic ultrasound appearance of a cyst is a round or oval, smooth, clearly outlined mass with no internal echoes and demonstrating posterior acoustic enhancement. Using these criteria, ultrasound is 98% accurate in diagnosing simple cysts.

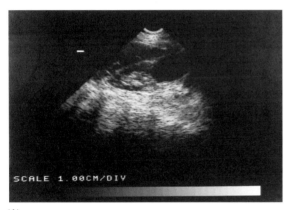

(A)

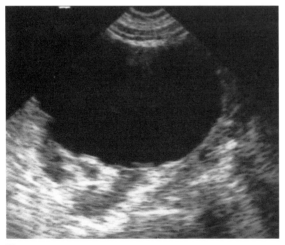

(B)

Fig. 9.12 (A) Simple cyst in lower pole of right kidney. (B) Large cyst occupying most of left kidney.

Box 9.2   Advice

Artefacts can be observed within a simple cyst if:

- the cyst is small and does not lie within the focal zone of the ultrasound beam
- there are reverberations from reflectors or skin–transducer interfaces superficial to the cyst especially when the kidney itself is relatively superficial
- the gain setting is too high and electrical or acoustic interference is evident
- echoes from adjacent tissues lie in the same part of the beam as the cyst if the cyst is small (the partial volume effect).

To avoid confusion and exclude any false artefactual echoes, it is essential to scan the cyst in different directions and to increase the frequency if possible. Acoustic enhancement may not be seen if the cyst is very small or if the tissue deep to the cyst is highly reflective or if the wall of the cyst is calcified. In this case there may be acoustic shadowing present.

If the cyst is considered to contain echoes, calcification (1–3% of simple cysts have some calcification in their wall and 20% of these are malignant) or solid components or has a collapsed or irregular wall, it should be followed up by further investigations and/or aspiration. Cyst aspirate should be straw coloured, fat and blood free. If cysts become symptomatic, they can be drained under ultrasound control and a sclerosant injected.

The appearance of a simple cyst may be imitated by other conditions such as a renal artery aneurysm (Doppler will help to identify this), parapelvic cyst which is usually solitary and protrudes into the renal sinus or an obstructed moiety of a duplex collecting system or a hydronephrosis (look for other evidence of obstruction).

Some simple cysts contain septa. The incidence of malignancy is very small when the septa are thin and no solid material is seen within the cyst.

Adult polycystic disease (Potter type III)

CLINICAL INFORMATION

Adult polycystic disease is an autosomal dominant trait affecting one in 1000 of the population and equal numbers of men and women. It often manifests itself after the third decade of adult life, although screening of families in which one member is known to have this condition has seen a higher detection rate in children. Presentation in children is uncommon. Cysts grow progressively, often unknown to the patient until masses are felt. Renal function becomes gradually impaired and chronic renal failure and hypertension develop. Cysts can also develop in the pancreas (10%), liver (30–40%), spleen (5%) and occasionally lungs and berry aneurysms of the cerebral arteries can develop owing to hypertension. Patients can live with hypertension-controlling medication or require a renal transplant, depending on severity.

ULTRASOUND APPEARANCES

If the disease has not become established, such as in the screening of child relatives of sufferers of this disease, the earliest sign will be a single or small number of renal cysts or an increase in the reflectivity of the renal parenchyma. This is due to the increased number of interfaces from the developing cysts that ultrasound sees (being 0.1–5 mm in diameter) and the inability to visualize them individually. If cysts are not seen by the age of 19–20, it is considered unlikely that the patient has inherited the disease so this is the age at which family members should be screened.

In cases of established disease when the patient presents with symptoms, both kidneys are usually enlarged and measure up to approximately 20 cm in the longitudinal axis. There are a large number of cysts of varying sizes on both kidneys measuring from a few millimetres to several centimetres in diameter and completely altering the normal shape and outline of the kidneys. The cysts are often irregular in shape owing to the fact that they are packed tightly together. The cysts may contain internal echoes if haemorrhage or infection has occurred. Focal areas of normal kidney can sometimes be seen in between the cysts.

Box 9.3   Advice

Scan the liver, pancreas and spleen to search for accompanying cysts.

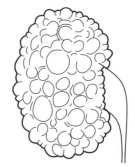

(A)

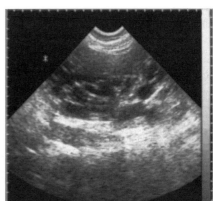

(B)

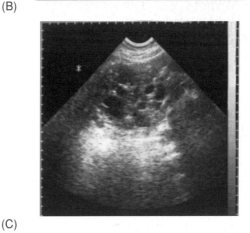

(C)

Fig. 9.13 (A) Diagrammatic appearance polycystic kidneys, (B) Longitudinal and (C) transverse section of polycystic left kidney.

Infantile polycystic disease (Potter type I)

CLINICAL INFORMATION

This is an autosomal recessive condition usually presenting in infancy or childhood or diagnosed *in utero* during an ultrasound scan. It is relatively uncommon and infants develop renal failure and compression of the lungs owing to massive enlargement of the kidneys. Fibrosis of the liver can also occur. The severity of the disease is relative to the age at which the condition presents.

If presenting at birth, the condition is rapidly fatal as 90% of the renal tubules are involved. At infantile presentation, the child is uraemic as 60% of the renal tubules are involved and life expectancy is short. Young children presenting with chronic renal failure and hypertension have 25% of their renal tubules involved. Late presentation in older children shows as hepatic fibrosis and portal hypertension; some small cortical cysts are sometimes seen.

ULTRASOUND APPEARANCES

Both kidneys are uniformly smooth and enlarged and highly reflective and the normal corticomedullary differentiation is lost. The multiple small cysts are approximately 1–2 mm in diameter, arising from the collecting ducts as fusiform dilatations. As they enlarge, they become more spherical. There can be a thin rim of normal, relatively hypoechoic tissue around the periphery of the kidneys. Diagnosis of the condition *in utero* can be made from the echogenic appearance of the kidneys and from the combined circumference of both kidneys measuring approximately 60% of the abdominal circumference instead of the normal 27–30%.

Multicystic dysplastic kidneys (Potter type II)

CLINICAL INFORMATION

This condition is relatively rare but is the most common cause of an abdominal mass in the neonate. It is usually caused by atresia of the proximal ureter and pelvis causing obstruction to drainage *in utero* and an accompanying hypoplastic renal artery. It presents in childhood as a renal mass and involves one kidney or a moiety of one kidney.

ULTRASOUND APPEARANCES

The kidney or moiety involved is enlarged and replaced with cysts of different sizes but not as varying as with adult polycystic disease. Between the cysts are often highly reflective, unresolvable, very small cysts. No normal tissue can be seen.

> **Box 9.4   Advice**
>
> Scan the contralateral kidney carefully as there is an increased risk of an accompanying obstruction to drainage such as a pelviureteric junction obstruction.
>
> If a neonatal multicystic dysplastic kidney is missed, the kidney will atrophy as it does not function and the cysts calcify.

Medullary cystic disease

CLINICAL INFORMATION

This is a rare autosomal dominant inherited disorder. It presents in the late teenage years and is associated with interstitial fibrosis leading to early onset of chronic renal failure.

Medullary cystic disease and juvenile nephronophthosis (see below) account for 10–25% of cases of end-stage renal failure in patients up to 30 years old.

ULTRASOUND APPEARANCES

The kidneys are small and of increased reflectivity and the corticomedullary differentiation is lost owing to many small cysts ranging in size from minute to approximately 1 cm in diameter (these being surrounded by echogenic material) in the medulla.

Juvenile nephronophthosis

CLINICAL INFORMATION

Similar to medullary cystic disease, juvenile nephronophthosis is a severe autosomal recessive inherited disease and presents at about the age of 11 onwards to middle teenage years. Patients present with loss of renal function, hypertension, proteinuria and loss of sodium resorption leading to uraemia.

ULTRASOUND APPEARANCES

The kidneys are normal size or small and are highly reflective, appearing similar to medullary cystic kidneys.

Medullary sponge kidney

CLINICAL INFORMATION

This is an uncommon and probably congenital condition in which there is cystic dilatation of the collecting tubules of the renal papillae. It may be found in a part of one kidney or throughout both kidneys. Patients present between the ages of 20 and 40 with abdominal pain, haematuria and pyelonephritis. About one-third of patients have hypercalcuria and develop calculi in the dilated tubules, leading to renal colic and infection. Renal function is not impaired.

ULTRASOUND APPEARANCES

The kidneys appear normal or have increased echogenicity in the region of the medullary pyramids from multiple small calculi.

Renal cysts in dialysis (acquired cystic disease)

CLINICAL INFORMATION

Patients on long-term dialysis risk developing renal cysts. The risk increases with time and eventually 70–80% of this group are affected after four years. The cysts are seen in small kidneys with severe change of renal tissue and are usually bilateral, measuring from minute to 3 cm. They are prone to haemorrhage and are also associated with a risk of renal carcinoma (10% of cases) as hyperplastic changes in the cysts lining would appear to be premalignant.

Box 9.5   Advice

When monitoring the appearance of long-term renal dialysis patients, pay careful attention to the size as enlargement is indicative of malignant change and malignant change in small cysts is very difficult to detect.

Benign tumours

Adenoma

CLINICAL INFORMATION

Small adenomas are often found at post-mortem, rather than in life. They arise from the renal tubules.

ULTRASOUND APPEARANCES

The appearance of a renal adenoma is non-specific and it can resemble a renal adenocarcinoma. It usually appears as a small (less than 3 cm), round, solid tumour. As only 4% of renal carcinomas are echogenic, a small echogenic tumour is usually benign. However, occasionally adenomas are echo poor. Exclusion of malignancy is by biopsy of the mass.

Oncocytoma (granular cell adenoma, eosinophilic adenoma)

CLINICAL INFORMATION

This is relatively rare and, until recently, was considered as a benign epithelial tumour and a variant of adenoma. It is now thought to be part of the group of renal cell carcinomas but without generalized malignant potential. It presents more commonly in males than females and between the ages of 50 and 60. Patients are often symptom free but can present with pain and bleeding. Oncocytomas can grow to a large size.

ULTRASOUND APPEARANCES

Oncocytomas are homogeneous, well defined and relatively highly reflective in appearance. The larger tumours contain a central, star-shaped scar of either higher or lower reflectivity which can be seen clearly on a CT scan.

Angiomyolipoma

CLINICAL INFORMATION

Angiomyolipomas are relatively rare tumours composed of smooth muscle, fat and large blood vessels. They are relatively uncommon in clinical practice, although, as with adenomas, they are not infrequently (11%) seen at post-mortem. Solitary angiomyolipomas are found more frequently in females over 40 but are often multiple in configuration and associated with multiple renal cysts in patients with tuberose sclerosis. Pain derived from haemorrhage may accompany this condition.

CLINICAL INFORMATION

Angiomyolipomas are commonly smoothly outlined, highly reflective and isoechoic to the renal sinus owing to the amount of fat within the mass, although they can be echo poor or of mixed echogenicity. A CT scan can help confirm diagnosis by demonstrating fat densities within the tumour if the slices are narrow, but this is difficult on small tumours and incidental findings of angiomyolipoma are often managed by follow-up ultrasound scans.

Urinoma

This is an anechoic fluid collection in the perinephric space which occurs secondary to obstruction and rupture of the pelvicalyceal system, calculi, trauma or surgical/radiological intervention. A small collection will track around the kidney, forming an anechoic rim. With an increase in size, the fluid moves inferiorly, displacing the kidney superiorly and anteriorly. Echoes are only seen within as a result of infection or haemorrhage.

Mesoblastic nephroma

CLINICAL INFORMATION

Mesoblastic nephroma or congenital Wilms' tumour is normally a benign hamartoma although it can be malignant. It is found in the neonate and young infant and can become quite large and in an infant less than one year old a large mass is more likely to be a mesoblastic nephroma than a Wilms' tumour.

ULTRASOUND APPEARANCES

Mesoblastic nephroma is a large tumour with a homogeneous echo pattern and relatively low-level echoes. Haemorrhage and necrosis can, like Wilms' tumours, give rise to echo-poor areas within the tumour.

Malignant tumours

Renal cell carcinoma

Also known as renal adenocarcinoma, clear cell carcinoma, hypernephroma or Grawitz tumour.

CLINICAL INFORMATION

Nearly all large renal tumours are malignant. Renal cell carcinoma is by far the most common renal malignancy, accounting for about 86–90% of primary renal malignancies and about 3% of all adult carcinomas. Five percent are bilateral although are not usually found at the same time. Early in their development they are small masses in the cortex which enlarge and invade the renal parenchyma. Later, patients present typically with loin pain and haematuria and a mass is often found in the flank, although one study found this classic triad in only 3.8% (4/105). Patients may also show evidence of a raised ESR, hypertension, malaise, anaemia, fever and hypercalcaemia. Occasionally a pathological fracture from a bone metastasis may occur.

Renal cell carcinoma is seen in the middle-aged or elderly patient in the ratio of 3:1 males:females. More small tumours have been found incidentally in the last decade during ultrasound or CT scans for other reasons such as metastatic disease.[1] With earlier incidental detection, some consider that the prognosis and overall survival rate of patients with renal cell carcinoma may be improved.[2] This may be because tumour confined within the renal capsule has a 70% 10-year survival but a poor prognosis if metastases are found at the time of diagnosis. Spread of the tumour is through the capsule into the pelvis via the ureters or via the renal vein into the IVC, producing secondaries in lungs and bone.

ULTRASOUND APPEARANCES

The appearance of renal cell carcinomas changes according to the size and spread of the tumour. If contained within the capsule, the tumour is often smooth and appears solid with a relatively echogenic homogeneous pattern. If larger and breaking out of its capsule, the mass is often large, irregular and heterogeneous with poorly defined borders, 80% having a relatively low reflectivity. Adenocarcinomas may grow rapidly or slowly. They may become so large that they replace the kidney altogether. As the tumours grow, haemorrhage and necrosis occur and produce an even more heterogeneous appearance; 6–20% contain calcium speckles, usually in the middle of the tumour. Adenocarcinomas can also be cystic in appearance, either unilocular or multilocular with a thickened irregular wall and containing internal echoes or calcification (Fig. 9.14).

The sensitivity of ultrasound in detecting masses smaller than 1 cm is 26%, 60% for 1–2 cm and 82% for 2–3 cm. However, the research revealing these figures is more than 10 years old and the sensitivity should now be greater with the availability of higher resolution equipment. Ultrasound is less specific when identifying pathology owing to the variety of appearances that other tumours have, both benign and malignant. Hypertrophic areas, focal inflammation and thickened columns of Bertin can all simulate an echo-poor renal cell carcinoma and other imaging modalities may have to be employed, such as a contrast-enhanced CT scan, in order to establish whether the apparent mass is normally functioning renal tissue or not.

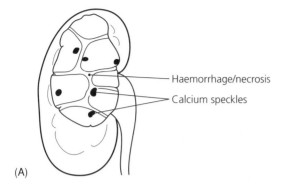

(A)

Haemorrhage/necrosis
Calcium speckles

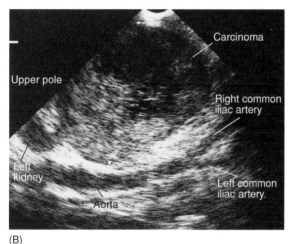

(B)

Carcinoma

Upper pole

Right common
iliac artery

Left
kidney

Aorta

Left common
iliac artery

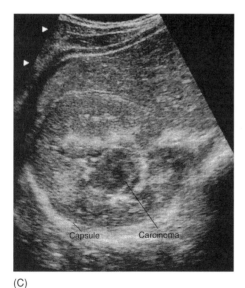

(C)

Capsule   Carcinoma

Fig. 9.14 (A–C) Examples of renal cell carcinoma.

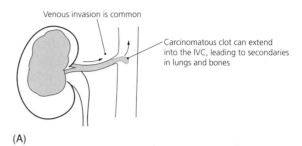

(A)

Venous invasion is common

Carcinomatous clot can extend
into the IVC, leading to secondaries
in lungs and bones

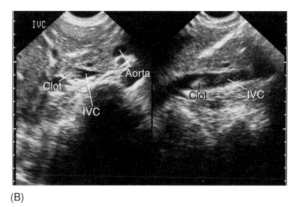

(B)

IVC

Clot

IVC

Aorta

Clot   IVC

Fig. 9.15 (A, B) Carcinomatous clot detachment from main tumour.

Box 9.6   Advice

If a renal mass is seen, you must investigate to the best of your ability the renal veins, IVC, the other kidney, liver, paraaortic region and the area around the kidney for tumour extension. Tumour within the renal vein (found in 4–30% of cases) causes widening of the vessel with internal echoes. Tumour within the IVC can also arise from a phaeochromocytoma of the adrenal gland or a malignant melanoma (Fig. 9.15).

Transitional cell carcinoma

CLINICAL INFORMATION

Transitional cell carcinoma is more frequently found in the bladder but patients with a transitional cell carcinoma at one site are at risk of developing a second tumour at another site within the urothelium. Patients can develop a transitional cell carcinoma from exposure to industrial carcinogens (see Bladder cancer, p. 188).

ULTRASOUND APPEARANCES

A papillary transitional cell carcinoma can fill the renal pelvis and obstruct the flow of urine to the bladder, causing dilatation of the collecting system. The mass is predominantly homogeneous and of relatively low echogenicity.

Metastases

CLINICAL INFORMATION

Renal metastases are uncommonly found during a scan but more often seen at autopsy. They are usually multiple and originate from breast, lung or the kidney itself.

ULTRASOUND APPEARANCES

Solitary metastases cannot be differentiated from primary renal tumours. They are usually solid and of varying reflectivity.

Wilms' tumour (nephroblastoma)

CLINICAL INFORMATION

Wilms' tumour is the most common malignant childhood tumour; 80% present in children under five with a mean presentation of three years. The mass is painless, often grows rapidly and is found in equal numbers of males and females. The child may present with a large abdominal mass, fever, raised blood pressure in 50% of cases, 33% have haematuria and a raised white cell count. The tumours can arise from any part of the kidney and are bilateral in 5–13% of cases. They are staged as follows.

- Stage 1: encapsulated and no metastatic spread.

- Stage 2: extracapsular infiltration.

- Stage 3: extension beyond the kidney with peritoneal and lymph node involvement.

- Stage 4: distant metastases (liver, lung).

- Stage 5: bilateral renal involvement.

Wilms' tumours are usually detected by ultrasound followed by contrast-enhanced CT of the chest and abdomen and treated by a combination of nephrectomy, radiotherapy and chemotherapy and survival rates are good. The majority of children, even those with metastatic disease, are cured.

ULTRASOUND APPEARANCES

Wilms' tumours appear large, solid and well circumscribed and heterogeneous in texture. Often, they have echo-poor areas of necrosis and haemorrhage, which may appear reflective if recent. If the tumour is large, it may be difficult to see any normal renal tissue and confirm that the tumour is renal in origin. The IVC may be displaced or compressed by the mass and tumour may extend into the renal veins and IVC. As this is echo poor, it may be difficult to see tumour in the IVC on grey scale and the only indication may be slight dilatation of the vessel. Colour Doppler may be required to confirm the presence of tumour in the IVC; tumour in the renal veins is often too small to see clearly owing to its compression by the mass.

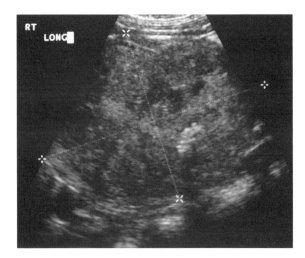

Fig. 9.16 Wilms' tumour.

Box 9.7 Advice

With any solid renal mass in patients of this age, a Wilms' tumour should always be suspected. Check carefully for free fluid suggesting a ruptured tumour, any evidence of enlarged lymph nodes, infiltration of the tumour into other organs, the contralateral kidney for evidence of bilateral involvement and the liver for signs of metastases which, if present, are usually echo poor.

Evidence of tumour invasion of the IVC and right atrium should be sought.

Nephroblastomas are frequently indistinguishable in appearance from neuroblastomas which arise from the adrenal gland (see Adrenal tumours, p. 211) except that they are sometimes less heterogeneous than neuroblastomas and, unlike neuroblastomas, rarely contain calcification.

Lymphoma

CLINICAL INFORMATION

Although primary renal lymphoma is rare, 41% of long-standing non-Hodgkin's lymphoma show renal involvement either in one or both kidneys in either a diffuse or multiple focal appearance.

ULTRASOUND APPEARANCES

The kidney is often enlarged with focal areas or patches of reduced reflectivity where the normal parenchyma is replaced by echo-poor solid material. The walls are indistinct and there is little or no shadowing posteriorly. When diffuse, the corticomedullary differentiation is often reduced or lost and the kidney can take on a more globular appearance.

Box 9.8   Advice

Do not confuse the echo-poor focal areas with simple cysts; look for posterior acoustic enhancement to confirm a simple cyst. In addition, search for evidence of splenomegaly and lymphadenopathy, especially around the aorta and porta hepatis.

Urinary tract infections and inflammatory conditions

CLINICAL INFORMATION

Infections of the urinary tract are common in adults and children and, if unchecked, can result in renal scarring leading to hypertension and renal failure. The role of ultrasound in the investigation of urinary tract infections is to confirm normality of number, size, position, texture and structure, exclude any masses or obstruction and detect abscess or scarring if present. Size is variable in these conditions. It used to be thought that kidneys enlarged during an acute phase on infection and shrank when the condition was chronic, but this is not reliable. The cortex often thickens in the acute stage and has reduced reflectivity on ultrasound or may increase in reflectivity, producing less or more of a corticomedullary differentiation respectively.

Although scarring is detectable by ultrasound, it appears that it is only seen at its more advanced stages when there is a thinning of the parenchyma as a result of fibrosis. Early stages of fibrosis often reveal a normal renal appearance. A DMSA (dimercaptosuccinic acid) radioisotope scan is required as a more sensitive diagnostic test to assess scarring. Doppler studies can help to define the flow in the renal vein and artery. Power Doppler examinations of the parenchymal flow pattern are considered insufficiently reliable and consistent to be used in diagnosis of diffuse conditions.

Urinary tract infections (UTIs) in adults are common in women but not in men. If not treated, they can lead to severe renal disease and ultimately end-stage renal failure. Infection comes usually from bacteria from the patient's own bowel which can enter the urinary tract either via the bloodstream, the lymphatics, by direct extension from a vesicocolic fistula or, more commonly, along the urethra. Bacteria reach the bladder by first colonizing around the urethra (causes have been given as lack of personal hygiene, the use of sanitary towels, bubble baths or soaps with a high chemical content). They then transfer along the urethra to the bladder during sexual intercourse or by catheterization. This is easier in the female as the urethra is short; males have a longer urethra which helps discourage bacteria from reaching the bladder and have added protection from the bactericidal properties of prostatic fluid. When the bacteria reach the bladder, they can establish there and pass up the ureters to the kidneys relatively easily owing to dilated hypotonic ureters and vesicoureteric reflux. Urine is normally sterile owing to bladder defence mechanisms that protect it against UTIs.

Pregnant women are more prone to urinary tract infections from obstruction of the ureters by the gravid uterus and from urinary stasis associated with dilatation and kinking of the ureters due to increased progesterone levels relaxing the smooth muscle within the ureters.

UTIs are common in children and infants. It has been found that 20% of children with a proven UTI have vesicoureteric reflux, 20% have another abnormality and in 60% there is no abnormality seen. The role of imaging in UTI is to exclude structural abnormality such as obstruction, duplex or pelvic kidney, exclude scarring and confirm or exclude vesicoureteric reflux. All children should be investigated after their first proven UTI.

The most vulnerable patients are children under one year as scarring occurs if there is an infection within the first six months of life. Ill babies with UTIs often vomit but are quiet. If they cry, the cause of the illness is not usually a UTI. Between one and four years, although vesicocolic reflux normally stops spontaneously by the age of four, renal scarring has already occurred and can progress especially if there is an accompanying abnormality such as a Hutch diverticulum. A normal DMSA radioisotope scan can exclude significant vesicocolic reflux. Over the age of four, a child with a first proven UTI will often have a DMSA scan only when there is a second UTI, providing the ultrasound scan reveals no abnormality.

The protocols for investigating children with UTIs have been the subject of debate. It is generally accepted that the investigations for those infants up to one year should be:

- ultrasound

- micturating cystourethrogram (MCUG)

- DMSA scan (some centres will request this if the above two investigations reveal an abnormality).

For those from one to four years the investigations should be:

- ultrasound

- DMSA scan

- MCUG if there is a second proven UTI, a family history of UTIs, clinical evidence of pyelonephritis or the other tests are abnormal.

Children over four years should have:

- ultrasound

- abdominal X-ray if there are lower urinary tract symptoms

- DMSA scan for those with systemic symptoms

- MCUG if the DMSA scan shows evidence of scarring.

DMSA scans, if available, are more sensitive than ultrasound in demonstrating renal scarring and give a low radiation dose to the patient.

Acute pyelonephritis

CLINICAL INFORMATION

Acute pyelonephritis is the term given to bacterial infection of the kidney, the majority ascending from the lower urinary tract but occasionally via the bloodstream. The affected kidney visually appears swollen and inflamed with streaks of pus in the parenchyma. Women between the ages of 15 and 40 are the most at risk and the condition is more commonly seen in females (90% females, 10% in males). Causes are linked to pregnancy, obstruction of the urinary tract, neuropathic bladder, immune suppression, calculi and diabetes.

Patients present with loin pain, frequency of micturition, fever, haematuria, offensive urine and dysuria. In 90% of cases, the culprit organism is *E. coli*; Proteus, Klebsiella and Pseudomonas share the remaining 10%. The reason for the ascending spread of infection into the renal papilla could be that *E. coli* produces a toxin that prevents ureteric peristalsis and allows the ureters to dilate. Some strains stick particularly to the epithelium. With treatment, the kidneys heal but the condition can recur, this process of repeated inflammation and healing leading to chronic pyelonephritis (Fig. 9.17).

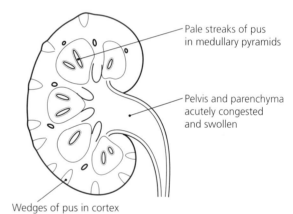

Pale streaks of pus in medullary pyramids

Pelvis and parenchyma acutely congested and swollen

Wedges of pus in cortex

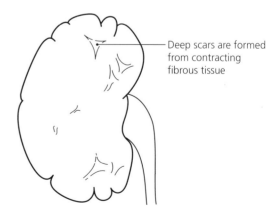

Deep scars are formed from contracting fibrous tissue

Fig. 9.17 Acute pyelonephritis.

ULTRASOUND APPEARANCES

If there is no medical history of urinary tract infection (UTI) in adult patients and if the patient recovers quickly with antibiotics, it is considered unnecessary to investigate the kidneys for structural abnormality as abnormalities are found in less than 1% of adult kidneys. The kidney is usually normal in size and appearance in these cases. Severe renal infection (acute bacterial nephritis) is considered when a fever and raised white cell count have lasted more than 72 hours despite antibiotic administration. When the UTI in adults is severe, the kidney often appears slightly larger and generally of a lower reflectivity. Ultrasound is also employed to try to ascertain the cause of the infection such as an obstruction, calculus or abscess.

In contrast, children with a UTI have a much higher incidence of structural abnormalities such as vesico-ureteric reflux and obstruction leading to urinary stasis which in turn can lead to infection. In severe cases, swelling of the infected kidney has been reported to increase its size by up to 75% over the unaffected kidney, especially in infancy.

With both children and adults, in severe infection, the reflectivity of the kidney is reduced compared to the unaffected one, the renal sinus appears all the more reflective and the corticomedullary differentiation is reduced. A return to normal appearances may take up to two months after severe infection. Scarring in adults is unusual compared with children.

Box 9.9 Advice

Scarring on ultrasound may only be seen in severe cases. Remember that the DMSA scan is more sensitive than ultrasound in demonstrating scarring and that scarring will probably have been present a long time before it is seen on ultrasound.

When describing reflectivity of the kidneys, a grading system has been proposed.

- 0 where the cortex is less reflective than the normal liver.

- 1 where the cortex is more reflective than the normal liver but less than the echogenicity of the sinus.

- 2 where the reflectivity of the cortex is iso-echoic to that of the sinus.

Chronic pyelonephritis

CLINICAL INFORMATION

Chronic pyelonephritis is the result of continuing healing and inflammation of the kidney and accounts for 15% of end-stage chronic renal failure. Chronic inflammation and scarring occur, resulting in the destruction of nephrons. The pelvicalyceal system is distorted and hypertension can occur. There are two types of chronic pyelonephritis: reflux associated and obstructive. In reflux-associated chronic pyelonephritis, reflux of urine up the ureters from the bladder causes recurrent inflammation leading to scarring. This often occurs in childhood and progressively leads to a reduction of renal function presenting in early adulthood.

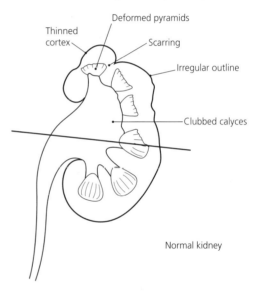

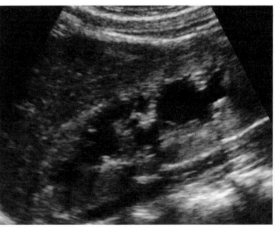

Fig. 9.18   Chronic pyelonephritis showing renal scarring.

In obstructive chronic pyelonephritis, obstruction in a lower part of the urinary tract from calculus or renal tract anomaly can lead to recurrent infection. Scarring occurs over a blunted, distorted, renal calyx and most commonly at the upper and lower poles of the kidneys.

ULTRASOUND APPEARANCES

Areas of increased echogenicity can be seen along with blunting of the calyces and thinning of the cortex. The size of the kidney is often reduced and the outline mis-shapen (Fig. 9.18).

Box 9.10   Advice

Ensure that the normal appearance of foetal lobulation is not mistaken for scarring. Foetal lobulation is smooth and regular.

Renal abscess

CLINICAL INFORMATION

Patients with a renal abscess or abscesses (as they can be single or multiple) usually present with pain in the flank, fever, dysuria and frequency. Abscesses can form after severe acute pyelonephritis or other diffuse infection and the same organisms are seen. There is an association with diabetes, calculi, recurrent pyelo-nephritis and drug abuse. Abscesses can lie within or around the kidney or under the capsule.

ULTRASOUND APPEARANCES

These are variable and can range from a simple, hypo-echoic appearance to a larger, complex one. The mass is usually irregular with thick walls, some through transmission of sound with distal enhancement although less than that of a cyst. There may be debris evident as reflective echoes within the mass and the abscess may contain gas which shows as a poorly defined reflective area with unsharp or 'dirty' shadow-ing distal to it. Abscesses are frequently drained under ultrasound control.

Box 9.11   Advice

The appearance of a renal abscess can be imitated by an infected or haemorrhagic cyst or lymphoma.

Pyonephrosis

CLINICAL INFORMATION

In pyonephrosis there is pus in the urine or an infected hydronephrosis. It can occur after obstruction by a stone in the urinary tract, malignancy or by extrinsic obstruction such as compression of the ureters by the uterus in the third trimester of pregnancy. It occurs in children secondary to anomalies such as vesico- or pelviureteric junction obstruction. Pyonephrosis may be suspected if the patient has a UTI which has not improved after treatment with antibiotics. Patients may have no symptoms and the condition may be discov-ered by the presence of pus in the urine or they may present with loin pain and fever.

ULTRASOUND APPEARANCES

There may be low-level echoes within the collecting system resting on the dependent parts and showing a fluid/debris level. However, the appearances can be normal with an anechoic appearance of the urine although with reduced distal enhancement. Aspiration may be required to confirm diagnosis.

Box 9.12   Advice

High gain settings can imitate echoes from pus within the urine. Blood within the urine and fungus within the collecting system can also imitate pus.

Xanthogranulomatous pyelonephritis

CLINICAL INFORMATION

This condition is caused by obstruction of the pelvi-calyceal system by calculi, often large, such as staghorn calculi. The kidney becomes infected and after a long period of infection, the calyces enlarge and become filled with pus/debris and the cortex is often reduced in size. The pain accompanying xanthogranulomatous pyelonephritis is less severe and acute than in pyonephrosis.

ULTRASOUND APPEARANCES

The appearances are similar to pyonephrosis with low-level echoes in the collecting system suggesting fluid and/or debris.

Fungal infection

CLINICAL INFORMATION

The most common fungal infection is *Candida albicans* which is associated with ill patients who have lowered immunity to infection, who are on steroids or antibiotics, who are diabetics or those who have a malignancy. It occurs in neonates who are premature, are being fed parenterally, have an umbilical catheter or patent ductus arteriosus or are on antibiotics.

ULTRASOUND APPEARANCES

The whole kidney may become infected by the fungus increasing its reflectivity. Multiple abscesses may appear and give the kidneys a highly reflective appearance if small or less reflective if the abscesses are larger. Fungus ball plugs may be seen in the collecting system which may fill it entirely eventually. The fungus balls are highly reflective but cast no acoustic shadow posteriorly.

Diffuse renal disease

Acute tubular necrosis (ATN)

CLINICAL INFORMATION

This is a common cause of acute renal failure caused by metabolic or toxic disturbances and is reversible if these disturbances are corrected. Ischaemic tubular necrosis occurs after impairment of renal perfusion or hypoxia as a result of hypotension and hypovolaemia in shock or after sudden blood loss, such as after major surgery and severe burns. Toxic tubular necrosis is uncommon and caused by heavy metal poisoning (lead, mercury), drugs, solvents and other toxins such as poisoned mushrooms, antifreeze, radiological contrast agents and weedkiller.

In the first week of ATN, glomerular filtration is reduced and the kidneys appear swollen as patients develop acute renal failure and oliguria. Within the next 2–3 weeks, the renal tubular epithelium regenerates but polyuria develops as the tubules have not developed sufficiently to be able to resorb electrolytes and water. Therefore fluid and electrolyte balance is carefully monitored. Renal function is restored as the tubular cells regain their normal function.

ULTRASOUND APPEARANCES

The kidneys often appear normal although some patients have kidneys with a greater renal size, especially the anteroposterior measurement. The medullary pyramids are well defined but are often of higher reflectivity than normal and appear swollen. Increased arterial resistance is seen with Doppler.

Interstitial nephritis

CLINICAL INFORMATION

Acute interstitial nephritis causes acute renal failure from inflammatory cell infiltration of the kidney's interstitial tissues. It is often started by drugs, especially analgesics and antibiotics, or various infections and is associated with tubular damage or atrophy. It is classified into drug-induced acute interstitial nephritis, where recovery occurs after withdrawal of the causative agent, drug-induced chronic interstitial nephritis where fibrosis, inflammation and atrophy of the tubules occur, analgesic nephropathy which can lead to chronic renal failure after long-term exposure and where the risk of developing urothelial carcinoma is greater, and radiation nephritis after the kidneys are included in the field of radiation when the patient is being treated for cancer by radiotherapy.

ULTRASOUND APPEARANCES

This condition is similar in clinical presentation and ultrasound appearances to acute tubular necrosis. The kidneys may be normal in size or enlarged, the cortex normal or increased in reflectivity. So a patient with acute renal failure with increased reflectivity may have interstitial nephritis.

Glomerulonephritis

CLINICAL INFORMATION

This is a term covering conditions caused by an abnormality of the structure of the glomerulus. Structural change to the glomerular basement membrane can lead to abnormal loss of protein in the urine or nephrotic syndrome. Damage to the glomeruli associated with proliferation of the endothelial cells leads to haematuria or nephritic syndrome. Damage to the glomeruli can be severe, leading to permanent scarring. If it is rapid, acute renal failure occurs. In chronic glomerulonephritis, the patient with chronic renal failure has kidneys where the glomeruli are hyalinized.

There are several types of glomerulonephritis, the three most common being as follows.

● Acute diffuse proliferative glomerulonephritis presenting as the nephritic syndrome, occurring mainly in adults. Infection is commonly strepto-coccal, glomerular filtration is reduced and blood pressure and blood urea and creatinine rise. With treatment, this resolves in 3–6 weeks although some can progress rapidly to renal failure or more slowly to chronic renal failure.

- Membranous nephropathy presenting with protein-uria and the nephrotic syndrome. This is mainly seen in adults who can present with fluid accumula-tion – puffy eyes and ankles – decreased urine output, raised blood pressure, proteinuria, loss of appetite, headaches and smoky urine. The basement membrane is thickened and abnormally permeable. In 50% of cases, chronic renal failure will occur over about 10 years, 25% develop stable but persistent proteinuria and the other 25% develop remission.

- Membranoproliferative glomerulonephritis (MPGN) has two types. Type I is seen mainly in adolescents and young adults and accounts for 90% of this condition. Renal function deteriorates over about 10 years, resulting in chronic renal failure. Type II accounts for 10% and is seen in children and young adults It may cause haematuria and nephrotic syndrome or nephritic/nephrotic syndrome. It has a poor progno-sis and chronic renal failure develops over many years. It can be seen to recur in transplanted kidneys.

ULTRASOUND APPEARANCES

There may be slight enlargement in the acute phase and in the chronic stages, the kidneys become small and shrunken as a result of nephron loss due to glomerular or vascular disease. Nephrocalcinosis can occur in patients with chronic glomerulonephritis. The pelvicalyceal system appears normal. However, ultrasound is often non-specific when it comes to assessing this type of pathology.

For further information on acute and chronic renal failure, refer to Appendix 4.

Diabetes mellitus

CLINICAL INFORMATION

The kidneys are affected by vascular changes in these patients and monitoring renal function is important. Diabetes is now one of the most common causes of end-stage renal failure. Diabetic kidneys are prone to bacte-rial infection. Acute pyelonephritis is a common complication of diabetes mellitus owing to the relative immune suppression that diabetics have. Papillary necro-sis, where the tips of the papillae are shed in the urine, can lead to acute renal failure. Ischaemia of the kidneys is caused by atheroma in the aorta and renal arteries.

ULTRASOUND APPEARANCES

Appearances are variable both in size and reflectivity. In the initial stages, the glomerular filtration rate increases and this is associated with a small increase in the size of the kidneys, both in volume and length. As the disease becomes chronic, the kidneys decrease in size but reflectivity stays about the same or slightly more echogenic.

AIDS

CLINICAL INFORMATION

Renal disease in AIDS patients is a frequent cause of mortality. Despite the patients being dialysed, there is almost 100% mortality within six months of the onset of uraemia. Renal biopsy has shown segmental glomerulosclerosis and focal glomerulonephritis. Acute tubular necrosis, interstitial nephritis and, more un-usually, focal nephrocalcinosis have also been seen.

ULTRASOUND APPEARANCES

Parenchymal changes are variable according to the renal conditions acquired by the patient, but many AIDS patients have been seen to have very large, reflective kidneys.

Vascular pathology

Renal vein thrombosis

CLINICAL INFORMATION

This condition is uncommon and occurs usually in the neonate after dehydration due to vomiting or diarrhoea. It has also been associated with the nephrotic syndrome, glomerulonephritis, trauma, pregnancy, the oral contraceptive pill, steroids or, most commonly in adults, tumour extension into the renal vein. The left renal vein is affected three times as much as the right owing to its length and position. Most cases present on one side only.

ULTRASOUND APPEARANCES

Sudden occlusion of the renal vein can cause a kidney to enlarge and the reflectivity is lower than normal.

The appearance of the renal sinus may be changed by haemorrhage. Within 1–2 weeks, the cortex can start to become more reflective, with focal echo-poor areas due to haemorrhage, and start to reduce in size. In 1–2 months, a small, highly reflective kidney can be seen. As the kidney contracts after about one month, the corticomedullary differentiation is lost. Doppler can show reduced or absent flow in the vein and renal parenchyma and demonstrate thrombus if present. The arterial waveform is highly pulsatile with reversed diastolic flow. Thrombus can sometimes be seen on real time in the renal vein or IVC (see Fig. 9.15). Left renal vein occlusion can show initially in the male as an acute left varicocoele.

Renal artery occlusion

CLINICAL INFORMATION

Sudden renal artery occlusion can be caused by aortic dissection, arterial plaque haemorrhage, trauma and emboli. As one kidney only is affected, this does not produce renal failure.

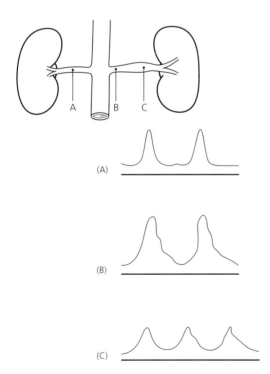

Fig. 9.19 Renal artery stenosis. (A) Normal Doppler flow. (B) Stenosis of renal artery giving increased peak flow and turbulence at stenosis site. (C) Distal to stenosis, systolic peak is lower and longer than (A).

ULTRASOUND APPEARANCES

After the occlusion, the kidney may be of normal or slightly larger size with normal echogenicity. Sometimes there is an echo-poor halo of tissue seen under the renal capsule, suggesting oedema from collateral vessels. After a longer period of time, it can slowly reduce in size but remains smooth in outline and the collecting system remains normal. A pulsed wave Doppler examination will reveal no flow in the relevant renal artery.

Renal artery stenosis

CLINICAL INFORMATION

Renal artery stenosis usually causes hypertension. It is rare in children, being a result of dehydration, umbilical artery catheterization in neonates and emboli from patent ductus arteriosus but in adults the most common causes are aortic aneurysm, atheroma, arteritis, emboli and trauma. It is often bilateral and is seen in 10–15% of patients requiring long-term dialysis.

ULTRASOUND APPEARANCES

When one kidney is affected, it usually appears normal or slightly smaller in size.

Pulsed wave Doppler can be used to assess the blood flow in 80% of patients and the examination is more easily performed on the right side than the left. If decreased or absent flow is seen in diastole, this may suggest partial or complete stenosis or there may be a failure to obtain a signal owing to technical factors. With stenosis, the peak flow is increased with turbulence at that site and beyond the stenosis, the systolic peak is lower and longer than normal. The stenosis is often adjacent to the aorta and is difficult to scan owing to position and to the presence of bowel gas anteriorly. If a normal signal is seen, this does suggest that a significant arterial flow is unlikely. In cases of an abnormal or absent signal, further investigations are required to confirm the diagnosis.

Obstruction

BACKGROUND

The obstruction of the flow of urine from the kidney can take place at any site in the urinary tract and from a number of causes. Depending on the side, site and severity of the obstruction, it usually causes a pelvicalyceal dilatation of lesser or greater proportions.

It is considered that if the pelvicalyceal dilatation is long-standing, causing the cortex to measure 1 cm or less, this is termed a hydronephrosis.

Common sites of obstruction and causes are:

- renal pelvis (calculi, tumours)

- pelviureteric junction (calculi, narrowing, compression by extrinsic mass)

- ureter (calculi, extrinsic masses such as fibroids or pregnancy)

- bladder (calculi, tumour near or around ureteric entry)

- urethra (calculi, stricture, prostatic hypertrophy).

As with the biliary system, strictures in the urinary system produce varying appearances according to the level of the obstruction (Fig 9.20).

- Obstruction of the urethra produces dilatation of the bladder to a lesser or greater extent, possible diverticulae and thickened bladder wall in long-standing obstruction, dilated ureters (megaureters) and a pelvicalyceal dilatation of both sides.

- A stricture at the lower end of a ureter can produce a dilated ureter (megaureter) and pelvicalyceal dilatation on one side.

- A high obstruction at the pelviureteric junction can cause a pelvicalyceal dilatation but without the associated megaureter.

Obstruction of the outflow of urine predisposes the patient to urinary tract infection and the formation of stones. It may be caused by soft tissue masses such as transitional cell carcinoma, fungus balls, sloughed papilla, blood clot or pyonephrosis, by

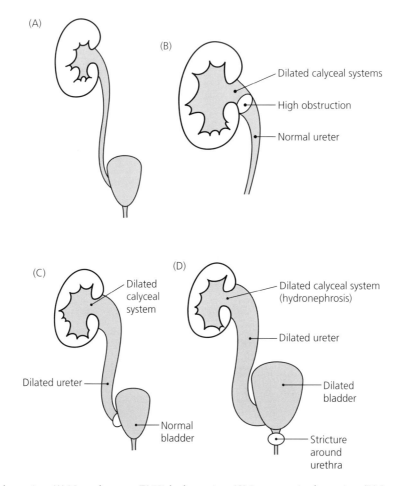

Fig. 9.20 Sites of obstruction. (A) Normal system. (B) High obstruction. (C) Low ureteric obstruction. (D) Low urethral obstruction.

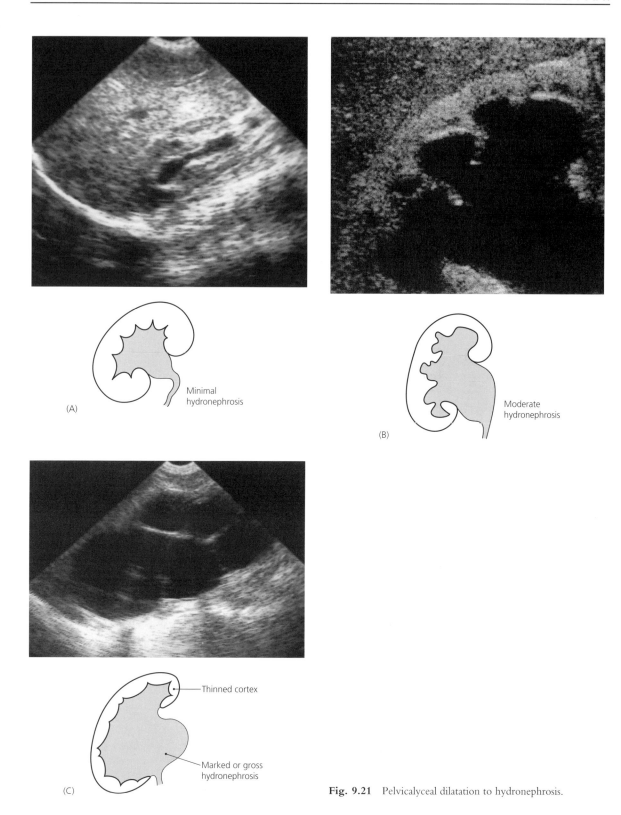

(A) Minimal hydronephrosis

(B) Moderate hydronephrosis

(C) Thinned cortex

Marked or gross hydronephrosis

Fig. 9.21 Pelvicalyceal dilatation to hydronephrosis.

fibrosis and consequent stricture or by urinary tract calculi.

ULTRASOUND APPEARANCES

The appearances of the results of obstruction, whether caused by a soft tissue mass or by urinary tract calculi, are similar. There are three recognized grades of pelvicalyceal dilatation, mild, moderate and marked, which describe the appearances ranging from a small, central dilatation to a large pool of urine and associated thinning of the cortex. A mild pelvicalyceal dilatation appears as an echo-free area, centrally positioned, within the renal sinus. In moderate pelvicalyceal dilatation, this collection to communicates with the peripheral calyces and in marked pelvicalyceal dilatation/hydronephrosis, the obstructed large calyces and sinus are easily recognized. The length of the kidney is often slightly increased and the cortex is thinned when the hydronephrosis is marked. Once the obstruction is relieved, the cortical thickness returns to normal (Fig. 9.21).

If the obstruction is in the region of the vesicoureteric junction, dilated ureters can sometimes be seen for a few centimetres distal to the renal sinus (seen by angling the probe anteriorly) and distally, viewed posterolateral to the full bladder. The middle part of the ureters is usually hidden behind bowel gas and cannot be seen.

The appearances of obstruction to the outflow of urine distal to the bladder are that of a large tense, anechoic bladder, with thickened wall if chronic, and possible diverticulae, the possibility of bladder stones and dilated ureters and collecting systems.

Box 9.13   Advice

A distended bladder in a patient able to void normally can cause a dilatation of the collecting system and so investigations of renal collecting systems must be performed when the bladder is empty. Even after micturition, the renal pelvis may remain dilated for a few minutes and sometimes longer in the elderly.

Pelvicalyceal dilatation can be differentiated from renal cysts in so far as the fluid collections communicate; cysts do not. There is also, even in the more extreme cases of hydronephrosis, a thin lateral border of renal parenchyma seen whereas with polycystic disease, it may be impossible to identify any normal renal component.

If a pelvicalyceal dilatation/hydronephrosis is seen, look for the cause of obstruction. This may not always be within the urinary tract but extrinsic masses such as pelvic masses, fibroids and enlarged lymph nodes may be the cause.

Neonates in the first 72 hours after birth are dehydrated and any attempt to confirm prenatal findings of a dilated collecting system must be delayed until they are rehydrated as the dehydration can mask a hydronephrosis.

Parapelvic cysts can be mistaken for a small hydronephrosis. In this case, look for any signs of obstruction during the scan.

Renal vessels entering the renal pelvis can sometimes be mistaken for mild obstruction and a Doppler examination may be used to confirm vascularity.

An extrarenal pelvis of less than 10 mm in anteroposterior diameter that is not accompanied by a pelvicalyceal dilatation is usually managed conservatively. However, a larger extrarenal pelvis with pelvicalyceal dilatation requires further exploration to assess function.

Obstruction in pregnancy

CLINICAL INFORMATION

In pregnancy, a mild pelvicalyceal dilatation can be seen from about the 12th week and can increase in severity throughout pregnancy, especially in the third trimester. This appearance is most marked at 28 weeks, the right side often being worse than the left. Patients are prone to urinary tract infections. After birth, the dilatation decreases but can remain for several months in minor form.

ULTRASOUND APPEARANCES

The appearances will be as previously described for pelvicalyceal dilatation. In advanced pregnancy, the size of the pregnant uterus displacing bowel upwards in the abdominal cavity can add to the amount of intestinal gas present around the area of the kidneys and make for a difficult scan. A pelvicalyceal dilatation can usually be seen well enough but looking for any other reason for obstruction, such as calculi in the upper or lower ureter, is often very difficult.

Obstructed moiety in duplex kidney

CLINICAL INFORMATION

Sometimes, a kidney will have a half-obstructed (usually the upper half), half-normal appearance. In this case, the cause is the obstruction of one moiety of a duplex kidney, usually by the ectopic insertion of a ureter into bladder, urethra, vagina or seminal vesicle.

ULTRASOUND APPEARANCES

The upper pole of the kidney appears dilated, often with thinning of the cortex which can be more reflective than usual, and a prominent renal sinus and calyces; the lower pole appears normal. There is often a thin band of normal renal parenchyma separating the

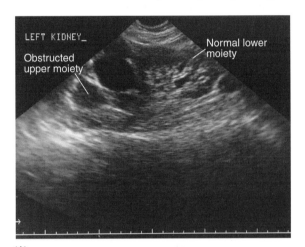

(A)

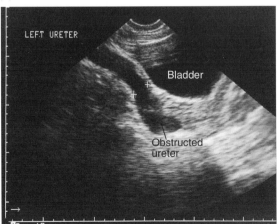

(B)

Fig. 9.22 (A) Obstructed upper moiety. (B) Dilated ureter to upper moiety.

upper and lower collecting systems. A dilated ureter can often be seen exiting from the upper moiety and entering the bladder. A ureterocoele (see Chapter 10) may be seen at the insertion of the dilated ureter into the posterior part of the bladder.

Reflux in children

CLINICAL INFORMATION

Pelvicalyceal dilatation can be caused by vesicoureteric reflux of urine from bladder to kidney. It can be caused by foreign body or calculi in the urethra, a failure of the vesicoureteric junction to develop or posterior urethral valves. Reflux can lead to infection and consequent scarring.

ULTRASOUND APPEARANCES

Reflux cannot be reliably seen with ultrasound unless contrast is used. Radionuclide examinations are often requested for diagnosis as a normal urinary tract might be seen with intermittent reflux. There may be mild or severe dilatation of the urinary tract on one or both sides. Scarring shows as a focal reduction of cortical thickness or change in normal shape although this is difficult to confirm when the kidney is lobulated. A kidney that has not grown compared to the other side is often a result of chronic reflux. If the difference between the size of one kidney and another is more than 10–15%, further investigations to confirm or exclude reflux should be requested.

Obstruction by posterior urethral valves

CLINICAL INFORMATION

See also page 191. Renal dysplasia in male infants is associated with posterior urethral valves.

ULTRASOUND APPEARANCES

The kidneys can be normal or small, highly reflective with little or no corticomedullary differentiation, possible small cortical cysts, a normal renal sinus or possible severe hydronephrosis, dilated ureters and a clubbed calyceal system.

Calculi

CLINICAL INFORMATION

It is said that about 2% of the population in the UK have a stone in the urinary tract at any one time but that the prevalence is much higher in the Middle East, probably owing to the higher temperature contributing to dehydration (see below). Males have a higher incidence of urinary tract calculi than women in a ratio of 2:1.

Renal calculi are composed of calcium oxalate, uric acid and urates or phosphate. Like gallstones, urinary tract stones are often mixed. Urate stones can be covered with oxalate and both oxalate and urate stones can develop an external layer of phosphates. It is thought that precipitates form in the renal tubules and pass into the renal pelvis where they grow.

Factors causing stones to form include:

- the pH of the urine (urate and oxalate stones form in an acid urine, phosphate stones in alkaline urine). The urine becomes alkaline in many cases of renal sepsis

- increased concentration of urine from frequent dehydration

- urinary stasis from obstruction which encourages the precipitation of salts

- renal tumours, parts of which necrose and calcify

- hypercalciuria and hyperphosphaturia from hyperparathyroidism, excessive vitamin D intake, excessive milk and alkaline from long-term stomach ulcer medication and immobilization leading to the reduction of calcium in the bones (disuse osteoporosis).

Small calculi passing down the ureter cause colic. The ureters are often injured, a stricture is formed and impaction of a subsequent stone becomes more likely. Large stones can impact at upper or lower ends of the ureter or within the pelvis, causing urinary stasis which can lead to hydronephrosis and infection, which in turn can lead to further stone formation.

Many people with urinary tract calculi have no symptoms. However, the most common symptom is pain, this being sharp, dull, present all the time or intermittent. Renal pain is worsened by movement and only relieved by analgesia. The pain is felt in the loins but sometimes radiates anteriorly, causing the patient to complain of abdominal pain. Patients often demonstrate renal pain by putting their hands on their waists, thumbs facing anteriorly and fingers spreading posteriorly between the 12th rib and the iliac crest.

When the stone is causing an obstruction, any increased fluid intake or diuretic such as tea, coffee or alcohol can make the pain worse. Patient movement can cause the stone to move and cause pain and sometimes haematuria. When a stone enters a ureter and obstructs it or causes spasm as it passes down, patients suffer a severe, intense pain. The patient with ureteric colic often has pallor, sweating and vomiting and is restless, trying to find a comfortable position. As the stone passes through zones of innervation of the ureter from T10 to L1, the referred pain can pass from loin to testis. If left untreated, the pain often subsides within hours.

Blood tests can show a calcium level which is either normal or high; urine tests can reveal traces of protein and blood. After having one renal stone, more than 50% of patients will have another stone or stones form within 10 years. The risk of recurrence increases if there is an untreated metabolic condition present which is a known causative factor in stone formation.

ULTRASOUND APPEARANCES

As with gallstones, renal calculi are seen as highly reflective masses with distal acoustic shadowing and are seen either within the renal parenchyma or in a dilated collecting system. If there is urine around the calculus and if the calculus lies within the upper part of the ureter, then it is seen relatively easily if large enough. Smaller stones, those less than 3–4 mm in diameter, can be seen if the kidney is scanned carefully and slowly. If the stone is causing an obstruction to the collecting system, it is more easily seen than if it is mobile and lying close to the calyces which have a similar reflectivity (Fig. 9.23).

If the stone is small, casts no shadow and lies within a non-obstructed collecting system or in the middle portion of a ureter, it may easily be missed. If the stone lies at the lower part of the ureter, it may be seen when scanning through the bladder. Colour Doppler or grey-scale B-mode imaging may be used to assess the entry of urine into the bladder at the ureteric orifice (see Fig. 2.1B).

Staghorn calculus

CLINICAL INFORMATION

This large, single stone is associated with ulceration and infection of the renal pelvis and calyces.

ULTRASOUND APPEARANCES

Staghorn calculi can fill up an entire dilated collecting system and, as they are as reflective as the calyces

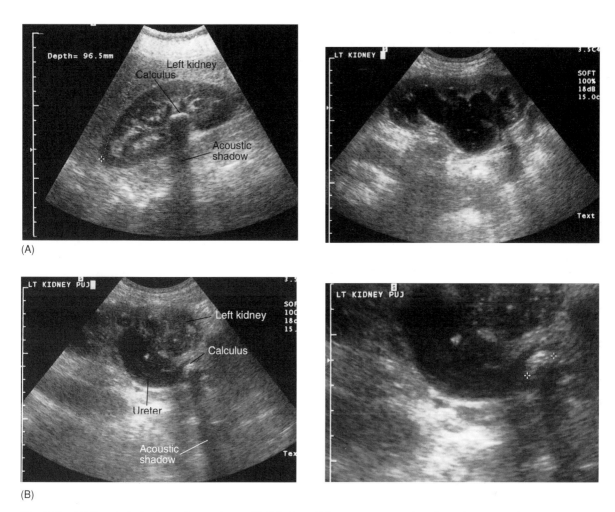

(A)

(B)

Fig. 9.23 (A) Renal calculus in renal parenchyma. (B) Calculus within upper ureter causing obstruction.

themselves, they are often not obvious. Strong shadowing from this area and a subsequent plain radiograph will confirm a staghorn calculus (Fig. 9.24).

Box 9.14   Advice

The highest frequency possible must be used when searching for calculi. Ensure the appropriate focusing zone is selected.

Highly reflective focal areas can be seen within the kidney if the patient has undergone recent extracorporeal shock wave lithotripsy (stone fragments) or has had a stent inserted or has recently had a percutaneous nephrostomy (air).

Nephrocalcinosis or medullary calcinosis

CLINICAL INFORMATION

This is caused by persistent hypercalcaemia or hypercalciuria as a result of primary hyperparathyroidism, excess vitamin D and Cushing's syndrome and causes calcification within the renal parenchyma. It is often found in the region of the medulla but can sometimes be found within the cortex. It is seen occasionally in patients with chronic glomerulonephritis and as a side effect of long-term frusemide therapy in very low birthweight premature babies requiring assisted ventilation. It can disappear when frusemide is stopped or when it is taken in combination with chlorothiazide.

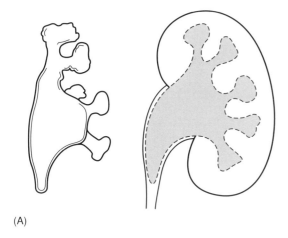

(A)

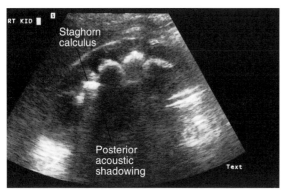

(B)

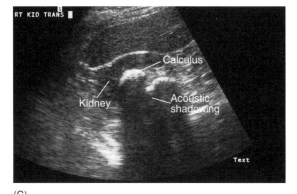

(C)

Fig. 9.24 (A) Diagram and ultrasound images of Staghorn calculus. (B) Longitudinal. (C) Transverse.

Highly reflective regions within the parenchyma are seen, especially in the medulla. Acoustic shadowing will only be seen when the calcification is sufficiently large but will not be present when it is smaller than the beam width. This condition can be confirmed by a plain abdominal radiograph if required.

Renal trauma

CLINICAL INFORMATION

Although the kidneys are relatively well protected by ribs, vertebrae and paravertebral muscles, trauma to the kidneys is a common occurrence with adults and children. Common trauma are penetrating injuries from stab wounds, deceleration or acceleration injuries from road traffic accidents and blunt injuries to the kidneys, to which children are more vulnerable than adults. The role of ultrasound in the trauma situation is to detect the result of trauma such as haematoma, vascular injury and laceration, assess any damage to the adjacent organs such as the liver, spleen, pancreas, stomach and colon, search for free fluid and confirm normal appearances of the contralateral kidney.

Patients with severe renal damage can present with gross haematuria, shock and flank pain. Classification of blunt injury trauma has been divided into four categories: small corticomedullary tears, larger tears with accompanying fracture of the kidney, shattered kidney with several separate pieces and disruption of the vascular pedicle with avulsion of the pelviureteric junction. With major trauma in the third category, patients can be treated conservatively with bed rest and antibiotics until the haematuria stops as long as the contralateral kidney is normal and the patient is clinically stable. This is why a careful assessment of the other kidney must be made. Traumatic damage to the kidney is often worse if there is an abnormality of the kidney already, such as hydronephrosis or tumour.

Haematomas can occur under the renal capsule (subcapsular haematoma), within the kidney (intrarenal haematoma) and around the kidney but outside the capsule (perirenal haematoma). In subcapsular haematomas, blood can spread around the kidney or collect in one place (focal haematoma). These may indent the cortex. Resolving haematomas can fibrose and compress the kidney, leading to hypertension.

Haematoma can either be echo poor when fresh or echogenic as it clots. As the haematoma liquefies, it becomes echo poor or anechoic or has a complex appearance.

Lacerations and splits in the renal parenchyma are seen as reflective thickened lines radiating from the periphery to the hilum. Colour flow Doppler can help in the exclusion of renal vascular disruption. Subcapsular haematomas can appear as echo-poor haloes around the kidney but deep to the capsule although if the haematoma is clotting, the reflective clot is harder to see close to the capsule itself. Intrarenal haematoma is generally seen as a focal area of low reflectivity. If echogenic, the haematoma may be missed if in the region of the reflective collecting system. Some renal haematomas can enlarge and in themselves cause enough intrinsic pressure that they can rupture the kidney. Perirenal haematomas are usually reflective by the time the patient is scanned and can expand into the anterior or posterior pararenal spaces. If the haematomas are large, they may contain blood and urine and possibly septa.

Renal transplant

Background

Apart from long-term renal dialysis, renal transplant is the only alternative for survival in those with chronic renal failure. Donor kidneys come from living related and unrelated donors once it has been established that they have two healthily functioning kidneys and are compatible with the recipient. Cadaveric kidneys can be preserved for up to 72 hours after death.

Ultrasound has an important role in the care of the renal transplant patient. It contributes towards the diagnosis of the disease, is used to guide biopsy needles to confirm a diagnosis prior to the transplant and is used, with Doppler ultrasound, to monitor the success or failure of a graft. It can be used to guide drainage tubes and catheters if this procedure is required. It is also a mobile technique which allows the scanner to be brought to the bedside of the patient.

The transplanted kidney is usually placed in an extraperitoneal pouch in the right or left iliac fossa anterior to the iliacus and psoas muscles. Right renal grafts are more commonly placed in the right iliac fossa but the left is sometimes used. Vessels can be anastomosed in two ways: end to side or end to end. With the end-to-side method, the renal vessels are anastomosed to the external iliac vessels. With the end-to-end method, the donor renal vein is anastomosed to the external iliac vein and the renal artery to the internal iliac artery. The former method is preferred as there is less chance of renal artery stenosis occurring. Lymphatic vessels are ligated to prevent leakage of lymph and the formation of a lymphocoele. Children of less than 20 kg receive the donor kidney into the abdomen and the renal vessels are connected to the abdominal aorta and IVC (Fig. 9.25).

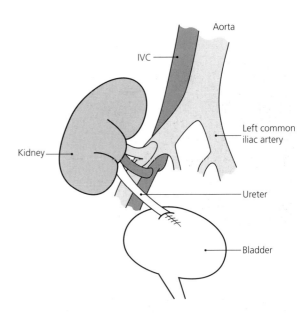

Fig. 9.25 Diagram of end-to-side renal transplantation.

The ureter from the donor kidney is implanted into the bladder through a submucosal tunnel designed to prevent reflux. This involves opening the bladder and the subsequent risk of infection. Alternatively, the recipient ureter is connected to the donor's renal pelvis or two ends of donor and recipient ureters are connected. The patient's own organs are left *in situ* whenever possible unless the patient has chronic vesicoureteric reflux, renal parenchymal infection or infected stones or has massively enlarged polycystic kidneys which need to be removed to make room for the transplant.

The patient is given cyclosporin A, an effective but expensive and nephrotoxic immunosuppressant. If rejection is going to take place, it will happen in the first few months following the transplant when the immunosuppressed patient can succumb to viruses normally controlled by the body's own immune system.

Equipment required

As the kidney lies superficially, a higher frequency probe (5–7.5 MHz) can be used. It is not advisable to use a sector probe as information will be lost closest to the skin surface owing to the sector shape and small footprint. Some high-frequency linear or curved linear probes have small footprints and here too, only a small amount of information would be seen at one time. If a small footprint probe is used, images should be taken on a split screen and the upper and lower portions of the organ 'joined together' to make one image. The best compromise is often a 5 MHz curved linear or linear probe. As with any postoperative ultrasound procedure, sterile gel should be used and infection control protocols adhered to.

Suggested scanning technique

The first scan is usually performed at about 18 hours after the transplant and then on every other day for the ensuing 2–3 weeks. Care must be taken when scanning to avoid infection spread and scanning over drains and dressings.

The lie of the transplanted kidney is variable as the size and length of the donor kidney and vessels are as varied as the size of the recipient. Blood vessels are often quite tortuous and are difficult to trace, although it is relatively easy to see the external iliac artery, the origin of the blood supply to the kidney.

Normal ultrasound appearances

The healthy transplanted kidney appears similar to a normal native kidney. The medullary pyramids are anechoic and the corticomedullary differentiation better is seen than with native kidneys. This is probably due to the higher frequency used and the better view afforded with the superficial kidney. The calyces are seen in better detail, possibly because there is a temporary mild obstruction at the insertion of the ureter.

The pulsed wave Doppler signal of the renal artery appears similar to that of the native kidney: a rapid rise

to systole and a slower flow continuing throughout diastole. Normal main renal artery blood flows at between 20 and 52 cm/s (mean 32 cm/s). The pulsatility index (PI) can be used as the indicator of resistance to blood flow and the PI of a normal healthy renal artery and branches is between 0.7 and 1.4. This demonstrates a low resistance to flow in the vascular bed. A PI of more than 1.5 suggests possible dysfunction. The resistive index (RI) is also used to measure resistance to arterial flow in the renal vascular bed but does not require accurate angle-corrected measurements. Normal RI is less than 0.7–0.8 and one of more than 0.9 indicates transplant dysfunction. Colour Doppler imaging allows rapid assessment of arterial renal perfusion and venous patency.

Box 9.15 Advice

Air can be seen within the kidney as a result of nephrostomy tube insertion and can produce a highly reflective gas pattern as a result. Ensure this is not mistaken for infarct or calculus.

A small amount of perinephric fluid is normal postoperatively but must be monitored. If the fluid does not resolve, drainage may be necessary.

Normal sizes

The transplanted kidney must be measured in all three dimensions post transplant. The healthy renal transplant increases in size in the first six months owing to hypertrophy. A normal increase in renal volume in the first two weeks after transplant is considered to be 16% (7–25%) and by 22% (14–32%) in the first three weeks.

Posttransplant complications

Complications of the renal transplant can be seen immediately (<1 week), early (1–4 weeks) and late (>1 month) and can be grouped as shown below.

Acute tubular necrosis (ATN)

CLINICAL INFORMATION

This condition has previously been described but is usually the result of lack of oxygen causing the necrosis of the renal tubules prior to the transplant. Severe ATN shows as anuria in the immediate postoperative

Pathology	Immediate (<1 week)	Early (1–4 weeks)	Late (>1 month)
Tissue	Acute tubular necrosis Acute rejection	Acute rejection	Acute > chronic rejection, cyclosporin toxicity, infection
Vascular	Renal vein thrombosis (RVT), renal artery stenosis (RAS)	RVT	RAS
Urological	Oedema of ureter	Urinoma	Lymphocoele
Iatrogenic	Haemorrhage		

period with high serum creatinine levels. ATN occurs in 20–60% of cadaveric grafts. The kidney can recover within a few days and produces urine. Vascular spasm and interstitial oedema reduce the size of the vascular bed and increase the impedance to the flow of blood. ATN is often a cause of transplant failure.

ULTRASOUND APPEARANCES

The kidney can appear normal but is often swollen, oedematous and of low reflectivity with the renal sinus echoes lost or compressed owing to swelling and loss of corticomedullary differentiation. The PI and RI measurements on pulsed wave Doppler examination are usually higher than normal. Biopsy may be required to exclude ATN.

Acute rejection

CLINICAL INFORMATION

Rejection is the process by which foreign tissues are immunologically destroyed. Rejection is likely if urine is not produced by 48 hours after the transplant and there is a fever and raised creatinine level. It can involve the renal cells (interstitial) or vessels (vascular). Rejection is divided into three areas:

- hyperacute rejection where the graft is irreversibly destroyed within minutes following the connection of blood vessels (rare)

- accelerated rejection, occurring during the first few days and leading to loss of the graft

- acute rejection, occurring during the first weeks or months and requiring immediate diagnosis and treatment.

ULTRASOUND APPEARANCES

Acute rejection is seen in a variety of ways. The kidney can become swollen. It should be noted that the AP

diameter of the kidney is normally less than the transverse diameter but renal swelling is suggested when the AP diameter is equal to or more than the transverse diameter. It has been seen that patients with acute rejection have an increase in cross-sectional area of >10%. Rejection is suggested when the renal volume increases by >20% in five days, >25% in 14 days and >30% in 21 days.

Medullary pyramids can become anechoic and enlarged, giving an increased corticomedullary differentiation. Sometimes the renal parenchyma can be of lower reflectivity than normal, reducing this differentiation. Central sinus echoes can be reduced. With pulsed wave Doppler, there is gradual decrease in diastolic flow related to the severity of the disease, leading to absent or reverse diastolic flow.

Box 9.16   Advice

The fever can be due to postoperative infected fluid collections such as haematoma, urinoma or lymphocoele and therefore ultrasound is used to exclude these.

A PI of more than 1.5 was at one time said to be 75% sensitive and 90% specific in the diagnosis of acute rejection but a PI level of 1.8 can also be found in acute tubular necrosis, acute venous obstruction and severe pyelonephritis. In addition, cyclosporin nephrotoxicity can reduce diastolic flow and Doppler appearances can be similar to acute rejection.

Chronic rejection

CLINICAL INFORMATION

Chronic rejection is the usual cause of long-term graft failure. There is no clear definition of the time taken for acute renal failure to become chronic renal failure. There is no cure for this except dialysis and another transplant, if possible.

ULTRASOUND APPEARANCES

After being of normal size initially, the transplanted kidney reduces in size and the renal pyramids increase in echogenicity with subsequent loss of cortico-medullary differentiation. The cortex fibroses and becomes more reflective.

Cyclosporin nephrotoxicity

CLINICAL INFORMATION

Cyclosporin nephrotoxicity is caused by high levels of cyclosporin A in the blood and is seen mostly in the second or third month after transplantation when drug doses are being altered to suit the needs of the patient. This condition is diagnosed when abnormal renal function, raised serum creatinine levels and elevated cyclosporin A levels coincide.

ULTRASOUND APPEARANCES

The appearances of the transplanted kidney are usually normal. A reduction in diastolic flow and a high PI level can suggest cyclosporin nephrotoxicity but they are also seen in other conditions.

Renal vein thrombosis (RVT)

CLINICAL INFORMATION

This is relatively rare (<1–2%) but is a surgical emergency and tends to occur within the first four weeks post transplant. It occurs as a result of kinking of the vein or extrinsic compression or from excess mobility of the graft.

Patients present with little or no production of urine and raised creatinine levels. Early detection of RVT is necessary as the transplant kidney has no collateral veins and there is a risk of venous infarction and rupture. The condition usually requires exploratory surgery.

ULTRASOUND APPEARANCES

Colour flow Doppler will show absence of flow in the renal vein and raised PI or RI in the renal artery with pulsed wave Doppler. When the renal vein is occluded, there is no forward flow in the renal artery in diastole, perhaps even reverse flow, and reduced systolic flow.

Renal artery stenosis (RAS)

CLINICAL INFORMATION

RAS is the most common vascular complication post surgery, developing in up to 12% of transplants and often occurring after the first month post transplant. The stenosis is often at or just distal to the site of anastomosis and is a result of intimal hyperplasia. It is more common in end-to-end anastomoses, hence the preference for end-to-side anastomoses. Acute onset of hypertension and a rise in creatinine often suggest a RAS. Treatment is by percutaneous angioplasty which is successful in opening the stenosis in 90% of cases and normalizing blood pressure in 75%. Surgical repair has a 5% graft loss.

ULTRASOUND APPEARANCES

The structure of the kidney is normal. With a pulsed wave Doppler examination, however, there is damping of systolic flow proximal to the stenosis, an increase in velocity and turbulence across the stenosis in systole and diastole and a reduced distal systolic velocity. The PI is either normal or increased proximal to and at the site of the stenosis and normal or decreased distal to the stenosis.

Fluid collections

CLINICAL INFORMATION

Small collections of fluid around the kidney are normally insignificant and commonly seen after a transplant. Larger collections may compress the kidney, ureter or blood vessels. Fluid collections are normally lymphocoeles but can be urinomas or haematomas.

- Lymphocoeles occur in 5–15% of transplant patients and are the main cause of ureteric obstruction. They usually occur within one year of the transplant and are caused by incomplete ligation of the pelvic lymphatics or after a previous episode of severe rejection. Patients present with a palpable mass, leg pain and oedema and reduced renal function owing to ureteric compression. Most lymphocoeles need no treatment, but can be aspirated percutaneously.

- Urinomas (collections of urine forming after a leak) usually present within three weeks after surgery, usually at the ureterovesicular or ureteroureteric anastomoses.

- Haematomas can occur from trauma during the operation or from a percutaneous biopsy of the transplanted kidney.

- All these fluid collections can become easily infected, as the patient is immunosuppressed, and subsequently form an abscess.

ULTRASOUND APPEARANCES

Fluid collections can grow and cause obstruction. If large enough, they can compress the ureter and dilate the renal pelvis.

- Lymphocoeles grow slowly and are anechoic except for occasional loculations. Urinomas are echo-free collections which may not be seen when small. They enlarge rapidly and can contain internal echoes when infected. Diagnosis is confirmed by aspiration and will show a high creatinine level.

- Haematomas contain echogenic clot. They are often found in subcutaneous tissues or around the operation site. They may have a number of internal echoes and be difficult to differentiate.

- Fluid collections can grow and cause obstruction to the kidney. They can be aspirated under ultrasound control to help form a specific diagnosis. Infected abscesses and lymphocoeles can be drained percutaneously under ultrasound control.

Box 9.17 Advice

A baseline scan performed after the operation is essential in order to monitor change. The bladder must be empty in order to avoid a false diagnosis of hydronephrosis. Some fullness is also usually present and can be ignored if seen during the baseline scan. Ensure that the bladder is not a fluid collection: either void or fill to confirm that the anechoic area is the bladder. If the patient has a fever, look for an abscess at the site where the native kidney lay (the nephrectomy site).

Interventional procedures

Drainage of the obstructed urinary system

If the lower part of the urinary system is obstructed, immediate relief is given by catheterizing the patient, either transurethrally or suprapubically. Small amounts of fluid in the upper urinary tract can be drained by ultrasound-guided puncture. This involves passing a fine (20 or 22) gauge needle under local anaesthetic along the line of the ultrasound beam into the collecting system and withdrawing the fluid. It can then be sent to the laboratory for culture and cytology tests. A drainage catheter and trocar can be inserted in a similar way for percutaneous drainage of larger amounts of fluid within the collecting system.

Transcutaneous renal biopsy

MAIN INDICATIONS

- Nephrotic syndrome.

- Unexplained renal failure.

- Failure to recover from assumed reversible acute renal failure.

CONTRAINDICATIONS

- When the patient has a single kidney only (except in renal transplant).

- Small kidneys.

- Haemorrhagic disorders.

- Uncontrolled hypertension.

PROCEDURE

- Clotting time assessed.

- Serum grouped and saved for crossmatching.

- Explanation to and consent from the patient.

- Patient lies prone, draped over a pillow.

- Kidney (usually the right as its lower position affords better access) is scanned under ultrasound control and the site localized.

- Track of the needle towards the kidney is anaesthetized.

- A sample of cortex is obtained during arrested breathing, thus avoiding damage on entering the renal tissue. Care must be taken not to puncture vessels at the renal hilum.

AFTERCARE

- Dressing applied to the puncture site.
- Bed rest for 24 hours.
- Pulse rate and blood pressure checked regularly.
- Strenuous activity is avoided for two weeks following the biopsy.

POSSIBLE COMPLICATIONS

- About 20% can have haematuria.
- Pain in the flank referred to the shoulder tip.
- Perirenal haematoma.
- Profuse haematuria demanding occlusion of bleeding vessel.
- Infection.
- Mortality rate is about 0.1%.

A concise account of urinary tract interventional procedures performed under ultrasound control has been reported.[3]

References

1. Dalla Palma L, Pozzi-Mucelli R, Magnaldi S, Pozzi-Mucelli F 1988 Diagnostic imaging of renal tumours of small dimensions. Radiol Med 76: 590–596

2. Porena M, Vespasiani G, Rosi P et al 1992 Incidentally detected renal cell carcinoma: role of ultrasonography. J Clin Ultrasound 20: 395–400

3. Crowe PM, Tudway DC, Banerjee AK 1997 Ultrasound assisted intervention in the genitourinary system. BMUS Bull 5: 12

Further reading

Blakeborough A, Irving HC 1995 Ultrasound in the assessment of renal transplants. BMUS Bull 3: 18–24

Broderick NJ 1995 Ultrasound in the investigation of urinary tract infection and vesicoureteric reflux in neonates and children. BMUS Bull 3: 6–17

Chen P, Maklad N, Redwine M 1998 Colour and power Doppler imaging of the kidneys. World J Urol 16: 41–45

Dubbins P 1994 Colour flow Doppler of the renal tract. BMUS Bull 2: 10–14

Mucci B, Macguire B 1994 Does routine ultrasound have a role in the investigation of children with urinary tract infection? Clin Radiol 49: 324–325

Swift S, Weston MJ 1998 Diagnosis of adult urinary tract abnormalities using ultrasound. RAD Magazine 24(281): 37–38

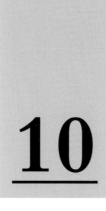

10

THE BLADDER

Anatomy
Scanning
Normal ultrasound appearances
Pathology

Anatomy

The bladder lies in the pelvic cavity posterior to the symphysis pubis. In males it lies anterior to the rectum, in females it lies anterior to the vagina and below and anterior to the uterus. Size depends on the amount of urine present in the bladder. When the bladder fills, it rises up and out of the pelvic cavity. It is not unknown for a bladder in an adult with retention to reach the level of the umbilicus. As the pelvis in children under three is relatively small, the bladder tends to lie intraabdominally even when empty.

The bladder is described as having a base, a superior surface and two inferolateral surfaces. The base faces backwards and downwards and is almost triangular in shape. The apex of the base is relatively fixed and called the neck. It is pierced by the internal urethral orifice and points towards the symphysis pubis. The inside of the bladder is lined by mucous membrane and is thrown into folds when empty except for the trigone, a triangular area which is smooth and does not expand with bladder filling.

The ureters are normally only 8 mm wide and run from the renal pelvis downwards and forwards and enter the bladder inferiorly on the posterolateral surface (see Chapter 9 for fuller description). They open at the upper angles of the trigone inside the bladder. The urethra opens at the apex of the trigone and the passage is controlled by internal and external urinary sphincters. In the male, the urethra runs through the prostate gland situated at the base of the bladder and is joined by ejaculatory and prostatic ducts (Figs 10.1, 10.2).

The shape of the empty bladder is described as pyramidal, as the superior surface is flat, and it becomes almost spherical when full. The average adult bladder can normally hold 400–500 ml but has been known to hold up to 1500 ml.

Blood supply

From branches of the internal iliac arteries.

Blood drainage

Via branches of the internal iliac veins.

Lymph drainage

Mainly via the external iliac lymph glands.

Nerve supply

Bladder control is activated by sympathetic and parasympathetic nerves which are responsible for the emptying reflex.

Relations

MALE

- Anterior – symphysis pubis.
- Superior – peritoneum, small intestine, sigmoid colon.
- Posterior – rectum, vasa deferentia (seminal ducts), seminal vesicles.
- Inferior – prostate and urethra.

FEMALE

- Anterior – symphysis pubis.
- Superior – peritoneum, uterus.
- Posterior – vagina and cervix.
- Inferior – pelvic fascia and urethra.

Palpation

The bladder can be felt with the flat of the hand when full as an easily compressed, rounded mass lying centrally above the symphysis pubis. It is confirmed as being the bladder by the patient when pressure is applied.

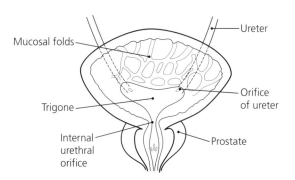

Fig. 10.1 Section of bladder as viewed from the front (male bladder).

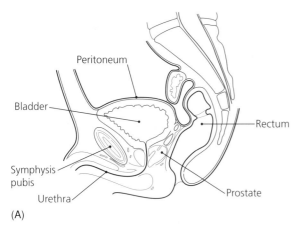

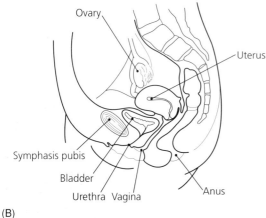

Fig. 10.2 (A) Sagittal section showing position of bladder in the male. (B) Sagittal section showing the position of the bladder in the female.

Scanning

Patient preparation

The bladder must be comfortably full, not over-distended otherwise a false hydronephrosis may appear. Ensure that the bladder is not distended and the patient is not in retention before asking the patient to drink. For an average adult, the fluid regime may be as follows.

- 1–1.5 litres of still, non-milky fluid one hour before the time of the examination. This allows time for the fluid to reach the bladder rather than the scan taking place while the fluid is in loops of bowel, complicating the appearances.

- If the patient is catheterized, the catheter can be clamped and fluid given one hour before the examination. If the bladder becomes too full, the clamp can be released until the patient is comfortable and then clamped again.

- For children, an assessment must be made of the health, size and age of the child before giving any fluid preparation. From >5 years of age, two glasses of squash drunk 30 minutes before the examination may be sufficient to fill the bladder. Infants can drink normally with no special minimum amount.

Equipment required

3.5–5 MHz sector or curved linear transducer, 7.5 MHz for babies. Suprapubic transabdominal ultrasound scanning using the above transducer is ideal for all assessments.

Suggested scanning technique

The TGC and overall gain must be adjusted so that anterior bladder wall reverberations are eliminated. Place the transducer longitudinally in the midline just above the symphysis pubis. From the midline, carefully scan longitudinally, moving from left to right so that the borders and contents of the bladder are observed. Turn the probe transversely and again, observing the borders and contents of the bladder, scan from the base of the bladder down towards the apex, observing an enlarged prostate if one is present (see Chapter 11), bladder wall thickness and contour.

The lower ureters can be seen in the bladder wall by scanning obliquely along the area of the trigone and angling laterally.

Suggested minimal sections

- For bladder volume estimation, the largest pre- and postmicturition (if residual urine is present) longitudinal and transverse sections must be taken.

- Two sections must be taken through any pathology with measurements and sections demonstrating the extent of pathology/focal wall thickening.

- In addition, a transverse section showing ureteric insertion and urine jets, if visible, should be taken.

Normal ultrasound appearances

BLADDER

The normal distended urinary bladder appears in longitudinal section as an almost triangular, anechoic structure and is approximately rectangular in cross-section. It is surrounded by an echogenic structure that represents the bladder wall. The ureteric orifices appear as small thickened areas at the base of the bladder and urine flowing into the bladder is frequently seen on real time as small jets entering the bladder with ureteric peristalsis. This appearance is apparently due to the difference in specific gravity between bladder and ureteric urine. It is often seen after patients have been given large quantities of fluid to drink. The average jet travels 3–5 cm and is seen on average 2–4 times per minute.

UTERERS

All that is usually seen of the ureters is a small length proximally and the entrance into the bladder distally, owing to the fact that they lie in front of the psoas muscles but behind gas-filled intestines. The normal lower ureter can sometimes be seen within the bladder wall (Fig. 10.3).

Normal sizes

When distended, the wall is smooth and thin, its thickness measuring approximately 2–3 mm in the adult and 5 mm when the bladder is empty. The bladder thickness measures proportionally more in infants.

Box 10.1   Advice

Large ovarian cysts and hydrocoeles have been mistaken for bladders. Large diverticula of the bladder can be conversely mistaken for ovarian cysts or other cystic pathology.

Bladder volume estimation

Several ways have been described in the literature for measuring the bladder volume and several ways are used by imaging departments at this time. One method, described by *Poston et al* and evaluated by *Kiely et al*, calculated the bladder volume using:

maximum length in sagittal plane × AP depth in sagittal plane × maximum width in transverse section × 0.7 ml (Fig. 10.4).[1,2]

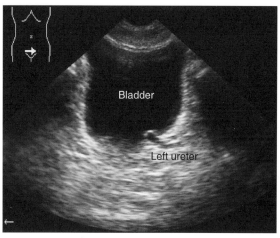

(A)

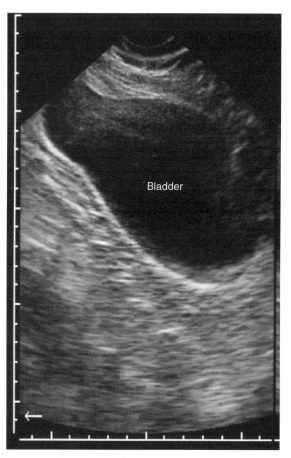

(B)

Fig. 10.3 Ultrasound appearances of the bladder and lower ureters. (A) Transverse and (B) longitudinal sections.

NB: Some centres measure both the AP depth and width on the transverse section.

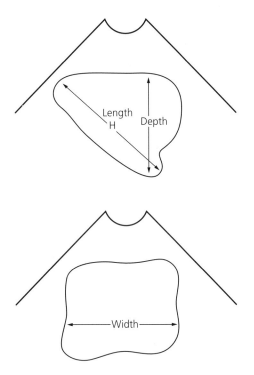

Fig. 10.4 Calculating bladder volume.

Measurements are taken before and after micturition, although some urologists only require postmicturition volumes to be estimated if significant. The above formula assumes that all bladders are the same shape and that they retain the same shape at different volumes, which they do not. Bladder shapes have been classified as cuboidal, ellipsoid or triangular prism. Therefore allowances have to be made regarding the accuracy of the exercise, especially where a monitoring series of scans is carried out.

In Kiely *et al*'s study of 34 bladder volumes, there was a wide range of errors (52% overestimation to 29% underestimation) and the method for estimating bladder volume was considered unsatisfactory. Bih *et al* (1998) suggested that the volume could be more easily calculated by using a correction coefficient for each type of bladder shape.[3] Whichever method of calculation is used, the accuracy is still considered unsatisfactory.

Ultrasound urodynamics

This is frequently requested, mostly in conjunction with the effects caused by the enlarged prostate in older men.

A uroflow examination demonstrates the maximum flow rate, the average flow rate, the amount of urine passed, the time taken to void urine and the time taken to reach the greatest flow rate.

There should be more than 200 ml urine in the bladder before measuring and voiding otherwise the results are inaccurate; voided volumes of less than this are considered to have little clinical relevance and smaller volumes adversely affect flow rate. Bladders that are overfull often inhibit micturition. After the full bladder is scanned, observed and measured, the patient urinates into a flow rate machine after being asked not to strain. The flow rate meter starts automatically from the first drop of urine passed. When the flow is finished, the patient is then scanned again to measure the residual volume. Patients having more than 100 ml residual urine are asked to void again and the residual volume measurement is taken once more. The normal maximum flow rate is between 30 and 50 ml/s. Over the age of 60, the peak flow may be only around 18 ml/s.

SUGGESTED PROTOCOL FOR ULTRASOUND URODYNAMICS IN MALE PATIENT

- Scan and measure bladder as described when full. If <200 ml, give patient more to drink, then rescan.

- Scan and measure prostate (see relevant section).

- Send patient for ultrasound cystodynamogram (uroflow).

- Scan bladder and measure residual volume if present. If residual volume is more than 100 ml, send patient to empty his bladder again.

- Scan kidneys; voiding the bladder before scanning the kidneys reduces the chance of false hydronephrosis from an overfull bladder and makes the rest of the examination more comfortable for the patient (Fig. 10.5).

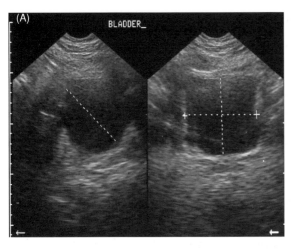

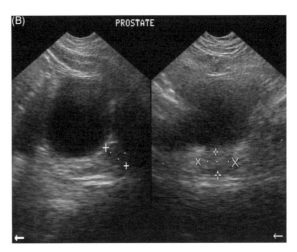

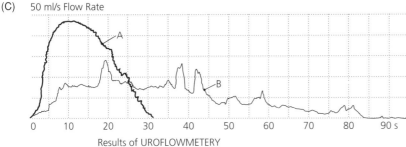

(C) 50 ml/s Flow Rate

Results of UROFLOWMETERY

Examples of:
A = normal flow
B = impaired flow

Voiding Time	T100	s
Flow Time	TQ	s
Time to Max Flow	TQmax	s
Max Flow Rate	Qmax	ml/s
Average Flow Rate	Qave	ml/s
Voided Volume	Vcomp	ml

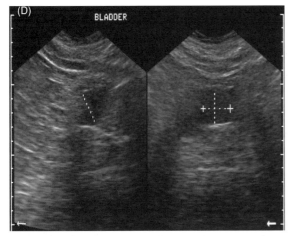

Fig. 10.5 Sequence of urodynamic examination. (A) Calculate bladder volume. (B) Measure prostate. (C) Uroflow meter. (D) Measure residual volume.

Box 10.2   Advice

Scan the aorta in men over 50 to exclude abdominal aortic aneurysm as this condition affects males of approximately the same age range and may not have been previously detected. Observe the prostate for general shape and texture and measure the size.

Pathology

- Bladder cancer
- Polyps
- Bladder calculi
- Foreign bodies

- Diverticulum
- Trauma
- Ureterocoeles
- Posterior urethral valves
- Ectopia vesicae
- Cystitis

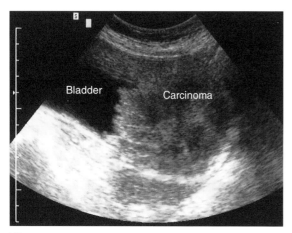

(A)

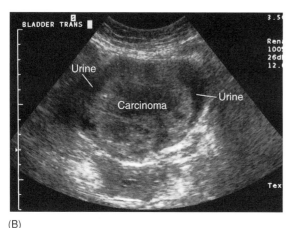

(B)

Fig. 10.6 Transitional carcinoma of bladder. (A) Longitudinal and (B) transverse.

Bladder cancer

CLINICAL INFORMATION

Bladder cancer (urothelial malignancy) is four times more common in men than in women. Ninety percent

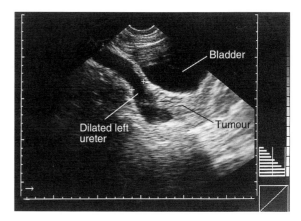

Fig. 10.7 Tumour at lower end of left ureter.

of bladder malignancies are transitional cell carcinomas, the remaining 10% being squamous or adeno-carcinomas. Transitional cell carcinomas are most common in men but are also found in women. They grow slowly, spreading by direct invasion at first and then by lymph node spread. The majority of transitional cell tumours have a papillary growth pattern and appear like a fronded, cauliflower-shaped lesion.

The patient presents with frequency, dysuria and often haematuria. Diagnosis is confirmed by abnormal urine cytology or by biopsy. Fifty percent of these malignancies will spread within three years and of those with malignant spread, there is only a 6–23% five-year survival rate compared to a 50–80% survival rate for those with localized malignancy. Transitional cell carcinomas are often the result of exposure to occupational or other carcinogens such as cigarette smoking, dyes and rubber, such as in car tyre production.

ULTRASOUND APPEARANCES

Bladder tumours are seen as masses intruding into the bladder lumen. Non-invasive tumours tend to be well bounded and do not deform the bladder wall. Those that spread into the wall of the bladder are usually seen as irregular, hypoechoic masses breaking up the usual smooth contour of the bladder wall. Solid tumour is difficult to differentiate from chronic cystitis and bladder wall oedema as a result of long-term catheterization (Figs 10.6, 10.7).

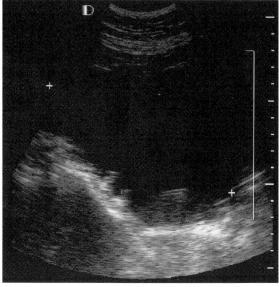

(A)

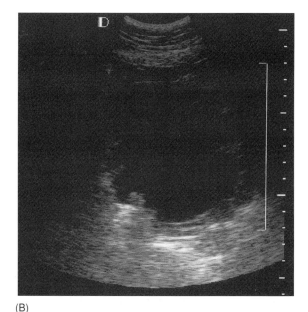

(B)

Fig. 10.8 (A) Longitudinal and (B) transverse sections through a bladder created from section of colon.

Box 10.3 Advice

Poor gain settings in the bladder region can mask small bladder wall tumours. Turn the gain settings down and avoid too many sound and reverberation artefacts.

If tumour is seen, look for tumour in kidneys and other evidence of malignant spread.

A consequence of a history of bladder malignancy is that the bladder (and the prostate in vesicoprostatectomies) may have been removed and a replacement bladder fashioned from a section of the large bowel. The internal folds give an unusual appearance of a bladder with irregular focal wall masses or trabeculation (Fig. 10.8).

Polyps

CLINICAL INFORMATION

There are various types of polyps ranging from benign outpouchings (hamartomatous polyps) to gland-like (adenomatous polyps) to those that are premalignant (dysplastic polyps). Polyps are seen incidentally or cause patients to present with painless haematuria. Cystoscopy is usually recommended as a further investigation.

ULTRASOUND APPEARANCES

Bladder polyps can appear as small tumours adherent to the bladder wall. They can be of higher echogenicity than the bladder wall and can be seen occasionally on a small stalk with posterior reverberation artefact (Fig. 10.9).

Bladder calculi

CLINICAL INFORMATION

Bladder calculi are often found in cases of urinary stasis following the patient's inability to empty the bladder completely. They are often seen, therefore, accompanying bladder diverticula (see below) or as a result of an enlarged prostate. They can be single or multiple and, owing to the urine acidity, are usually smooth in shape.

ULTRASOUND APPEARANCES

Bladder calculi appear as mobile, echogenic masses within the bladder lumen that move with change in posture and cast posterior acoustic shadows.

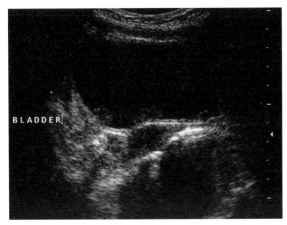

(A)

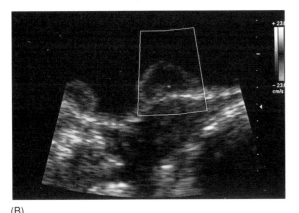

(B)

Fig. 10.9 (A) Transverse section of bladder showing bladder polyps. (B) Enlarged detail of polyp.

As stones are associated with outflow obstruction, assess the kidneys for stones or an obstructive picture and examine the prostate at the time of the scan. The bladder muscle is often trabeculated in cases of long-term distension.

Foreign bodies

CLINICAL INFORMATION

For reasons known only to themselves, people insert objects into orifices. The urethra is no exception and there have been reports of nails, pins, ball point pen refills, feathers, etc., etc., etc. being found in the bladder.

ULTRASOUND APPEARANCES

Foreign bodies are usually of a relatively hyperechoic shape with some distal shadowing. As the patient may be under investigation for urinary tract obstruction or haematuria as a result of the foreign body insertion, this may be an unexpected finding.

Diverticulum

CLINICAL INFORMATION

A bladder diverticulum is an acquired or congenital, thin-walled herniation of the bladder wall mucosa between the bundles of detrusor muscle. It often occurs as a result of long-standing outflow obstruction or neurogenic bladder. It can be variable in size and, as it contains little muscle in the wall, it can increase in size during the action of micturition as the normal outflow is reduced. Eighty-five percent lie lateral and superior to the ureteric insertion; 5% are associated with a transitional cell tumour.

ULTRASOUND APPEARANCES

Diverticula are seen as anechoic, fluid-filled structures in close proximity to the bladder. They can contain debris, blood clot or stones.

Box 10.4   Advice

Bladder tumours can calcify, become encrusted with calcium salts and superficially appear similar to stones but of course are fixed in position. Move the patient to confirm mobility.

Blood clot and small foreign bodies can also appear similar to stones. Read the patient's history in the notes first and ensure that the kidneys and prostate are examined carefully if there is the possibility that it could be a blood clot from a tumour.

Box 10.5   Advice

Ovarian cysts or ascites can be mistaken for a diverticulum.

Trauma

CLINICAL INFORMATION

Trauma to the bladder is more common in children than in adults and can be caused by blunt abdominal trauma, pelvic fracture as a result of a road traffic accident or a penetrating injury.

ULTRASOUND APPEARANCES

Fluid may be seen around the external area of the bladder or within the peritoneum.

Ureterocoeles

CLINICAL INFORMATION

A ureterocoele is a dilated part of the distal ureter that has pushed through into the lumen of the bladder at the vesicoureteric junction. There is often a stenosis of the distal ureter that causes this dilatation. Ureterocoeles can form in other places, usually where there is an ectopic insertion of a double ureter or a ureter from the upper moiety of a duplex kidney into the bladder.

ULTRASOUND APPEARANCES

A ureterocoele is seen as an anechoic rounded structure with a thin wall protruding into the bladder. It is often described as a 'cobra-head deformity' owing to its shape or as a cyst within a cyst and is seen as being continuous with the dilated ureter (Fig. 10.10).

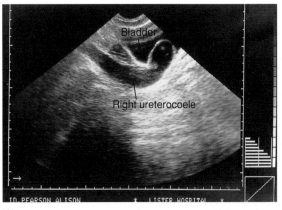

(A)

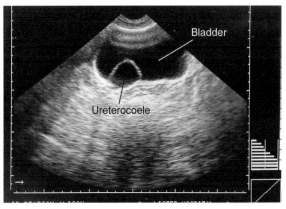

(B)

Fig. 10.10 Right-sided ureterocoele. (A) Longitudinal section and (B) transverse section showing ureterocoele within bladder.

> ### Box 10.6 Advice
>
> Ureterocoeles are often associated with a dilated upper urinary tract and especially with the upper half of a duplex collecting system so a careful scan of the kidneys should be made to exclude full or partial obstruction. Observation of the ureteric jets should be made by colour Doppler or B-mode to exclude stenosis (see Fig. 2.13 in chapter 2).

Posterior urethral valves

CLINICAL INFORMATION

Bladder outflow obstruction caused by urethral valves causes distension of the posterior urethra. This is the most common form of obstruction to the lower urinary tract in boys but is very rare in girls. This condition can cause renal dysplasia (see Chapter 9).

ULTRASOUND APPEARANCES

Attention is often drawn to obstruction of the bladder during antenal scans. Posterior urethral valves can cause the bladder wall to become thicker than normal (often more than 5 mm thick) and the upper urinary tract to be dilated. The posterior urethra appears as a thin anechoic structure distal to the base of the bladder. It is only seen in 50% of cases when the bladder is scanned at rest and scanning during micturition would be required to see the dilated urethra clearly.

The appearance of the kidneys accompanying this condition is described in Chapter 9 but the appearances can range from severe hydronephrosis and dysplasia to near normal.

Ectopia vesicae

CLINICAL INFORMATION

This congenital abnormality in which the bladder opens out onto the anterior abdominal wall is usually detected antenatally and repaired soon after birth. The role of ultrasound prior to the repair is to confirm the presence and normality of the kidneys. Postoperatively when the bladder has been resited within the abdomen and the anterior abdominal wall sewn up, ultrasound is used to exclude any complications such as a hydronephrosis due to kinking of the ureters.

Box 10.7   Advice

Ensure that the risk of infection is kept to an absolute minimum by the use of sterile coupling gel and correct technique.

Cystitis

CLINICAL INFORMATION

Inflammation of the bladder can be caused by radiation therapy, drugs, infection or trauma from surgery or from the presence of a urinary catheter. It is common in pregnancy and in males presents secondary to prostatic obstruction or urethral stricture. Infection in the non-obstructive state is usually caused by *E. coli* and in the obstructive state by Proteus and Staphylococcus.

In 20–30% of children with proven urinary tract infections, vesicoureteric reflux is found. Radiographic micturating cystograms are often performed during the work-up of investigations.

ULTRASOUND APPEARANCES

The bladder will often appear normal but can have a significantly thicker wall due to oedema.

Box 10.8   Advice

Bladder ultrasound should be combined with flow rate measurement and a post micturition scan to assess bladder emptying.

Urinary catheters

ULTRASOUND APPEARANCES

Urinary catheters such as a Foley balloon catheter can be seen easily with ultrasound as long as the catheter has been clamped and the bladder is adequately filled. The high reflectivity of the walls of the catheter and

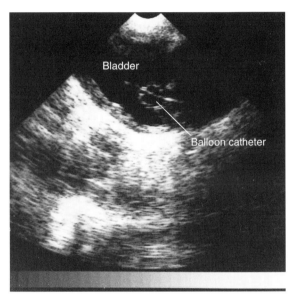

(A)

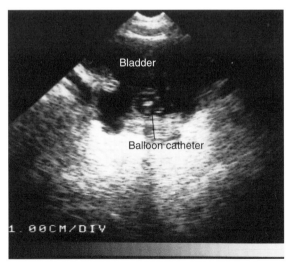

(B)

Fig. 10.11   (A) Balloon catheter in longitudinal and (B) transverse section.

the outline of the balloon can be seen in transverse and longitudinal sections in contrast to the anechoic urine. Visualizing the catheter can help in positioning or assessing a non–emptying catheter (Fig. 10.11).

Ultrasound is valuable in the assessment and guidance of a suprapubic catheter insertion when the patient is obese and it is difficult to palpate the bladder to find a site for insertion or assess the amount of urine in the bladder.

References

1. Poston GJ, Joseph AEA, Riddle PR 1983 The accuracy of ultrasound in the measurement of changes in bladder volume. Br J Urol 55: 361–363

2. Kiely E, Hartnell GG, Gibson RN, Williams G 1987 Measurement of bladder volume by real-time ultrasound. Br J Urol 60: 33–35

3. Bih LI, Ho CC, Tsai SJ, Lai YC, Chow W 1998 Bladder shape impact on the accuracy of ultrasonic estimation of bladder volume. Arch Phys Med Rehabil 79: 1553–1556

11

PROSTATE

Anatomy
Scanning
Normal ultrasound appearances
Pathology
Focal disease
Diffuse disease

The prostate is a male accessory sex gland that opens into the urethra just below the bladder. It normally measures $3 \times 2.5 \times 3.5$ cm.

During ejaculation it secretes an alkaline fluid that forms part of the semen.

Anatomy

The prostate is a chestnut-shaped gland which lies at the base of the bladder behind the symphysis pubis and surrounds the first part of the urethra. It has a base facing upwards and an apex facing down. It is covered with an outer capsule of fibrous tissue. Ducts from the glandular portion of the prostate open into the prostatic urethra (Figs 11.1, 11.2).

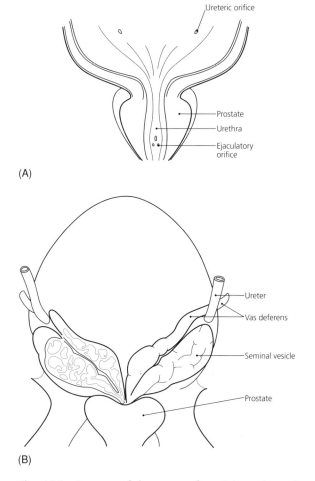

(A)

(B)

Fig. 11.1 Anatomy of the prostate from (A) anterior and (B) posterior aspects.

Blood supply

From the inferior vesicular artery, a branch of the internal iliac artery.

Blood drainage

Into the prostatic plexus of veins circling the prostate and then into the internal iliac veins.

Lymph drainage

Into the internal and external iliac and sacral lymph nodes.

Nerve supply

The prostate is supplied by the prostatic plexus that branches off from the hypogastric plexus.

Palpation

Digitally per rectum. The dorsal surface of the prostate can be felt and its approximate size and smoothness or lumpiness assessed.

Relevant tests – normal values

The PSA (prostate-specific antigen) test is offered after an abnormal digital examination. Please note: there can be a difference of 30% between tests as several PSA tests are used. There is no standardisation at present. It is possible to have a raised PSA level with a normal prostate and vice versa. The significance of the raised RSA level depends on the type of PSA in the blood, the prostatic size (PSA density = RSA value/prostate volume), the PSA velocity (= change of levels over a period of time), the man's age and whether ejaculation has occurred within the last 24 hours.[1]

Hybritech test	0–4 ng/ml
Acid phosphatase	1–5 U/l
Alkaline phosphatase	25–115 U/l

Scanning

Patient preparation

For transabdominal examinations of the prostate, the patient is required to have a sufficiently full bladder,

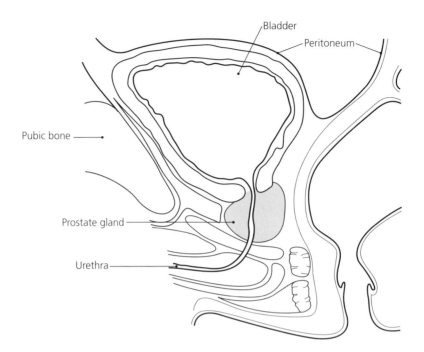

Fig. 11.2   Sagittal section through bladder and prostate.

bearing in mind, though, that the reason for the scan often causes difficulty in emptying the bladder. In other words, do not expect the patient to drink much if the bladder is often quite full anyway. Ensure that sufficient coupling gel is applied to the suprapubic area.

Equipment required

A 3.5–5 MHz sector transducer is better than a curved linear transducer for acute suprapubic caudal angling.

Suggested scanning technique

Transabdominal and transperineal approaches to scanning the prostate only will be mentioned. There are several descriptions of transrectal prostatic scanning available.[2–4]

TRANSABDOMINAL SCANNING

Ensuring that the bladder is sufficiently full in order to act as an acoustic window, place the probe on the lower part of the patient's abdomen and scan longitudinally in the midline with the probe angled down towards the feet. It may be necessary to press slightly but not uncomfortably on the bladder in order to

obtain the best images. Measure the length and thickness in this section then turn the probe around 90° and angle down towards the feet. Obtain an image of the greatest width and measure the width.

TRANSPERINEAL SCANNING

If the bladder cannot be sufficiently filled, this approach can be used. The patient should remove his underpants and a towel used to lift the scrotum and penis up and out of the way. The patient is asked to lie with his legs apart. The probe is placed between the legs posterior to the scrotum and angled up and down and to left and right sides in order to visualize the whole gland. Transverse and longitudinal images should be measured in order to obtain a volume calculation.

Practically, in order to obtain a transverse section of the prostate in this way, the transducer needs to be held upside down and the image inverted as most transducers are too large to allow the cable and connection to be positioned between the patient's perineum and the top of the couch unless a specialized couch with lithotomy stirrups is used. The latter is not practical or desired considering the age of most of these patients.

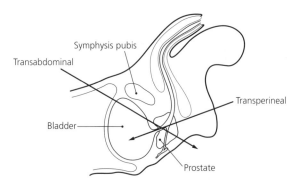

Fig. 11.3 Scanning planes – transabdominal and transperineal.

Ensure that the correct right–left orientation is set when the image is inverted (Fig. 11.3).

Suggested minimal sections

Transverse and longitudinal sections of the largest dimensions of the prostate in these sections, any invasion into the bladder wall and protrusion of the hypertrophic gland into the urine-filled bladder. Sections showing effect of prostatic pathology such as a dilated upper urinary tract.

Normal ultrasound appearances

The normal prostate should appear as a small, rounded, homogeneous structure containing low to mid-level echoes at the base of the bladder surrounded by a thin, echogenic capsule (Fig. 11.4).

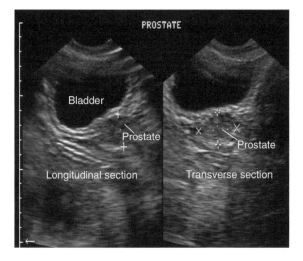

Fig. 11.4 The normal prostate (transabdominal scan).

Normal sizes

The adult prostate normally measures approximately $3 \times 2.5 \times 3.5\,\text{cm}$.

Volume of prostate

This can be estimated using the measurements obtained.

$$\frac{(L \times W \times T)}{2}$$

where L = length, W = width of transverse diameter, T = thickness or anteroposterior measurement (Fig. 11.5).

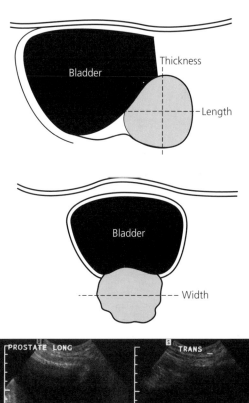

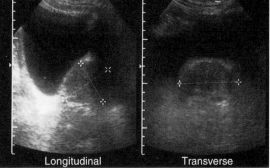

Fig. 11.5 Measuring the prostate.

The normal volume of the prostate is <20 g.

As the specific gravity of the prostate is 1, a direct translation of volume to grams can be made.

Box 11.1   Advice

An irregularly shaped prostate may be mistaken for a bladder tumour. A careful scan in the longitudinal position should exclude a tumour.

Seminal vesicles are best seen on a transverse scan.

NB: Transabdominal scans of the prostate are made only for an estimation of size and contour. A close examination of the prostate requires a transrectal scan.

Pathology

Focal:

- carcinoma of the prostate
- benign prostatic hyperplasia or hypertrophy
- abscess
- cyst
- calculi

Diffuse:

- prostatitis

Focal disease

Carcinoma

CLINICAL INFORMATION

Prostate cancer is the sixth most common malignancy in the UK, the fifth most common cause of male death and the second most common cause of death from cancer in males in the USA. It is rarely seen before the age of 55 but its prevalence increases after that. The most common type is the adenocarcinoma but squamous cell and transitional cell carcinomas are also seen.

Cancer spreads directly from the prostate to the pelviprostatic tissue and via the lymphatic system where it invades the pelvic nodes and subsequently the abdominal chain. There can be retrograde spread to the vertebral veins and so vertebral metastases are common. Pelvic and femoral bony metastases can also occur.

As cancer usually originates in the periphery of the prostate, the disease is often well established by the time any symptoms such as difficulty with micturition present. The first sign may result after compression of the spinal cord from a vertebral metastasis. Rectal examination may reveal a hard, irregular gland. Acid phosphatase levels rise and if bony metastases are present, alkaline phosphatase levels rise also. Many carcinomas rely on testosterone for growth and so the condition is treated by either orchidectomy or oestrogenic drugs.

ULTRASOUND APPEARANCES

Typical prostatic cancers seen on a transabdominal scan are hypoechoic, although 15–20% are isoechoic or hyperechoic compared to the normal tissue. The majority (>70%) are seen in the periphery of the gland. Areas of low reflectivity are commonly seen in the central zone and are usually not significant, usually being focal areas of inflammation. Most predominantly echo-poor areas situated in the peripheral zone are proven to be carcinoma. An irregular outline often signifies invasion of the prostatic capsule. The malignant potential of prostate carcinoma correlates with the tumour size: tumours >1.5 cm in diameter are more

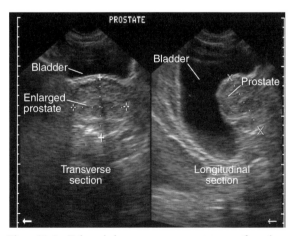

Fig. 11.6 Enlarged heterogeneous prostate confirmed at biopsy to be carcinoma.

liable to metastasize. Hypertrophy of the gland often accompanies a carcinoma (Fig. 11.6).

Box 11.2 Advice

If a prostatic mass is seen that could possibly be a carcinoma, examine the paraaortic area for enlarged lymph nodes.

If the prostatic mass is large, examine the renal tract for any evidence of obstruction.

Seminal vesicles can be confused with prostatic tissue but they lie lateral and slightly superior to the prostate. The fact that they are bilateral structures is easily confirmed on a transverse scan.

Benign prostatic hyperplasia

CLINICAL INFORMATION

Benign prostatic hyperplasia (BPH) is the most common disorder of the prostate as it increases in size in the middle-aged and elderly. BPH is less common in Africans and Asians, is unknown in eunuchs and does not occur in patients suffering from hepatic cirrhosis. The prostate enlarges within the central zone and tends to increase the anteroposterior dimension of the gland, changing its shape from chestnut to more spherical but it often appears asymmetrical. The enlarged prostate may reach up to 100 g in weight. BPH stretches and distorts the urethra, obstructing the outflow of urine. In order to overcome the obstruction, the pressure within the bladder must be higher than usual in order to micturate. This can result in a dilated and hypotonic bladder with reflux of urine. The bladder muscle can become trabeculated.

Patients present with frequency, nocturia, difficulty in micturating, delay in commencing micturition, reduced force of the urinary stream and post-micturition dribbling. Pain in the region of the bladder may arise from bacteria or from the formation of bladder calculi. Flank pain can be caused by a dilated upper urinary tract.

ULTRASOUND APPEARANCES

The enlarged prostate is usually seen indenting the bladder at its base. It is often seen, especially when grossly enlarged, as a homogeneous, rounded structure

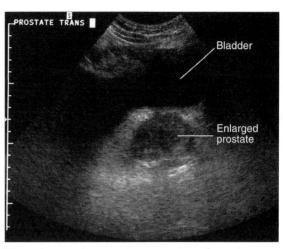

(A)

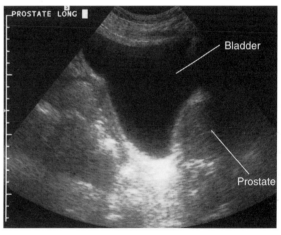

(B)

Fig. 11.7   Benign prostatic hypertrophy. (A) Longitudinal and (B) transverse sections.

with mid-grey echoes at the base of an enlarged bladder with possible bilateral hydronephrotic kidneys seen after chronic or acute retention (Fig. 11.7).

Box 11.3 Advice

After surgical treatment by means of a transurethral resection of the prostate (TURP), there is usually a U-shaped defect seen at the bladder where the urethra enters the prostate.

Prostatic abscess

ULTRASOUND APPEARANCES

The prostatic abscess is seen as a cystic area within the central zone containing low-level echoes.

Prostatic cyst

CLINICAL INFORMATION

These are rare and usually symptomless although they can result in urinary retention if large enough.

ULTRASOUND APPEARANCES

A prostatic cyst will appear as a rounded, echo-poor structure, usually within the central zone, with some distal acoustic enhancement.

Prostatic calculi

CLINICAL INFORMATION

Prostatic calculi have no clinical significance except that, on digital examination, they can feel hard like a neoplasm if large enough.

ULTRASOUND APPEARANCES

Calculi are seen as high-level echoes within the prostate. There may be evidence of acoustic shadowing but not always. They are typically described as being formed in a wing-like pattern and are found between the central and peripheral zones or within the length of the urethra.

Diffuse disease

Prostatitis

CLINICAL INFORMATION

An inflamed prostate is tender on examination, enlarged and soft on palpation.

ULTRASOUND APPEARANCES

With acute prostatitis, the prostate becomes enlarged, although not always, and the normal shape changes. The capsule becomes less distinct than normal and hypoechoic areas can be seen within the gland. Calculi, if present, show as echogenic foci. After treatment, the prostate usually returns to normal in size and shape but the echo-poor areas often remain for some time. With chronic prostatitis, the echo pattern is often heterogeneous and of relatively high echogenicity with calculi situated around the periphery and posterior to the urethra.

Box 11.4   Advice

The patchy areas of low reflectivity may be mistaken for malignancies.

References

1. Herschman JD, Smith DS, Catalona WJ 1997 Effect of ejaculation on serum total and free prostate-specific antigen concentrations. Urology Aug: 50(2): 239–43

2. Rickards D, Garber S 1993 The lower urinary tract. In: Cosgrove D, Meire H, Dewbury K (eds) Abdominal and general ultrasound, vol 2. Churchill Livingstone, Edinburgh, pp. 543–569

3. Rickards D 1993 Transrectal ultrasound: current applications. BMUS Bull 1: 25–28

4. Carey BM 1996 Prostate ultrasound. RAD Magazine 22: 29–30

12

THE ADRENAL GLANDS

Main functions
Anatomy
Scanning
Normal ultrasound appearances
Pathology

The adrenal or suprarenal glands are two small, flat, brownish-yellow, endocrine organs situated in close contact with the upper pole of both kidneys. They lie in the retroperitoneum and consist of an outer cortex (90% of the gland), composed of three layers of cells, and a reddish medulla (10% of the gland), composed of chromaffin cells which are derived from the sympathetic nervous system. In the adult, the adrenal glands are about one-thirteenth of the size of the associated kidneys; in the neonate, they are about one-third of the size.

Main functions

The adrenal cortex secretes:

- glucocorticoids (the major one being hydrocortisone [cortisol])
- mineralocorticoid (aldosterone)
- sex hormones (androgens and oestrogens).

The adrenal medulla secretes adrenaline (epinephrine) 80% and noradrenaline (norepinephrine) 20%. Epinephrine acts on the nerve endings of the sympathetic nervous system and prepares the body to meet a situation of excitement or stress. It increases the heart rate, dilates skeletal and cardiac vessels, constricts vessels of skin and intestines, decreases gastric and intestinal motility, dilates the pupil, relaxes the muscle of the bladder, stimulates sweating and dilates the bronchi.

Norepinephrine is not completely understood but is connected with the raising of blood pressure.

Production of hydrocortisone and androgens is controlled by adrenocorticotrophic hormone (ACTH) secreted by the pituitary gland; aldosterone is controlled by the production of renin from the kidneys.

Anatomy

The adult adrenal glands are approximately 3–5 cm long, 2–3 cm wide and 2–6 mm thick. The right gland is almost pyramidal in shape and is smaller and lies more inferiorly than the left gland which is crescentic in shape. The adrenal glands have an anteromedial ridge with a lateral and medial wing extending posteriorly. These wings straddle the anteromedial aspect of the upper pole of the kidneys.

Combined, the two glands weigh between 7 and 20 g, usually 5–8 g each. They are surrounded by fatty areolar tissue and lie within tight, fibrous capsules. Small accessory glands can be found surrounding the main glands. The adrenal glands must be described separately owing to their different positions and shapes.

Right adrenal gland

The right adrenal gland is pyramidal in shape and lies against and behind the IVC and in front of the upper pole of the right kidney and right hemidiaphragm. Part of the anterior surface is in contact with the bare area of the liver and causes an impression on its posterior surface. The superior part of the posterior surface is attached to the hemidiaphragm, the crus of the diaphragm lying medial to the adrenal gland.

Left adrenal gland

The left adrenal gland is crescent shaped and lies between the spleen, the upper pole of the left kidney and the aorta and behind the tail of the pancreas. Its concave surface is attached to the upper pole of the left kidney and it extends almost to the renal hilum. The upper anterior part of the gland is in contact with the stomach and the lower anterior part with the pancreas and splenic artery. The posterior surface of the left adrenal gland rests against the left crus of the diaphragm and laterally against the left kidney.

The right adrenal gland is more difficult to remove at surgery because of its position behind the liver and because the short adrenal vein and even the IVC itself can be lacerated.

Blood supply

The adrenal glands are usually supplied by three substantial arteries:

- superior adrenal artery originating from the inferior phrenic artery
- middle adrenal artery branching from the aorta
- inferior adrenal artery originating from the renal artery.

The arteries branch before entering the gland (Fig. 12.2).

Blood drainage

One central adrenal vein drains the gland. The short right adrenal vein runs medially to drain into the IVC.

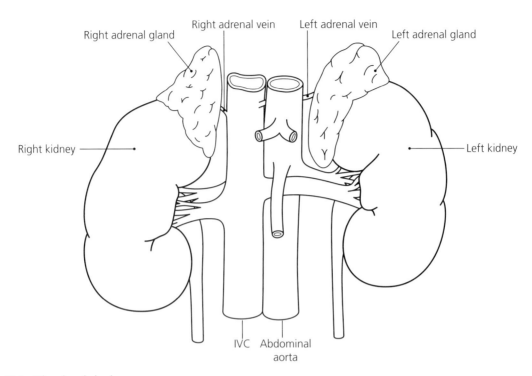

Fig. 12.1 The adrenal glands.

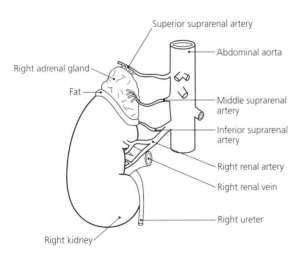

Fig. 12.2 Blood supply to the adrenal gland.

The left adrenal vein is longer and either joins the left inferior phrenic vein, which then enters the IVC, or empties directly into the IVC.

Lymph drainage

Lymph is drained along the path of the adrenal veins to the highest nodes of the lumbar chain.

Nerve supply

The nerve supply is mostly from preganglionic sympathetic fibres, derived from the splanchnic nerves. They pass through the cortex and innervate the medulla only.

Relevant tests – normal values

Plasma cortisol	0.15–0.7 µmol/l
Blood electrolyte levels:	
Potassium [K⁺]	3.5–5.0 µmol/l
Sodium [Na²⁺]	135–145 mmol/l

Scanning

Patient preparation

The normal upper abdominal preparation is suggested in order to reduce food artefacts and intestinal gas. Patients should practise holding their breath to avoid the image blurring during breathing.

Equipment required

As the position of the adrenal glands requires intercostal scanning, the transducer must have a small footprint and a compromise should be made between the highest possible frequency and the amount of penetration required to scan the subject. The appropriate focal zone should be chosen.

Suggested scanning technique

The right adrenal gland should ideally be seen in 80–90% of patients, the left seen in 60–75%, this being reduced because of the proximity of stomach and bowel gas. Adrenal glands are seen less often in the elderly. Because of the small size of the structures, the field size should be enlarged.

RIGHT ADRENAL GLAND

The patient should lie supine. Using the liver as an acoustic window, the transducer should be placed in the ninth or 10th intercostal space in the anterolateral aspect and positioned transversely. Angle the transducer towards the head, moving upwards from the renal hilum as far as 2–3 cm above the kidney. Observe the region posterior to the IVC and lateral to the right crus of the diaphragm. The upper part of the gland is shown as a linear or curved linear structure, the middle part as an inverted V or Y shape and the inferior part as a horizontal band.

The transducer should then be turned 90°. Find the upper pole of the right kidney and angle medially. Look for a Y- or V-shaped structure posterior to the IVC (Fig. 12.3).

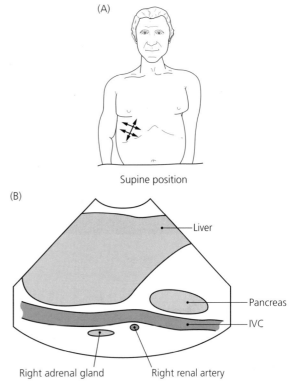

(A)

Supine position

(B)

Liver

Pancreas

IVC

Right adrenal gland   Right renal artery

Fig. 12.3 (A) Positioning for the right adrenal gland. (B) Section showing right adrenal gland.

LEFT ADRENAL GLAND

The left adrenal gland is more difficult to scan than the right. It is considered that the best position for the patient is in the RLD position and the optimum scanning plane is the longitudinal plane.

Scan longitudinally with the transducer in the intercostal space where the spleen and the upper pole of the left kidney can be seen, usually in the eighth or ninth intercostal space. The approach must be sufficiently posterolateral to avoid gas in the stomach or intestine. Angle the transducer until the aorta is seen longitudinally. The normal left adrenal gland can be seen as a triangular or V-shaped area when the spleen, upper pole of left kidney and aorta can be seen at the same time. It should have straight or slightly concave edges. The transverse section is then obtained by rotating the transducer through 90° (Fig. 12.4).

(A)

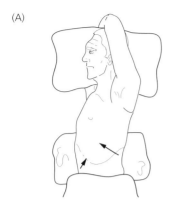

Right lateral decubitus position

(B)

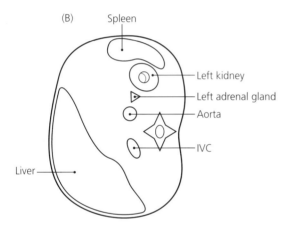

Spleen

Left kidney

Left adrenal gland

Aorta

IVC

Liver

(C)

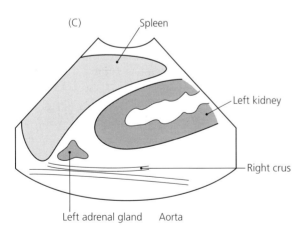

Spleen

Left kidney

Right crus

Left adrenal gland   Aorta

Fig. 12.4 (A) Positioning for the left adrenal gland. (B) Direction of sound when demonstrating left adrenal gland. (C) Section showing left adrenal gland.

Normal ultrasound appearances

The edges of the adrenal gland should be straight or concave. The cortex is hypoechogenic while the medulla is seen as being of slightly higher echogenicity within the cortex. The whole of the gland should be examined as small masses can affect only a part of the gland, leaving the rest normal in appearance.

The neonatal adrenal gland is easily seen as it is proportionately larger than that of the adult and there is less perirenal fat in the neonate. Because of the subject's smaller size, a higher frequency can be used. It has an echo-poor cortex and reflective medulla. At 5–6 months, the gland becomes smaller and by one year old, the gland is similar to that of the adult (Fig. 12.5).

> **Box 12.1   Advice**
>
> Often, the fat around the adrenal glands is clearly seen and thought to be the adrenal gland itself. Perinephric fat can be mistaken for it, as can the crus of the diaphragm on the right. The tail of pancreas, splenic vessels and stomach have all been mistaken for the left adrenal gland.

Pathology

- Cysts
- Haemorrhage
- Tumours: cortical, adenoma
- Carcinoma
- Metastases
- Myolipoma
- Phaeochromocytoma
- Neuroblastoma

CLINICAL INFORMATION

Too much or too little secretion from the adrenal glands has a dramatic effect on the patient. Some syndromes are attributed to over- or undersecretion of adrenal hormones.

Cushing's syndrome is an excess of glucocorticoids from a pituitary adenoma, adrenal adenoma, adrenal cortical carcinoma or overadministration of corticosteroids. This leads to high blood sugar levels and consequently diabetes mellitus, a depressed immune system, muscle

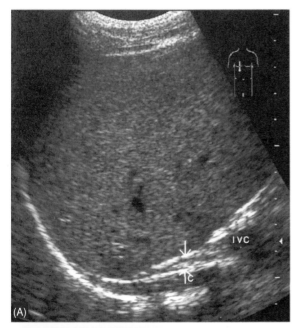

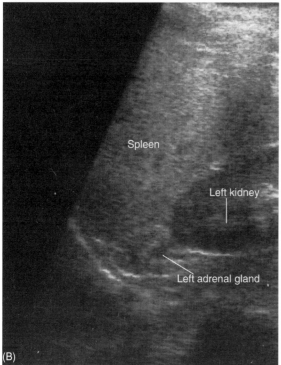

Fig. 12.5 Normal appearances. (A) Right adrenal gland. The medial (anterior arrow) and lateral (posterior arrow) wings of the gland lie just anterior to the crus 'C'. (B) Left adrenal gland. (Reprinted from Clinical Ultrasound, Bates, p 186, Fig 8.7a, 1999, by permission of the publisher, Churchill Livingstone.)

atrophy and weakness, severe osteoporosis, bruising, poor wound healing, redistribution of fats to face (moon face), neck and abdomen, suppression of growth hormone and emotional disturbance such as euphoria or depression. Diagnosis is from clinical features and raised plasma cortisol level. Too little leads to low blood sugar, depressed immune system, weight loss, loss of appetite, nausea and vomiting and increased skin pigmentation (the 'dusky complexion') from elevated ACTH levels.

Conn's syndrome is an excess of aldosterone leading to elevated sodium levels, lowered potassium, alkalosis, high blood pressure, weakness of skeletal muscles and acidic urine. Diagnosis of Conn's syndrome is from blood electrolyte levels (high sodium, low potassium).

Addison's disease is the converse of Conn's syndrome in so far as the sodium levels drop, potassium levels are raised, the patient has acidosis, blood pressure drops and excessive amounts of urine are passed, the patient suffers from vomiting and loss of appetite and becomes dehydrated and the skin has a brown pigmentation.

It must be remembered that the alteration of sodium and potassium levels has a profound effect on the electrical properties of cells.

An excess of androgens in women can cause hirsutism, acne, breast tissue atrophy and irregular periods but the sex drive is increased. In males, an oversecretion can cause precocious puberty. Too little and pubic and axillary hair is reduced.

Cysts

CLINICAL INFORMATION

The most common cyst associated with the adrenal gland is the endothelial cyst. Endothelial cysts are usually asymptomatic and are found incidentally in about 6% of patients at post-mortem and more frequently in women than in men. They can grow to quite a large size and occasionally calcify. They can be mistaken for renal, pancreatic and splenic cysts so care has to be taken when identifying their origin.

ULTRASOUND APPEARANCES

The cysts have thin walls, are round in shape and are echo free.

Haemorrhage

CLINICAL INFORMATION

In the neonate, it is not uncommon for the relatively distended vessels in the adrenal gland to haemorrhage up to one week after birth. This can be a result of a traumatic birth, stress or anoxia and is frequently seen in babies with diabetic mothers. It is said that it is more commonly seen on the right, with 10% bilateral, but this may be a result of technical factors.

ULTRASOUND APPEARANCES

The appearances can vary depending on whether the bleed is fresh (high reflectivity) or a few days old where the haemorrhage becomes less reflective and develops echo-poor areas. The mass can calcify with the borders becoming highly reflective and producing distal acoustic shadowing. Alternatively, a few calcified flecks can be left.

In adults, haemorrhage of a hypertrophic adrenal gland caused by ACTH therapy or as a result of stress can be seen. It is usually echo free but fibrin strands as a result of the haemorrhage resolving can increase the echogenicity. Again, the cyst can calcify or remain as a residual cyst.

Tumours – general

CLINICAL INFORMATION

Adrenal tumours can measure anything between 0.5 cm and 20 cm.

ULTRASOUND APPEARANCES

The adrenal gland is easier to see with a mass inside; the borders of the gland can become convex and the mass will appear to have a lower reflectivity than the surrounding fat. Tumours of the adrenal gland will tend to elevate the IVC as they grow. Large adrenal masses can tilt the kidney from its usual angle so that the upper pole moves laterally or the whole kidney can be pushed inferiorly.

Tumours tend to show focal areas of haemorrhage or necrosis and will therefore appear as heterogeneous masses while smaller masses tend to remain relatively echo poor. Adrenal tumours can be differentiated from renal tumours by the demonstration of an interface between the adrenal gland and the kidney.

Cortical adenoma

CLINICAL INFORMATION

Cortical adenomas tend to be small (1–2 cm in diameter) and can be found in 2% of the population.

Most do not produce steroids so only a very few cause Cushing's or Conn's syndrome. An adenoma causing Conn's syndrome may be active despite being small in size.

ULTRASOUND APPEARANCES

Cortical adenomas appear as smooth, round, well-circumscribed, homogeneous masses of relatively high echogenicity.

Carcinoma

CLINICAL INFORMATION

Carcinoma of the adrenal gland is rare. Nearly all cases produce glucocorticoids and sex steroids and patients present with the features of Cushing's syndrome and excess androgen. By the time that patients present, adrenal carcinomas are often large with invasion of the adrenal vein and IVC and subsequent blood-carried metastases are common. The liver is a frequent site of metastases from the adrenal gland.

ULTRASOUND APPEARANCES

Carcinomas usually have a relatively low echogenicity but can be echogenic. They are often bilateral. Larger right adrenal masses can appear like hepatic tumours and care must be taken to differentiate the two.

Box 12.2 Advice

If a carcinoma is suspected, the liver, IVC, renal vein and peritoneum should be examined for spread of tumour.

Metastases

CLINICAL INFORMATION

The adrenal glands are the fourth most common site in the body (after lungs, liver and bones) for metastases to occur. As such, in patients with a known primary, the adrenal glands must be carefully examined. Common primary sites are the lung, bronchus and breast. The adrenal glands are often associated with non-Hodgkin's lymphoma.

ULTRASOUND APPEARANCES

Appearances can vary and metastases can become quite large (5–8 cm in diameter). They are often oval or round in shape and are of low reflectivity.

Myolipoma

CLINICAL INFORMATION

This cortical tumour is rare and is composed of fat and bone marrow. It does not become malignant and does not disturb the endocrine system.

ULTRASOUND APPEARANCES

The ultrasound appearance of a myolipoma is of a highly reflective mass in the area of the adrenal gland caused by the fat in the mass.

Phaeochromocytoma

CLINICAL INFORMATION

Phaeochromocytomas are masses of the epinephrine- and norepinephrine-secreting cells of the adrenal medulla. They are uncommon in children. Phaeochromocytomas cause uncontrollable hypertension and bad headaches, they are found in up to 1% of patients with hypertension. Most are benign but between 5% and 10% are said to be malignant. Diagnosis is by catecholamine levels (epinephrine and norepinephrine) in the urine. Even small phaeochromocytomas (1–2 cm) can cause hypertension (Fig. 12.6).

ULTRASOUND APPEARANCES

Phaeochromocytomas appear as well-defined, solid, round or oval, homogeneous masses. As they enlarge, the homogeneity is often lost because of necrosis or haemorrhage. They can appear in extraadrenal sympathetic tissue, often in the retroperitoneal area next to the abdominal aorta.

Neuroblastoma

CLINICAL INFORMATION

Neuroblastomas are common paediatric adrenal tumours. They account for more than 20% of abdominal masses in children and 30% occur within the first year of life. Most originate from the adrenal gland but can occur in the chest, neck, pelvis or in the retroperitoneum. Children with a neuroblastoma look pale and ill and the prognosis is often poor.

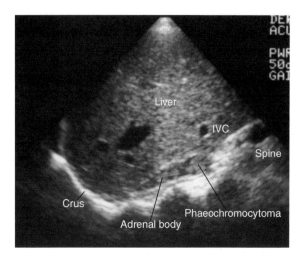

Fig. 12.6   Phaeochromocytoma.

Box 12.3   Advice

In patients with changed secondary sex characteristics, especially young girls, if the adrenal areas appear normal, a careful study of the ovaries must be made to exclude an ovarian tumour.

Adrenal glands must be differentiated from hepatic, pancreatic, splenic and renal masses.

The crus of the diaphragm can be mistaken for the adrenal gland.

If an adrenal carcinoma is suspected, the liver, IVC, renal vein and peritoneum should be examined for spread of tumour.

Much of the literature on adrenal gland scanning technique and appearances appears to be relatively old, the newest articles concerning pathological appearances in dogs and cats or the use of endoscopic ultrasound. Gunter et al describe the successful role of ultrasound in detecting small tumours but as it is an old article using lower resolution equipment, the success in visualizing the adrenal gland itself rather than just the surrounding fat is minimal.[1] Dietrich et al suggest the use of a combination of transabdominal and endoscopic ultrasound to examine both adrenal glands fully.[2]

Most neuroblastomas appear as large, heterogeneous masses situated at the upper pole of the kidney. They appear echogenic owing to fine calcification within the tumour. The borders may be indistinct as they can wrap themselves around the aorta and IVC and elevate them away from the spine. They rarely invade the kidney on which they are situated but can rotate or displace it because of their size. They can be accompanied by large lymph node masses and can metastasize to the liver bone marrow, skin and lymph nodes in later stages. Neuroblastomas can appear rather like Wilms' tumours, but enlarged lymph node masses and the wrapping around of the aorta and IVC are rare with Wilms' tumours.

The IVs neuroblastoma is a specific type which occurs in the early neonatal period and has a better prognosis. On ultrasound the liver is massively enlarged (so much so that breathing difficulties can occur) with a mixed echo pattern. An accompanying small adrenal primary tumour may be present but this is often extremely difficult to see.

References

1. Gunter RW, Kelbel C, Lenner V 1984 Real-time ultrasound of normal adrenal glands and small tumours. J Clin Ultrasound 12: 211–217

2. Dietrich CF, Wehrmann T, Hoffman C et al 1997 Detection of adrenal glands by endoscopic or transabdominal ultrasound. Endoscopy 9: 859–864

13

BOWEL

Main functions
Anatomy
Scanning
Normal ultrasound appearances
Pathology

Gas in the bowel has long been a reason for abandoning an ultrasound examination owing to the anterior position of the bowel and gas lying between the probe and the structures of interest. With recent technology and continued interest and research into the ability of ultrasound to image new areas, bowel is becoming an anatomical area to scan rather than just a nuisance.

Main functions

Small intestine

The greatest amount of digestion and absorption of food matter occurs in the small intestine. The mucosa secretes water, electrolytes and mucus to protect its internal wall from acidic chyme and digestive enzymes and to act as a lubricant to aid the passage of chyme. The smooth muscle in the small intestine produces segmental and peristaltic contractions which help to mix and propel the contents respectively at about 1 cm/minute. Chyme takes about 3–5 hours to enter the ileocaecal junction from the pylorus. Most of the water entering the digestive system is absorbed by the small intestine.

Large intestine

Chyme entering the colon is converted into faeces (water, undigested food, microorganisms and sloughed off epithelial cells) and expelled within 18–24 hours normally. The conversion involves the absorption of more water and salts, secretion of mucus and the action of microorganisms. Only about 10% of the chyme is converted and expelled, while 90% is absorbed. Bacteria in the colon and the type of food eaten (especially beans which contain complex carbohydrates) contribute to the production of flatus. Peristaltic waves move the chyme along the ascending colon. Peristaltic contractions (mass movements) occur in the transverse and descending colon and propel the faeces at about 20 cm at a time towards the anus. Mass movements are common after meals, being caused by the gastrocolic reflex.

Anatomy

The small intestine is approximately 6 metres in length extending from the pyloric orifice of the stomach to the ileocaecal valve where it continues with the large intes-

tine. The small intestine consists of the duodenum, jejunum and ileum and generally lies in the mid-abdomen, beneath the stomach and as far inferiorly as the pelvis. The large intestine is approximately 1.5 metres in length, is wider than the small bowel and is gathered into characteristic sacs or haustra. It consists of the caecum, ascending, transverse, descending and sigmoid colon and rectum. The large intestine lies around the small intestine (Fig. 13.1).

The first part of the duodenum, jejunum, ileum and transverse colon is covered in peritoneum while the second and third parts of the duodenum, ascending and descending colon and rectum are retroperitoneal.

Blood supply

The small intestine, caecum, ascending colon and proximal two-thirds of the transverse colon are supplied by the superior mesenteric artery and the rest of the large intestine as far as the anal canal is supplied by the inferior mesenteric artery.

Blood drainage

Via the corresponding superior and inferior mesenteric veins which eventually carry their enriched, nutrient-packed blood into the portal vein and into the liver.

Lymph drainage

From the colon into the superior and inferior mesenteric lymph glands and from the lower half of the rectum downwards into the inguinal lymph nodes.

Nerve supply

From branches of the sympathetic and parasympathetic chains of the autonomic nervous system.

Relations

The bowel is important when considering its relations to other structures that are to be examined. Knowing where the bowel lies is essential in working out how to avoid gas when scanning. Bowel is an anterior structure and as such will always lie between the probe and the interesting parts beneath. The duodenum has relevance as it curves around the head of the pancreas, often obscuring that part of the gland, and in addition the first part of the duodenum lies anterior to the lower part of the common duct, making it difficult to

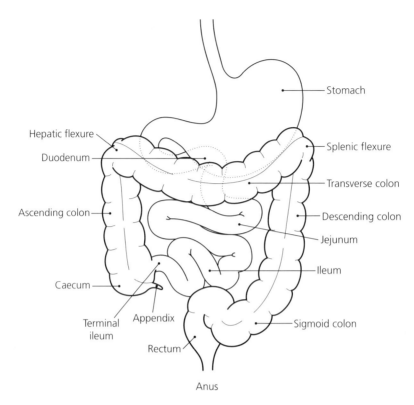

Fig. 13.1 General layout of the bowel.

search for pathology there. The jejunum tends to lie around the umbilical region and is of greater diameter than the ileum which lies in the hypogastrium and pelvis.

The mass of small bowel in the mid to lower abdomen can contain gas which can prevent access to the aorta and IVC. The large intestine often contains pockets of gas which appear at the hepatic and splenic flexures, making it difficult to visualize the lower half of the kidneys.

Surface markings

The ileocaecal junction is found at a point where the transtubercular plane (the line level with the iliac crests) crosses the lateral plane (a vertical line halfway between the midline and a vertical line drawn at the level of the anterior superior iliac spine) on the right. The appendix can be found just below this.

The ascending colon passes up from the transtubercular plane to the upper ninth costal cartilage where it turns

medially, becoming the transverse colon, and crosses the midline at the level of approximately the second lumbar vertebra, often crossing the second part of the duodenum above the umbilical plane. It crosses to the ninth or eighth costal cartilage where it turns downwards (the descending colon) to the level of the iliac crest before running medially and posteriorly on the way to the rectum.

Variations in normal anatomy

The position of bowel in different body types can be seen in the section on body types (see Chapter 1).

Ensure that you have access to the patient's history as there may have been a resection of the small bowel or other operative procedure that has altered the normal ultrasound appearance. Resection of one-third or a half of the small intestine is compatible with a normal life and it has been known for a patient to survive with only 45 cm of small intestine preserved.

Palpation

As a result of obstruction, the colon can become grossly distended with faeces. Faecal masses are obviously found in the flanks and epigastrium. Faeces are firm or hard but indentable, the dent persisting after releasing pressure on the mass. Faeces may be seen as multiple separate masses in the region of the colon, but can merge together to form one large mass.

Relevant tests – normal values

Haemoglobin	Male 130–180 g/l, female 115–165 g/l
Mean corpuscular volume (MCV)	80–94 fl
Mean corpuscular haemoglobin concentration (MCH)	1.7–2.0 fmol
White cell count (WCC)	4–11 × 10/l

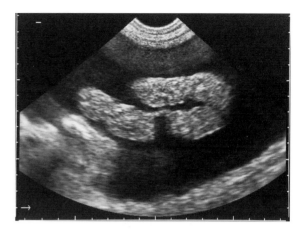

Fig. 13.2   Bowel outlined by ascites.

Scanning

Patient preparation

If the bowel is to be scanned in particular, a low-residue diet can be given for 24 hours before the examination and clear fluids can be taken at any time. More often, the imaging of the bowel will be part of a general scan for which the normal upper abdominal preparation will have been given or, more likely, it will be a part of an urgent scan for which no preparation will have been given. Patients requiring an urgent scan tend not to have hearty appetites but will be taking sips of clear fluids only.

Equipment required

Focusing zones and gain settings appropriate for the region under investigation:

- adult – 5 MHz curvilinear or linear transducer
- child – 5–7.5 MHz curvilinear or linear transducer.

Suggested scanning technique

Gas in the bowel is the reason we use acoustic windows to see other structures. This time there is no acoustic window. When scanning the large intestine, align the transducer along the estimated direction of the bowel and follow its course in longitudinal sections. Turn the transducer and scan in cross-section

along the course of the bowel. Gentle pressure may have to be applied but not if it causes pain. This may disperse some gas and offer better detail. The quality of the image improves dramatically when the patient has ascites (Fig. 13.2).

Normal ultrasound appearances

Appearances of normal bowel depend on contents, distension and position. It may be collapsed with a small amount of mucus or distended and containing gas or fluid. Bowel can show a target appearance with a highly reflective centre of mucus and trapped gas surrounded by the echo-poor bowel wall. This appearance is seen at the oesophagogastric junction, pyloric antrum and duodenum but seldom in the rest of the small and large bowel (Figs 13.3, 13.6).

Peristalsis can often be seen, especially after fluid intake, as in the sequence of images of the duodenum shown in Figure 13.4. Observation of peristalsis is useful when excluding other pathology in the abdomen.

When distended with fluid, bowel is much easier to visualize, appearing tubular in its long axis and circular in its short axis. The part of the bowel being scanned is recognized by the position within the abdomen, especially when filled with fluid or outlined by ascites, by the haustra of the colon, the valvulae conniventes of

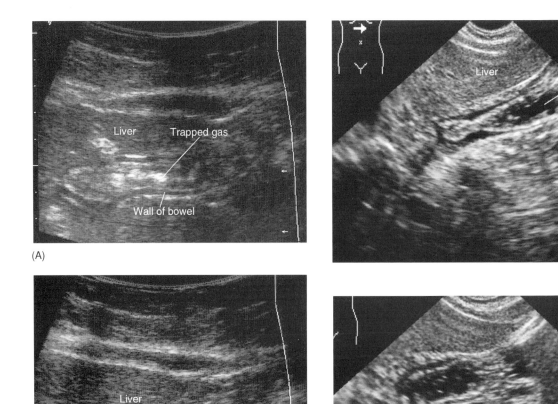

(A)

(B)

Fig. 13.3 (A) Longitudinal and (B) transverse sections of duodenum.

the jejunum or the smooth walls of the duodenum (Fig.13.5).

Generally small and large bowel appearances are complex, containing small amounts of fluid and gas even when fasting. Although seen better with endoscopic ultrasound, high-resolution ultrasound can occasionally demonstrate the five layers of the bowel. The reflective inner and outer layers correspond to the interface between the bowel wall and the lumen or serosal surface. Beneath this, adjacent to the lumen lies the echo-poor mucosa and the muscularis mucosa and the more reflective submucosa, then the echo-poor muscularis propria.

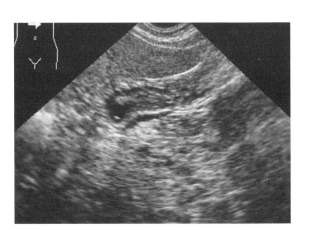

Fig. 13.4 Sequence of peristalsis in the duodenum.

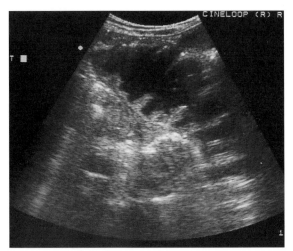

Fig. 13.5 Fluid-filled in a case of ileus.

GAS PATTERN

Gas can obscure areas of interest deep to the bowel. Reverberation echoes (tapering or comet-tail artefact (Fig. 13.6) allow distinction from shadowing.

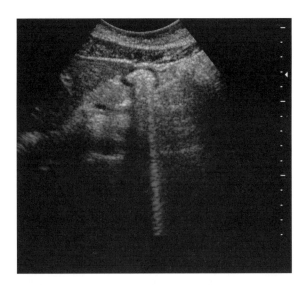

Fig. 13.6 The comet-tail artefact from gas in the duodenum.

NORMAL SIZES

Normal thickness of bowel wall in a distended state is 3 mm, 5 mm when non-distended.

Pathology

The most common conditions which are examined by ultrasound (excepting the use of endoscopic ultrasound) are as follows.

- Crohn's disease
- Obstruction
- Intestinal tumours
- Carcinoid tumour
- Malabsorption syndrome
- Appendicitis
- Intussusception
- Pyloric stenosis
- Bezoars
- Other appearances – 'peritoneal cake', inguinal hernia

However, many institutions will not consider looking at the bowel with ultrasound.

Crohn's disease

CLINICAL INFORMATION

Crohn's disease affects the terminal ileum mostly but can be seen in other segments of bowel. This is an inflammatory disease which causes the intestinal wall to thicken and the lumen to narrow. It usually occurs in young adults. These patients present with a painful mass in the right iliac fossa, abdominal cramps and diarrhoea and can have weight loss, malaise, fever or malabsorption syndrome (see page 221) and leucocytosis WCC $>10^9$/l.

SUGGESTED TECHNIQUE FOR SCANNING THE TERMINAL ILEUM

Scan the ascending colon in transverse section and move inferiorly and medially until the terminal ileum with associated peristalsis is seen entering the caecum.

ULTRASOUND APPEARANCES

The folds of the inflamed bowel tend to be absent. The terminal ileum can reveal bowel wall up to 1.5 cm thick. Peristalsis is reduced but fluid can be seen proximal to the area of reduced lumen. The involved loops of bowel can clump together, suggesting a solid mass. Abscesses can be seen as a complication of Crohn's disease, showing as a complex, irregular fluid-filled mass which can contain gas shadows. Ultrasound can be helpful in the drainage of abscesses prior to surgery and in the monitoring of the bowel after treatment where remission can be inferred from the thickness of the bowel wall. Fistulas can occur but are extremely difficult to see on ultrasound. They can connect the colon with the bladder and produce the appearance of gas artefacts in the bladder (pneumaturea). Gentle pressure on the bladder and release can move the gas artefacts and confirm diagnosis.

Box 13.1 Advice

With Crohn's disease the entire gastrointestinal tract should be scanned to search for other affected segments of bowel. Also renal stones and biliary tract pathology are commonly found.

Intestinal obstruction

ULTRASOUND APPEARANCES

Ultrasound is useful in observing peristaltic movement which is increased initially when there is mechanical obstruction and reduced or absent when there is an ileus. If bowel loops are fluid filled proximal to the obstruction, the site of obstruction is easier to see. When loops of bowel that are both dilated and normal are seen, this is a strong indication of mechanical bowel obstruction. With small bowel obstruction, dilated loops are usually anechoic or contain low-level echoes. Obstructed large bowel usually contains more highly reflective echoes. There is a suggestion of bowel pathology such as tumours or inflammatory disease if the bowel has central, highly reflective or complex echoes and a thickened halo around the bowel wall. This appearance can look like an ectopic kidney, dermoid cyst, normal colon or gallstones in a thick-walled, contracted gallbladder.

Intestinal tumours

CLINICAL INFORMATION

Carcinomas are usually seen in older patients or those with ulcerative colitis or Crohn's disease. They can be found at any point in the gastrointestinal tract but the small intestine is relatively resistant to malignancy, having an occurrence of less than 1% of all malignant lesions owing to its fast transit time (reducing the time

of exposure to potential carcinogens) and relative sterility of small bowel contents. Carcinomas are more common in the colon and are seen more frequently in the rectosigmoid area. After invading the blood vessels and lymphatics, they can spread quickly to the liver.

Clinically, patients may have a painful abdominal mass, melaena, anorexia, diarrhoea, constipation and/or weight loss. Carcinoma of the caecum can grow to a relatively large size but remain asymptomatic. The patient may present with only an iron deficiency anaemia.

BLOOD TESTS FOR IRON DEFICIENCY ANAEMIA

Haemoglobin (Hb)	Less than 8.1 mmol/l in males, 7.1 mmol/l in females
Mean corpuscular volume (MCV)	<80 fl
Mean corpuscular haemoglobin concentration (MCH)	<1.7 fmol

ULTRASOUND APPEARANCES

Bowel pathology appears as a variation to the normal bowel patterns. Carcinomas appear as circular or ovoid target masses of relatively low echogenicity (the tumour or oedematous wall) with a centre of higher reflectivity (the mucosa). The bowel wall may be thickened and measure more than 5 mm (Fig. 13.7).

Neoplasms are said to produce short segments of thickened bowel compared with inflammatory processes that produce long segments of thickened bowel, although this is not a hard and fast rule. Ultrasound cannot differentiate between different types of tumour and a carcinoma may appear like a large inflammatory mass. The usefulness of ultrasound in identifying colonic abnormalities is described in an article by Truong et al.[1]

Box 13.2 Advice

If a mass is found, look for peristalsis; carefully scan the liver and spleen for secondary masses, the adjacent organs for infiltration, the abdomen for free or enclosed fluid and paraaortic and mesenteric areas for lymph node enlargement.

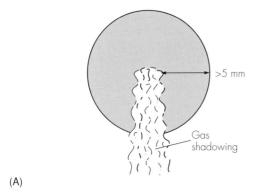

(A)

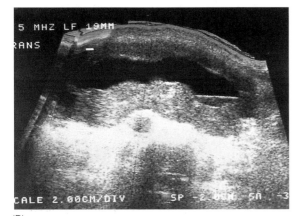

(B)

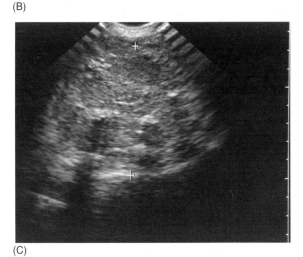

(C)

Fig. 13.7 (A) Typical ultrasound appearance of cross-section of cancerous bowel: wall is thickened to more than 5 mm, central reflective mucosa with gas shadowing. (B) Colonic carcinoma demonstrating thickened bowel wall and mucus/fluid level. (C) 7 cm heterogeneous mass situated distal to obstructed bowel, probably carcinoma.

Carcinoid tumours

CLINICAL INFORMATION

Carcinoid tumours can be found anywhere in the gastrointestinal tract but are more usually found in the appendix, small intestine or rectum.

ULTRASOUND APPEARANCES

They are usually less than 1.5 cm in diameter and appear as lobulated, hypoechoic masses with clearly identifiable margins lacking acoustic enhancement, appearing like lymphomas.

Malabsorption syndrome

CLINICAL INFORMATION

Malabsorption syndrome is the impaired digestion of food and subsequent malabsorption owing to the malfunction of the action or absence of the pancreas, liver or intestinal mucosa. Patients with malabsorption present with weight loss, abdominal distension and loose, bulky stools. If fat is not absorbed, the stools are pale, offensive in smell and float in water. The most common causes of malabsorption are chronic pancreatitis, coeliac disease, a resected ileum or stomach, Crohn's disease or liver/biliary disease preventing bile from entering the gut.

ULTRASOUND APPEARANCES

The appearances of bowel are complex. There is often fluid and gas distension of the small bowel. The contents are unusual with highly reflective masses and multiple reverberation echoes throughout the bowel loops.

Appendicitis

ULTRASOUND APPEARANCES

Appendicitis is most common in children and young adults but may occur at any age. Patients present with pain around the umbilicus that localizes in the right lower quadrant (McBurney's point), rebound tenderness (tenderness more severe when pressure released rather than when applied), anorexia, nausea, diarrhoea and vomiting, fever and a WBC count above 10^9/l (leucocytosis).

The appendix arises from the posteromedial aspect of the caecum, about 2.5 cm below the ileocaecal valve. It ranges in length from 1.2 cm to 22 cm and is very variable in position. Seventy-five percent lie behind the caecum and colon, making ultrasound access to the appendix very difficult, 5% lie medial to the caecum, in front or behind the terminal ileum and 20% lie medial to the caecum below the ileum or extending into the pelvis. The lumen of the appendix is very narrow in the elderly and very wide in the infant and as obstruction of the appendix is usually the cause for appendicitis, this condition is rare at both ends of the lifespan. The normal appendix measures 3–4 mm in cross-section and is seen as a blind-ended, non-peristaltic loop of bowel originating from the medial lower end of the caecum and sometimes containing a small amount of fluid that compresses with ease (Fig. 13.8).

SUGGESTED TECHNIQUE FOR SCANNING THE APPENDIX

Graded compression may be used for any part of the bowel although it is usually linked with the standard technique used for the evaluation of the appendix. Compression is applied to the abdomen with the probe in a transverse position, starting at the hepatic flexure and then working down towards the caecum. Compression helps to displace bowel gas and bowel contents and bring the structures close to the probe within the focal zone that has been set. The highest frequency possible must be chosen. Patient discomfort is minimized by release of the compression from time to time. Release carefully to minimize any rebound

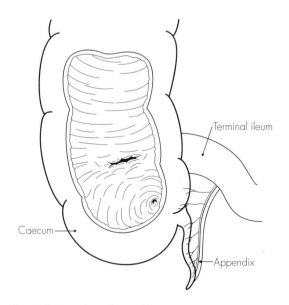

Fig. 13.8 Location of appendix.

tenderness. If the patient is asked to point to the area of maximum tenderness, scan down to that point. Scan in transverse section from the umbilicus to the point of maximum tenderness, identifying any normal/ abnormal appearances seen. Then turn the probe 90° and scan over the region of the appendix to see it in transverse section.

ULTRASOUND APPEARANCES

Normal appearances are seen in 30% of cases. The appearances of appendicitis are usually divided into three categories: acute appendicitis, gangrenous appendicitis and perforated appendix.

Acute appendicitis

Graded compression at the site of maximum tenderness reveals a non-compressible, sausage-shaped structure demonstrating no peristalsis. Non-compressibility is diagnostic of appendicitis. Usually there is no fluid within the lumen. Very occasionally there is some gas in the appendix which makes for difficult interpretation. In cross-section, it gives a target appearance measuring over 6 mm in diameter, usually between 7 mm and 10 mm. The wall thickness of the appendix in this state can be 3 mm or more.

Gangrenous appendix

With progression of the appendicitis, the lumen fills with fluid and distends even more – up to 2 cm in diameter – and the wall thickens. The lumen will not compress when pressed. Often an appendicolith (stone within the appendix) is seen with acoustic shadowing posteriorly. This is more commonly seen in children. The whole appendix must be visualized as sometimes the appearances of acute appendicitis are focal and localized to the tip of the appendix. This is often difficult depending on the position of the appendix anatomically.

Perforated appendix

The appendicular wall may rupture, producing a fluid collection or abscess in the right lower quadrant. The appearances now change, with a hyperechoic projection surrounded by echo-poor abscess. There may be thickened loops of adjacent bowel around the area and enlarged mesenteric lymph nodes in the right lower quadrant. Inflamed, highly reflective omentum may be seen around the appendix (Fig. 13.9).

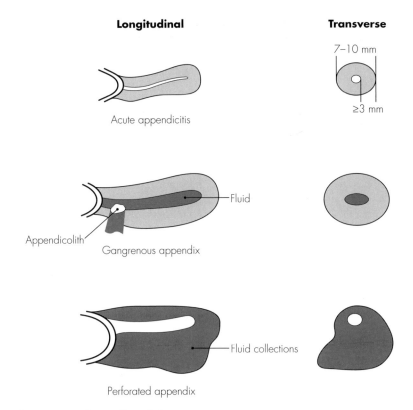

Longitudinal

Transverse

7–10 mm

≥3 mm

Acute appendicitis

Fluid

Appendicolith

Gangrenous appendix

Fluid collections

Perforated appendix

Fig. 13.9 Ultrasound appearances of appendix pathology.

Box 13.3 Advice

Obesity can prevent a satisfactory examination as inadequate compression may occur.

The external iliac artery and vein can be mistaken for the appendix but are pulsatile and compressible respectively. Use Doppler to show flow if in any doubt.

Normal bowel loops can be confused with the appendix but demonstrate peristalsis whereas the appendix does not. If right lower quadrant pain is present and the appendix appears normal, scan the pelvis in females and the biliary and renal system in all patients.

Evidence of enlarged lymph nodes and right iliac fossa pain can also indicate appendicitis.

Intussusception

CLINICAL INFORMATION

Intussusception is the most common childhood emergency and is usually spontaneous in onset. It occurs in a ratio of about 75% boys, 25% girls with the highest incidence in spring and autumn. In this condition, one portion of bowel telescopes into another distal portion of bowel, creating a mass of coiled bowel that causes obstruction. Peristaltic waves push the proximal bowel into the distal segment. The terminal ileum can prolapse into the caecum. It can be seen in adulthood but is usually secondary to a tumour.

Intussusception usually involves the colon (50% being in the transverse colon near the hepatic flexure). As it is superficial, it is palpable in 70% of cases. In the paediatric abdomen, it is a relatively large structure, measuring 3–6 cm diameter (Fig. 13.10).

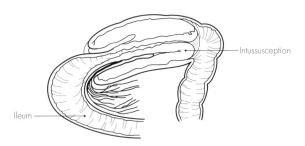

Fig. 13.10 Intussusception.

Patients present with sudden onset of pain and straining with 65% passing a redcurrant jelly stool (blood and mucus). There may be bile-stained vomiting. In time, if not resolved, ischaemic necrosis of the intussusception and intestinal obstruction may occur.

Intussusception can be reduced either under radiological control with barium or air or under ultrasound control using saline. The more severe cases require surgery. It is said that radiological reduction becomes harder the longer it is left because mesenteric vessels become constricted and venous obstruction occurs.

SUGGESTED TECHNIQUE FOR SCANNING INTUSSUSCEPTION

A 7.5–10 MHz linear or curvilinear probe should be used. A normal caecum in the right iliac fossa should be sought. If it is absent, an intussusception should be suspected but this may be due to malrotation. The large bowel should be scanned carefully in its entirety, looking for a mass.

ULTRASOUND APPEARANCES

Intussusception appears like a thick, hypoechoic ring inside another, with echogenic layers in between each ring representing the mucosa. In cross-section it looks like a doughnut. In longitudinal section, it can appear like a kidney; care must be taken not to confuse the two. The more echo poor and thicker the outside of the doughnut, the more oedematous the intussusception as, since the mesenteric vessels are dragged into the mass, they become constricted, leading to venous obstruction. There is always a tumour at the head of the intussusception in adults.

> **Box 13.4 Advice**
>
> Intussusception can appear like Crohn's disease, an appendicular abscess and ulcerative colitis and can occasionally be mistaken for a kidney.

Hypertrophic infantile pyloric stenosis (HPS)

CLINICAL INFORMATION

Hypertrophic infantile pyloric stenosis is the over-growth of the pyloric muscle which leads to narrowing of the pylorus. This is a frequent cause of persistent vomiting in infants. There is a random occurrence of three in 1000, the male to female ratio being 5:1. There have been noted increases in renal anomalies associated with HPS. The condition usually presents in previously healthy infants at around six weeks. Occasionally the symptoms start postnatally or up to five months after. Classically, there is projectile vomiting, free of bile, or it can be stained with blood from the rupture of gastric mucosa capillaries. The precise cause of pyloric muscle hypertrophy is still not clearly understood. The patient becomes dehydrated and peristalsis is clearly seen during feeding. The hypertrophic muscle can be felt as an olive-shaped firm mass in the right upper quadrant.

The indication for diagnostic imaging is when symptoms are present but the mass cannot be felt, although ultrasound is often requested in any case.

SUGGESTED ULTRASOUND TECHNIQUE FOR SCANNING HPS

The patient is usually very small, wriggling about, and has a stomach filled with air from crying, is upset at being prodded about by the paediatricians, being in a colder environment and having the clothing pulled up for the application of acoustic gel. If the baby has tried to feed, there is the possibility that at any time during the scan it will let loose a projectile vomitus.

To alleviate some of these problems, the room should be warm, the baby not uncovered unnecessarily for too long and the parents told about the procedure. It goes without saying that warm gel should be applied. The baby should be scanned at the beginning of the morning, when possible without being fed, but should be allowed water or dextrose to avoid dehydration. If this timing is not possible the scan should be performed at least two hours after a feed.

A 7.5 MHz sector or micro footprint linear probe should be used and attention should be paid to focusing and gain settings in order to obtain an optimum image.

Some centres pass a nasogastric tube and remove milk curds then feed with 60–100 ml of water so that the antrum is well outlined. Many would feel this to be excessive and allow the baby's natural tendency to take water or dextrose at the time of their normal feed, which is normally sufficient. The person accompanying the baby should be covered with paper or an incontinence pad to reduce the effect should the baby vomit.

With the baby cradled in the supine position, the stomach and pylorus should be sought by scanning in the transverse plane. This will, after some angulation, demonstrate the longitudinal section of the stomach and pylorus. Turning the baby to the right allows the fluid in the stomach to flow against the pylorus so it can be identified and images taken. The flow of fluid through the pylorus can also be assessed if present. The length and cross-section of the pylorus and muscle wall thickness must be imaged and measured, the cross-section through the pylorus being obtained by turning the probe at right angles and scanning longitudinally. Clinical ultrasound assessment can be accurate in up to 90% of cases.

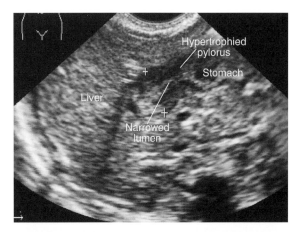

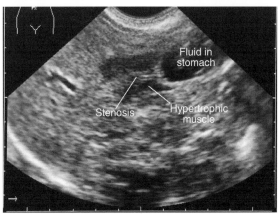

Fig. 13.11   Ultrasound images of pyloric stenosis.

ULTRASOUND APPEARANCES

The pylorus appears on cross-section as an echo-poor rounded structure with the highly reflective centre which is the narrowed lumen, with a central echo-poor appearance if water is passing through the lumen. When scanning transversely, the fluid in the gastric antrum will be seen as an echo-poor area to the patient's left. The length of the pylorus is seen as the distance between one end of the echogenic lumen and the other (Fig. 13.11).

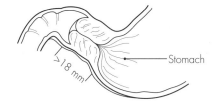

MEASUREMENTS SUGGESTING HYPERTROPHIC INFANTILE PYLORIC STENOSIS

Pyloric length	18 mm or more (normal 10–13.5 mm)
Pyloric diameter	15 mm or more (normal 7.5 mm ± 2.2 mm)
Pyloric muscle thickness	4 mm or more in cross-section (normal 2 mm ± 0.7 mm)

(Fig. 13.12.)

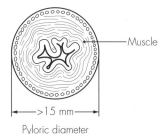

Fig. 13.12   Measurements suggesting pyloric stenosis.

Pyloric volume (V_p) has been used to assess muscle mass:[2]

$$V_p = [\pi (D_p^2).L_p]/4$$

where D_p is pyloric diameter and L_p is pyloric length. $V_p > 1.4\,\text{ml}$ is the cut-off point for normality.

Box 3.15   Advice

These measurements have to be taken with consideration of the patient's condition and size. They do not apply to premature babies. The diagnosis is often made from ultrasound appearance and clinical findings. Often, at least two of the above three measurements are required before a confident diagnosis is made. A pylorus that does not relax to let fluid pass through during the length of the scan is seen far more indicative of hypertrophic infantile pyloric stenosis. It is essential that the measurements are not taken during a pylorospasm as falsely exaggerated measurements will occur.

Bezoars

CLINICAL INFORMATION

Bezoars are accumulations of foreign material within the stomach or small intestine. They are classified and named after the most common contents: trichobezoars (hair and decaying food material), phytobezoars (vegetable matter) and concretions (antacids in adults and cow's milk in infants). Phytobezoars are the most common.

Bezoars are found more frequently in those who have undergone gastric surgery (the incidence after surgery being 10–25% and increasing 5–10 years after surgery), those with hypoperistalsis or those who do not chew their food sufficiently, either because they are young children or because they have inadequate dentition.

Trichobezoars must present, presumably, in those who eat hair for one reason or another, similar to the furballs expelled by cats at odd intervals.

Patients can present with symptoms similar to obstruction or peptic ulceration, including nausea, vomiting and abdominal pain. A bezoar that migrates to the duodenum or further can cause obstruction. Bezoars can be removed endoscopically or attempts can be made to dissolve the bezoar with medication if it is soluble.

ULTRASOUND APPEARANCES

Bezoars appear as highly reflective masses within the stomach or duodenum with strong posterior acoustic shadowing. The bowel proximal to the obstructing bezoar is often dilated and contains fluid.[3]

Box 13.6   Advice

If a bezoar is seen, check that the patient has not eaten prior to the scan. Ensure that the bezoar-containing bowel is not a gallbladder containing a large calculus.

Other appearances

'PERITONEAL CAKE'

This has been described as a clay or putty-like mass in the abdomen around the bowel in peritoneum and omentum, often seen in patients with ascites, especially in conjunction with metastatic spread from ovarian cancer, colonic carcinoma and tuberculosis.

INGUINAL HERNIA

This appears as gas-filled loops of bowel within the inguinal canal next to the testis. Appearances can be misleading if this condition is not taken into account when scanning the testes (see page 230).

References

1. Truong M, Atri M, Bret PM *et al* 1998 Sonographic appearance of benign and malignant conditions of the colon. Am J Roentgenol 17: 1451–1455

2. Westra SJ, De Groot CJ, Smits N *et al* 1989 Hypertrophic pyloric stenosis: the use of pyloric volume measurements in early ultrasound diagnosis. Radiology 172: 615–619

3. Bülent Y, Gönül G, Dogan A, Gülay T 1996 Ultrasonographic diagnosis of small intestinal phytobezoar. J Clin Ultrasound 24: 213–216

Further reading

Haller JO, Cohen HL 1986 Hypertrophic pyloric stenosis: diagnosis using US. Radiology 161: 335–339

Neilson D, Hollman AS 1994 The ultrasonic diagnosis of infantile hypertrophic pyloric stenosis: technique and accuracy. Clin Radiol 49: 246–247

14

MUSCLE

Rectus abdominis
    Scanning
    Normal ultrasound appearances
    Pathology
Psoas
    Scanning
    Normal ultrasound appearances
    Pathology
Diaphragm
    Scanning
    Normal ultrasound appearances
    Pathology

The muscles relevant to the abdomen are:

- rectus abdominis
- psoas
- diaphragm.

Rectus abdominis

Anatomy

The anterior abdominal wall consists of six layers.

- Skin
- Subcutaneous fascia
- Paired muscles (the external oblique, internal oblique and transversus abdominis laterally and the rectus abdominis medially)
- Transverse fascia (the lining of the abdominal cavity separating the muscles from the peritoneum)
- Preperitoneal areolar tissue and fat
- Peritoneum

The rectus abdominis muscle is one of the largest in the body and is paired. It lies in the midline of the abdomen, the two paired sides separated by the linea alba. It attaches to the costal cartilages of the fifth to seventh ribs, the lateral borders of the sternum and xiphisternum and to the symphysis pubis. The lateral muscles named above join at the lateral margin of the rectus abdominis and enclose it (Fig. 14.1).

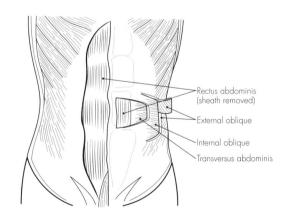

Rectus abdominis (sheath removed)

External oblique

Internal oblique

Transversus abdominis

Fig. 14.1 Diagram of rectus abdominis muscle.

Scanning

Patient preparation

No preparation is required.

Equipment required

Use the highest frequency possible (>7.5 MHz) to identify the superficial structures. Linear array transducers are better for scanning linear structures such as muscles. The transducer must have a good near-field resolution. Use of a gel block may be required to reduce near field reverberations. The transducer should be focused in the near-field.

Suggested scanning technique

As with any paired muscle, examine the normal side first in order to compare normal with abnormal. Scan longitudinally from the midline laterally, then turn the probe 90° and scan the muscle transversely from superior to inferior aspects. The transducer should be held at right angles to the muscle.

Normal ultrasound appearances

Subcutaneous fat is of mixed reflectivity, fat lobules appearing as echo-poor regions.

The muscles appear as low-level echoes with reflective linear fibrous strands. The rectus sheath which encloses the muscle appears as a reflective capsule around it.

Box 14.1   Advice

Reflective linear fibrous strands become less clear when the incident sound does not hit the muscle at right angles. The reflectivity of the muscle is reduced and can appear almost like fluid.

Masses or lumps arising from the abdominal wall must be scanned to ensure that their origin is muscular rather than from an intraabdominal organ.

Pathology

- Rectus sheath haematoma
- Hernia
- Abscess

Rectus sheath haematoma

CLINICAL INFORMATION

As the rectus muscles are enclosed in a fibrous sheath, blood may be trapped and a haematoma formed following injury. Haematoma may result from trauma or a predisposition to bleeding and is seen occasionally as a chronic, minor condition in pregnancy and when ascites is present. It can also occur spontaneously in muscular men and in old ladies. On palpation, the mass is tender and palpable and it is difficult to differentiate between a deep or superficial mass.

ULTRASOUND APPEARANCES

There may be a focal or general enlargement of the whole muscle at first. The haematoma can appear highly reflective in the early stages (days 2 and 3) and then as an echo-free mass with irregular margins and solid focal areas (clot) as it retracts by about day 14. The shape of the haematoma is defined by the borders of the rectus sheath muscle and can often appear as a wedge.

Hernia

CLINICAL INFORMATION

Herniation of bowel into the scrotum through the inguinal canal or the abdominal wall, especially at the incision site of a recent operation, is not unusual. Hernias can sometimes only be seen when the patient stands up or when internal pressure is increased, such as in coughing. When herniation occurs into the scrotum, a hydrocoele may be present (Fig. 14.2).

ULTRASOUND APPEARANCES

A hernia is seen as a gas- or fluid-filled sac with gas reflections and perhaps fat situated in the groin/scrotum abdominal wall.

Abscess

CLINICAL INFORMATION

Abscesses can be felt as a mass on the anterior abdominal wall. The abdominal wall can be inflamed around the site of the abscess, the patient may have a variable temperature and the white cell count may be raised.

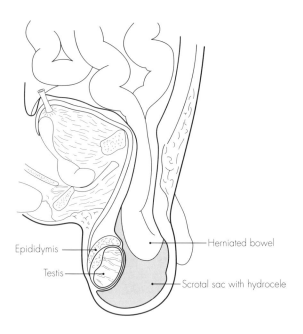

Fig. 14.2 Diagram of bowel protruding through the inguinal canal.

ULTRASOUND APPEARANCES

Abscesses can be seen on ultrasound within the rectus sheath and appear as ill-defined areas with thick irregular borders and mixed internal echoes, septa and debris, perhaps with small gas reverberations.

Psoas

Anatomy

The psoas major muscle, along with the iliacus and quadratus lumborum muscle, forms the posterior abdominal wall. Psoas major is used in the flexion of the hip joint and in flexing the lumbar spines laterally. Psoas minor is absent in about 30% of people; when present, it assists the psoas in its functions.

The psoas muscle arises from the transverse processes of the 12th thoracic vertebra (T12) and the bodies of T12 and L1–4. It passes downwards and laterally, becoming tendinous, and inserts eventually into the lesser trochanter of the femur (Fig. 14.3). It is normally clearly seen on a correctly exposed plain abdominal radiograph.

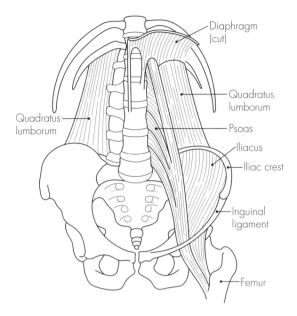

Fig. 14.3 Position of psoas muscle.

Relations

The psoas muscle lies posteromedial to the kidneys.

Scanning

Patient preparation

No preparation is required.

Equipment required

Use a curved linear or sector transducer of 3.5 MHz for an adult because a posterior abdominal structure is being scanned from the front. Focus posteriorly at the psoas muscle level. If scanning from the posterior aspect, a 5 MHz curvilinear or linear transducer can be used with appropriate focusing.

Suggested scanning technique

Scan the right kidney using the liver as an acoustic window. The scan plane should be slightly oblique and the transducer angled slightly medially. The left psoas muscle can be scanned in a similar way using the left kidney and spleen as an acoustic window. The left side is usually not so clear owing to gas in the stomach and a smaller acoustic window.

Both muscles can be scanned from the back. With the patient in the prone position, draped over some pillows in order to reduce the lumbar lordosis and the thickness of the erector spinae muscle, scan obliquely along the lie of the psoas muscle with the transducer placed lateral to the lumbar vertebrae and angling in to the psoas muscle. Scan both sides in turn.

Normal ultrasound appearances

The normal striated psoas muscle (similar to all other muscles) can usually be seen. The muscle appears as low-level echoes with reflective linear fibrous strands within and covered with a reflective fibrous sheath (Fig. 14.4).[1]

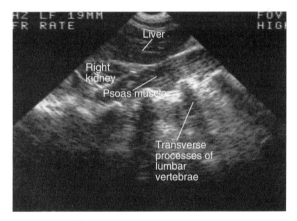

Fig. 14.4 Ultrasound image.

Pathology

- Psoas muscle abscess
- Psoas muscle haematoma

Psoas muscle abscess

CLINICAL INFORMATION

Abscesses form quite often in the psoas muscles. Historically, this was caused by pus from a tubercular infection of the lumbar vertebrae passing laterally into their sheath but the main cause of psoas muscle abscess is now renal pathology and appendicitis.

Patients present with pain on one side, hip or back pain which is worsened by the movement of the hip on that side. When lying supine, the affected side is often flexed to avoid further pain (Fig. 14.5). Children may also present with a palpable tender mass in the abdomen. There is often an accompanying raised temperature, ESR and white cell count.

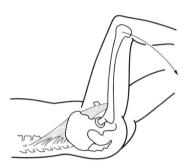

Fig. 14.5 Psoas muscle pathology causing pain on extension.

ULTRASOUND APPEARANCES

The psoas outline becomes enlarged and rounded and contains low-level echoes. The whole muscle may become echo poor if the abscess is diffuse.

Psoas muscle haematoma

CLINICAL INFORMATION

This is quite common in haemophiliacs, patients on anticoagulants and those with a leaking abdominal aortic aneurysm. It often occurs spontaneously and compares with haematoma in the perirenal space which usually occurs following trauma. Large psoas haematomas can cause constipation, fever and frequency of micturition if they are large enough to put pressure on the bladder. They can encroach on the femoral nerve and cause loss of sensation on the anterior part of the thigh and even paralyse the quadriceps. In haemophiliacs, therefore, it is important to diagnose and treat with factor VIII to prevent the femoral nerve being trapped.

ULTRASOUND APPEARANCES

A fresh haematoma may contain very few echoes and appear like a cyst. An older, chronic haematoma often develops septa and reflective debris which shifts with patient movement. Older haematomas may calcify or appear like a solid mass.

Box 14.2   Advice

Psoas muscle haematoma can appear like lymphadenopathy and retroperitoneal tumour invading the psoas muscle. Scan carefully for evidence of other enlarged lymph nodes and tumours.

There has been some research into the ultrasound of wasting muscle diseases by scanning the quadriceps muscles in a relaxed position using a 3.5 or 5 MHz linear array probe.[2] With Duchenne muscular dystrophy, the echogenicity of the muscle is increased, it sometimes becomes bulkier and gives the appearance of ground glass. Congenital muscular dystrophy gives a highly reflective appearance and sometimes the echo from the femur is absent.

Diaphragm

Anatomy

The diaphragm is a fibromuscular dome, concave inferiorly. It separates the thoracic and abdominal cavities. The muscular fibres of the diaphragm contract during inspiration, pulling the central tendon inferiorly. This in turn flattens the dome shape of the diaphragm and increases the volume of the thorax.

There are three major openings within the diaphragm. They allow entry into the abdominal cavity for the IVC, the oesophagus and the aorta at the level of T8–9, T10 and T12 respectively. There are three groups of muscular fibres which pass inwards and are inserted into the central tendon of the diaphragm. The sternal fibres arise from the back of the xiphisternum, the costal fibres from the costal cartilages and lower six rib shafts and the lumbar fibres from the arcuate ligaments that originate from L1 and the 12th rib and from both crura of the diaphragm that originate from L2–3 (Fig. 14.6).

Blood supply

The blood supply to the diaphragm is via the left and right superior and inferior phrenic arteries.

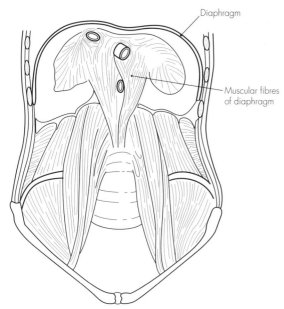

Fig. 14.6 The diaphragm.

Blood drainage

The blood drainage to the diaphragm is via the left and right superior and inferior phrenic veins.

Nerve supply

The diaphragm is supplied by the right and left phrenic nerves.

Scanning

Patient preparation

None required unless part of a general abdominal scan.

Equipment required

Curved linear or sector transducer of 3.5 MHz for an adult or 5 MHz for a thin adult or child.

Suggested scanning technique

- Right hemidiaphragm – with the patient in the supine position, place the transducer in the right

axillary line and scan intercostally along the line of the ribs, using the liver as an acoustic window. It may be possible to scan using a subcostal approach and angling acutely up towards the head.

- Left hemidiaphragm – again with the patient supine and using the spleen as the acoustic window, place the transducer in the left axillary line and scan intercostally along the line of the ribs.

Normal ultrasound appearances

The normal diaphragm appears as a highly reflective, curvilinear structure often with distal reverberation (Fig. 14.7). The crura are seen as tubular muscular structures above the level of the coeliac axis and lying anterior to the aorta and posterior to the IVC.

Movement of both hemidiaphragms can be assessed by scanning transversely with the transducer in the sub-xiphisternal position and angling upwards.

Paralysis of the phrenic nerve prevents movement of the diaphragm when the patient sniffs.

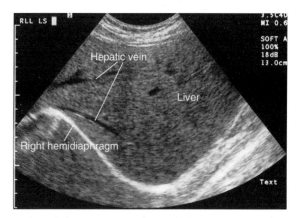

Fig. 14.7 The right hemidiaphragm as seen on ultrasound.

Pathology

- Pleural effusion
- Subphrenic abscess
- Diaphragmatic and hiatus hernia
- Eventration

Pleural effusion

CLINICAL INFORMATION

A pleural effusion can either be transudate (excess fluid containing less than 30 g/l of protein) passing through normal vessel walls or exudate (excess fibrin-containing fluid with a higher protein level of more than 30 g/l, passing through damaged vessel walls).

Transudate is often caused by cardiac failure; exudate by infection, tumour or infarction.

ULTRASOUND APPEARANCES

Pleural effusions show as anechoic areas situated superior to the diaphragm with posterior acoustic enhancement. Fibrin deposits can produce septa which float characteristically within the exudate and there is usually reduced diaphragmatic movement (Fig. 14.8).

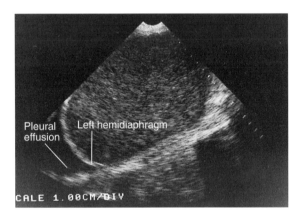

Fig. 14.8 Left pleural effusion seen above left hemidiaphragm and enlarged spleen.

Subphrenic abscess

CLINICAL INFORMATION

Subphrenic abscesses are caused commonly by appendicitis, perforated ulcer and, iatrogenically, by surgery. The subphrenic area is a common site in the peritoneal cavity for an abscess to form, appearing more frequently on the right than the left. The patient presents with fever, malaise and pain in the right or left hypochondrium and in the shoulder tip.

ULTRASOUND APPEARANCES

Subphrenic abscesses show as fluid collections between the diaphragm and the liver or spleen. They may be complex masses containing debris or gas which appear as echogenic areas with characteristic gas artefacts. Again, the diaphragmatic movement is reduced as seen when scanning with the patient breathing and sniffing.

Box 14.3 Advice

It is often difficult to differentiate between a hepatic and a subphrenic abscess.

For more information on abscesses, please see Chapter 15.

Diaphragmatic hernia

CLINICAL INFORMATION

These are congenital posterior (and usually left-sided) Bochdalek hernias, the less common and smaller, anterior, Morgagni hernias or acquired (traumatic and hiatus hernias).

Oesophageal hiatus hernia, in which a herniated portion of the stomach slides up through the diaphragm, is the most common diaphragmatic hernia, occurring in up to 30% of people over 50 years of age. Patients often present with symptoms of reflux oesophagitis where stomach acid produces inflammation of the oesophageal mucosa. The resultant heartburn is made worse by bending over or lying down and the patient may be taking antacids to relieve the pain.

ULTRASOUND APPEARANCES

With a diaphragmatic hernia due to trauma, bowel loops may be seen within the thorax. These will contain gas and often obscure the diaphragm. A pleural effusion makes identifying bowel loops within the thorax that much easier.

Hiatus hernias are often difficult to see unless outlined by fluid. If the patient is scanned erect to avoid the reflux of acid secretions, gas can rise in the stomach to above the level of the diaphragm and cause a confusing picture. The patient may be able to drink still fluid to help outline the stomach relative to the diaphragm if necessary but a barium swallow is still the main diagnostic test for confirming the condition (Fig. 14.9).

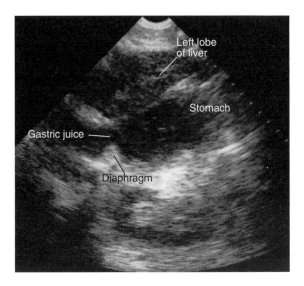

Fig. 14.9 Ultrasound image of hiatus hernia.

Eventration

CLINICAL INFORMATION

Eventration is a congenital weakness of the diaphragm allowing the stomach, bowel or liver to pass through.

ULTRASOUND APPEARANCES

Liver or bowel may be seen within a localized bulge in the diaphragm.

References

1. King AD, Hine AL, McDonald C, Abrahams P 1993 The ultrasound appearance of the normal psoas muscle. Clin Radiol 48: 316–318

2. Heckmatt J 1993 Ultrasound imaging of muscle. BMUS Bull 1: 28–31

15

FLUID COLLECTIONS

Scanning
Normal ultrasound appearances
Pathology
Interventional procedures

An essential part of any general abdominal scan should be to recognize normal fluid appearances and to exclude the presence of an abnormal fluid collection.

Scanning

Suggested ultrasound technique

With the patient in the supine position, the following areas particularly should be observed closely.

- Left and right subphrenic spaces (check the movement of the diaphragm)
- Subhepatic space (Morrison's Pouch)
- Left and right perirenal spaces
- The psoas muscles (check for pain in this area when the leg is moved)
- Both paracolic gutters
- The lesser sac of the omentum between stomach and pancreas
- The female pelvis (pouch of Douglas) or rectovesicular pouch in men
- The rectus sheath muscle

These areas should be scanned in longitudinal and transverse sections. Fluid will tend to collect first in the most dependent part of the patient, which is Morrison's pouch or the pelvic areas when lying supine (Figs 15.1, 15.2).

Normal ultrasound appearances

Areas of black signifying fluid can be seen in healthy patients in the gastrointestinal (GI) tract, the urinary bladder and the gallbladder. The latter two structures should be easily identified by all but the most inexperienced. The urinary bladder can, however, contain diverticula (see Chapter 10) which can alter its appearance.

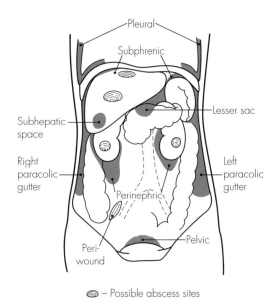

Fig. 15.1 Fluid collection and possible abscess sites.

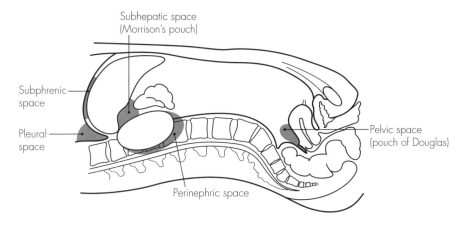

Fig. 15.2 Position of free fluid in supine female subject.

Box 15.1   Advice

Peristaltic action should help to indicate whether the fluid is within the GI tract or not although there may be little action when there is pathology involving the bowel. The position of the fluid should help to identify the part of the bowel in which it is contained (such as in the right or left lateral sides of the abdomen for the ascending and descending colon). If there is a fluid collection within the colon, a mass distal to the collection should be sought. Fluid in the stomach can imitate a splenic or left renal cyst.

A small fluid area in the mid to lower abdomen is usually fluid within the small bowel and this can imitate small cysts on the ovaries in females as the small bowel can lie around the upper parts of the female pelvic organs. Again, peristalsis should be observed to confirm that the fluid is within the bowel and to exclude pathology. This appearance is commonly seen in patients who require a full bladder preparation, who have taken a large quantity of fluid recently rather than 1–2 hours previously and whose small bowel has not yet absorbed the fluid. A small amount of fluid can also often be seen in the pouch of Douglas after ovarian follicles have ruptured during ovulation. This is absorbed relatively soon after.

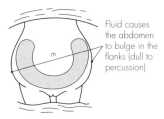

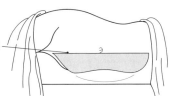

Fig. 15.3   Clinical examination of ascites.

Pathology

CLINICAL INFORMATION

When patients with a relatively large amount of free fluid lie supine, the fluid will run down with gravity and settle in the flanks, producing lateral bulging of the abdomen. On clinical examination, these bulges are dull to percussion. If the patient turns onto the side, the fluid will flow to the lowest point and its new position may also be found by percussion. This is called shifting dullness and demonstrates fluid in the peritoneal cavity (Fig. 15.3).

Abnormal fluid collections seen within the abdomen include:

- postoperative fluid collections/abscesses/haematomas
- fluid from the GI or renal tracts as a result of trauma, disease process or unsuccessful graft or transplant

- ascites
- blood vessel leakage
- fluid exudate post inflammation.

Postoperative fluid collections

CLINICAL INFORMATION

Postoperative wound infections will often present about five days after the operation. Infections can be limited or can progress to become abscesses by about day 10. Patients with abscesses often present with a spiking temperature, a raised white cell count and local pain. Postoperative collections can develop near the original incision site. Patients more at risk of developing abscesses are diabetics, those with connective tissue disorders or cancer and those who are immunosuppressed. Collections of fluid are mainly abscesses or haematomas.

ULTRASOUND APPEARANCES – ABSCESSES

Abscesses demonstrate the typical pattern of a thick, irregular border containing mixed echoes demonstrating solid and fluid contents with the possibility of gas seen within the mass (Fig. 15.4).

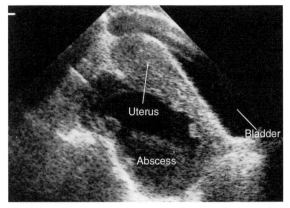

(A)

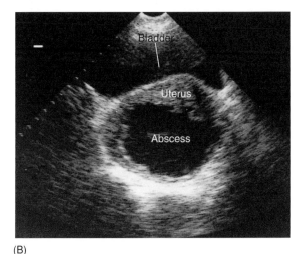

(B)

Fig. 15.4 (A) Longitudinal section and (B) transverse section of female pelvis showing retrouterine abscess.

ULTRASOUND APPEARANCES – HAEMATOMAS

Haematomas when fresh are usually echo free. After a few hours, they become more highly reflective owing to fibrin formation which produces multiple interfaces within the haematoma. After approximately 48 hours their reflectivity starts to decrease.

Fluid as a result of trauma, disease process or unsuccessful graft or transplant

- Urinomas – these are fluid collections free of internal echoes, usually secondary to obstruction, calculi or surgery.
- Lymphocoeles – much less common except in association with renal transplant (see Chapter 9).

- Seromas – again, much less common, associated with renal transplantation.

Ascites

CLINICAL INFORMATION

Ascites is an excess of plasma exudate in the peritoneal cavities. Often the whole abdomen is enlarged and obesity can mask ascites or gaseous distension. Ascites in thinner people is easier to spot clinically especially when there is much fluid present and the abdominal skin is stretched. It can accompany chronic cardiac failure (look for dilated hepatic veins and pleural effusion), cirrhosis, blood from a leaking aneurysm or vessel trauma and infection such as tuberculosis and pyogenic peritonitis.

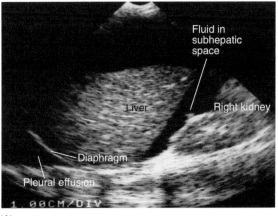

(A)

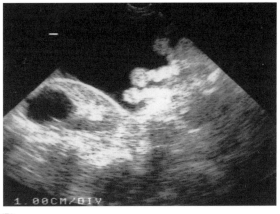

(B)

Fig. 15.5 (A) Free fluid in the upper abdomen around the liver and (B) anterior to the right kidney.

ULTRASOUND APPEARANCES

Ultrasound can detect as little as 10 ml of fluid in either Morrison's pouch or in the pelvic cavity. Fluid accumulates in the subhepatic space, then in the pelvis, then in the right paracolic gutter in turn (Fig. 15.5).

If the patient is moved around, the fluid can be more difficult to identify as it spreads itself around the surface of the organs, rather than settling in a deeper recess. With gross ascites, bowel loops will often be surrounded with fluid, as will the broad ligament in the female pelvis (Fig. 15.6).

Ascites can help in visualizing some structures by providing an acoustic window but can prevent the visualization of others especially when, in gross ascites, bowel tends to float to the anterior and central part of the patient and obscures deeper structures by means of the gas which it contains. Uncomplicated ascites appears as an echo-free area with acoustic enhancement and bowel moving freely within the fluid.

If segments of bowel are separated from each other or tethered to the abdominal wall, malignancy or infection is suggested. The presence of ascites may reveal peritoneal metastases. Internal echoes or mobile particles (possibly blood or pus) in the fluid suggest infection or malignancy. If infection has occurred previously, a cobweb-like appearance of septa within the fluid may be seen. This appearance can also be seen in malignant cases.

Blood vessel leakage

CLINICAL INFORMATION

Major leakages from blood vessels are usually a result of trauma and are diagnosed clinically. Ultrasound has only a minor role here, to detect or exclude a fluid collection; most patients will proceed immediately to surgery. Minor leakages may be difficult to detect according to their position although Doppler ultrasound can significantly increase the detection rate and is used extensively in the follow-up of transplant and graft operations.

Fluid exudate post inflammation

CLINICAL BACKGROUND

Fluid exudate from inflamed organs such as the gallbladder and pancreas is described under the relevant organs. Ultrasound is used for monitoring the reduction of fluid as it reabsorbs. In the case of pancreatic pseudocysts, it can be used to guide a needle into the appropriate pool of exudate for aspiration.

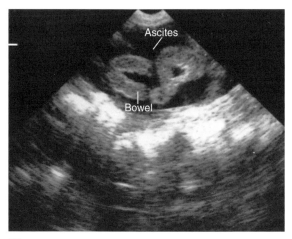

(A)

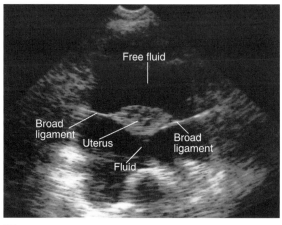

(B)

Fig. 15.6 (A) Free fluid outlining bowel and (B) around uterus.

Box 15.2   Advice

Scan from the lateral aspect when searching the paracolic gutter for fluid to avoid scanning through bowel gas. Patients may have to be flexibly scanned in order to move bowel gas from in front of the structures under investigation.

The acoustic enhancement from ascites can make the organs deep to the fluid 'brighter' than usual (see Fig. 15.5B). Ensure that this is not the real appearance of the organ by comparing it to the reflectivity of a neighbouring organ. Both should appear comparatively brighter.

does not lie between the needle and the lesion. Fine needles can cross through bowel without too much trauma in order to obtain a specimen and drain a small amount of fluid but a catheter cannot be inserted through the bowel to remain *in situ* whilst draining a large amount of fluid. Eighteen gauge needles can drain small lesions and have been reported as 95% successful while catheter drainage of large amounts is considered between 70% and 85% successful.

Reference

1. Spencer P, Spencer RC 1988 Ultrasound of post-operative wounds – the risks of cross infection. Clin Radiol 39: 245–246

Interventional procedures

Abscesses can be drained by percutaneous needle aspiration providing they can be seen clearly and bowel

16

MISCELLANEOUS INFORMATION

Role of US in trauma/emergency situation
Problem solving
Rule of thumb – abdominal pain
System for abdominal scanning
Reporting and report wording
Planning the ultrasound room

Role of ultrasound in the trauma/emergency situation

Ultrasound scanning of traumatized organs or systems can be found under the relevant chapters. But how much of a role does ultrasound play in the management of the trauma patient?

It has been said that approximately 10% of deaths from physical trauma among young people are due to abdominal injury. Eighty-three percent of those presenting in the trauma room have multiple injuries and the seriousness of some of the trauma may mask some abdominal injuries. These injuries tend to be fragmentation, intracapsular and extracapsular haematoma and laceration. The most frequently found injuries are to the spleen (the most frequently injured organ), liver, kidneys, retroperitoneum and pancreas. With blunt abdominal trauma, ultrasound is able to easily exclude a haemoperitoneum. A quick, single right subcostal or intercostal view of the liver and right kidney in patients with blunt abdominal trauma can exclude intraperitoneal blood with a sensitivity, specificity and accuracy of 81.8%, 93.9% and 90.9% respectively in most patients.

In a 1993 Dutch study[1] a scan of normal duration was reported to be able to correctly identify haemoperitoneum and intraperitoneal parenchymal damage with a sensitivity of 92.8%, specificity of 100% and accuracy of 99.4%.

Other research appears to agree with findings on detecting fluid but finds scanning for parenchymal damage to be less accurate. In a Swiss study of 312 patients with blunt thoracic or abdominal injuries carried out by surgeons using a mobile ultrasound unit, pathology was demonstrated in 113 (36.2%) cases: 47 had a haemothorax, 11 had pericardial effusions, 52 had free abdominal fluid, 24 had organ lesions and 10 had retroperitoneal haematoma. Of 14 patients with negative physical findings, five were referred for surgery based on positive ultrasound findings whereas none of the 66 patients with negative sonographic findings but positive clinical findings were referred for surgery. The sensitivity of ultrasound in detecting intraabdominal fluid was 98.1%, but only 41.4% in detecting organ lesions. Overall sensitivity of the ultrasound examination was 90% and specificity was 99.5%.[2] Further research from 1997 supports the view that free fluid can be accurately imaged but not solid organ trauma.[3] In addition, pelvic fluid is shown to be difficult to image in the trauma situation.[3,4]

Ultrasound has also been shown to be of use in the planning of treatment. An American study of the impact of systematic ultrasound carried out at the bedside of ITU patients[5] concluded that in 22% of patients (33 of 150), ultrasound findings influenced the diagnosis and had a direct impact on the therapeutic plan.

Problem solving

Scanning the abdomen is not purely a question of obtaining images of normal or abnormal organs or systems. When reading the request form, determine whether there is a problem and think how to solve the problem. Information written on the request form should not necessarily be taken as the absolute truth and you should take a brief history from the patient to see whether it matches what is on the request form. The examination depends on the clinical information to a great extent although there are some who prefer to have no information so that they are completely unbiased and free from a suggested diagnosis when performing the scan. However, most sonographers and radiologists look at the patient and automatically make a judgement based on the colour of the skin and sclera, shape of the abdomen, scars from previous operations, rigidity of the abdomen and general condition. All this, together with written information, is useful when scanning and underlines the necessity of having as much information available as possible prior to the scan as part of the preparation process.

Questions for the sonographer to ask:

- What is the cause of the pain?
- Why am I scanning the patient?
- What is useful to the referring clinician?

Rule of thumb – abdominal pain

Pain in	Relates to
Right hypochondrium + above diaphragm	Gallbladder, liver, right kidney
Left hypochondrium	Stomach, spleen, left kidney
Central abdomen	Pancreas, aorta, retroperitoneum
Right iliac fossa	Bowel (appendix), ovary, uterus
Left iliac fossa	Bowel (diverticulitis), ovary, uterus

Pain in both left sides and right = cancer.

System for abdominal scanning

It is sometimes difficult at first to adapt a system for scanning the abdomen in order to perform a general survey. The following may help in establishing some routine. This is, of course, flexible and should be adapted to suit the person performing the scan, the patient and the departmental protocols.

Supine position

TRANSVERSE

Scan transversely in the epigastrium looking for the pancreas. Adjust the angle to obtain the longest axis.

Scan the rest of the mid abdomen in the transverse plane looking to exclude abdominal aortic aneurysm (so that pressure can be applied to move duodenal gas out of the way of the pancreas if required). Angle up under the xiphisternum to view the liver in transverse section and the confluence of hepatic veins draining into the IVC.

Move to the right lateral side and scan subcostally on inspiration to see the right kidney in transverse section. Briefly scan transversely between the higher intercostal spaces to see if there is any free fluid in pleural, sub-phrenic or subhepatic spaces. Move down the right flank looking for fluid in the right paracolic gutter. Reach over and scan the left paracolic gutter, moving down to the pelvis, again looking for free fluid.

LONGITUDINAL

Scan through the right rib spaces to see the liver and right hemidiaphragm and assess texture of liver. Look for gallbladder through the rib spaces using the liver as an acoustic window if the patient is obese.

Scan the liver and right kidney subcostally and assess for structure, texture and size. Assess the IVC and aorta in longitudinal sections and the adrenals if possible. Reach over to the patient's left side and attempt to scan the spleen in gentle respiration through the lower ribs. Approach from the posterolateral position to avoid gas in the stomach and bowel which should have risen anteriorly with the patient in this position. Measure if possible. Attempt to see the left kidney.

LPO 45° position

OBLIQUE

Scan in a longitudinal oblique position at right angles to the right lower costal margin for further coverage of the liver and an assessment of the gallbladder which on thinner patients should lie more anteriorly, towards the midline and away from gas-containing bowel. Find the long axis of the gallbladder and proceed to scan trans-versely down its length. Use a longitudinal coronal oblique scan to view the aorta in its 'rosethorn view' and the IVC. Return to the lower costal margin and scan at right angles to it in order to view the common duct, hepatic artery and portal vein triad as it passes through the porta hepatis. Exclude lymph node enlargement at the porta hepatis.

LLD position

If not previously seen well, scan the right kidney longitudinally and transversely, the liver, gallbladder and the aorta.

RPO 45° position

This allows gas to move from the head of the pancreas towards the stomach. Scan transversely to view the pancreas again. Attempt to see the spleen scanning parallel to and between the lower rib interspaces if not seen clearly before.

RLD position

Scan longitudinally to see the left hemidiaphragm, spleen, left kidney, aorta through the left kidney and the tail of pancreas through the left kidney. Scan the left kidney in transverse section.

Return to supine position to rescan the pancreas if attempts have been futile up to now. If still difficult, see below.

Erect position

Scan transversely on inspiration to see the pancreas and the gallbladder if not seen clearly before.

Reporting and report wording

In the UK at present, general abdominal ultrasound scan reporting is an essential but politically contentious part of the scanning procedure for those non-medically qualified sonographers such as radiographers.[6] It is accepted that sonographers are accountable for the reports that they issue. At present, non-medically qualified sonographers should not write a diagnosis in the report unless it forms part of a scheme of work agreed by the employing authority, sonographers and medical staff. Without agreement, the report should contain only the recording and interpretation of observations. Legally, both the report and the accompanying images are public documents and part of the hospital medical records.

Reporting of abdominal scans by sonographers in the UK is carried out in different ways but for the most part is either in the form of free reporting, sometimes authorized by a radiologist, or by a ticked proforma with sufficient room for comments to be made. The report should certainly be made by the person who has performed the scan. The United Kingdom Association of Sonographers (UKAS) has produced *Guidelines for Professional Working Standards – Ultrasound Practice*[7] which contains examples of free written reporting on normal and abnormal scans and of report proforma worksheets which they recommend. Sonographers who have not seen this document should do so as it is a useful guide to reporting for those who are starting or wish to update their protocols. The relevant parts to this document are reprinted with kind permission of UKAS in Appendix 5.

The report may be a response to a question that has been asked and should be given even if it is not clear cut. However, usually, requests do not have specific questions to answer and for those prepared to accept requests to perform a general scan of the abdomen, the proforma can be a useful guide to whether everything has been checked during the scan.

Among the advice given is that if the report is written in freehand, it should be written in a way that is understood by the originator of the request, clearly and unambiguously, using technical language only when necessary to assist in the diagnosis. It is pointless using acoustic language to explain the visual appearances of a mass to someone who does not understand the significance of 'acoustic enhancement' (for example) unless it is explained.

Planning the ultrasound room

The siting of an ultrasound room may be wholly convenient for the service it provides, such as those situated within the obstetric or urology department, or inconvenient as, for example, the obstetric scanning service being provided by the radiology department situated far away from the obstetric department, causing heavily pregnant mothers to trail from one department to another. The siting of the department may be historical or political and the department may be well planned in advance with interdepartmental cooperation or situated haphazardly with no thoughts of patient convenience at all.

Finance is usually the major dictator when it comes to the sizing of an ultrasound room. As the size of the equipment has decreased since static B scanners were used, the rooms used to house the minimal equipment required have similarly become smaller. Sonographers have experience of working within the confines of old broom cupboards or ex-lavage rooms. As lights are usually fairly low within the room for the duration of the scan, the rooms are often windowless, providing a gloomy and airless working environment for the sonographers.

It is not within the remit of this book to tell experienced planners how to plan an ultrasound department but it may be useful to consider some practicalities for those in the enviable position of having sufficient space and funding to be able to plan an ultrasound department from scratch. This will be limited to a general medical ultrasound service.

Pre-planning stage

As the ultrasound department will have to meet the needs of the local community not only in the near future but for as long as can be envisaged, the following questions are important.

- What are the plans for the local area?

- Are there plans for population expansion, the move of light industries to the locality or the creation and growth of new industries? The foreseen increase in patients will have to be catered for.

- What are the strategic plans for the hospital? There may be plans to amalgamate two or more local smaller hospitals onto a preexisting or new site in which case it may be economical to wait until this happens before spending on a new department within the existing set-up. Or there may be plans to devolve the large hospital into smaller, community-based, patient-focused sites.

- What are the strategic plans for the department? Does it have to contend with a planned increase in outpatients clinics, new specialisms (such as a regional renal transplant centre), new consultants requiring additional ultrasound support (increase in interventional work under ultrasound control) and will it be provided with new equipment or have to use existing equipment which is perhaps not suitable for the workload?

Planning stage

If a department has to be expanded in size from what is already there, thought has to be given to:

- need for expansion
- room for expansion
- cost of expansion – use of existing materials/equipment
- convenience for patients and staff.

If designing a department from the beginning, the following will have to be considered.

- Where the department will be situated (close to other imaging rooms, to main source of patients).
- Size of room/rooms.
- Electricity, water, ventilation, drainage sites, health and safety regulations.
- Siting away from other sources of electrical interference (lifts, theatres, laser operation, etc.).
- Where the patients change for their ultrasound examinations. Do they change into a gown and dressing gown outside the department and bring their clothes with them in a basket or do they change in an area within the department?
- Clerical facilities including computer terminals, film/file storage, report generating.
- Waiting facilities (accommodation, drinking water, toilets).
- Staff accommodation if the department is away from other staff areas.
- Method of recording images (thermal paper only or the space and other facilities required for the installation of laser printers or dry laser printers).
- Storage facilities (consumables: laser film, acoustic coupling gel, paper towels and sheets). Being aware that buying in bulk can win financial discounts, it is obvious that there must be a place to store the bulk but the cost of storage space can sometimes be more than the discounts saved.

Privacy is extremely important. The reception/ administration area should not be sited in such a position that the public can see, by accident or design, any information belonging to any other patient that is either written or on computer. Similarly, any information given verbally to the staff by the patient must not be within earshot of other patients waiting for their scan, therefore the ultrasound room must have a door that closes and the waiting area must be far away enough for any conversation between staff and patients to remain confidential. Ultrasound rooms that consist of a couch and scanning machine which are constructed in the form of a cubicle with curtains do not afford a private environment. Even when waiting patients are far enough away from these cubicles, it is easy to overhear information from the adjacent cubicle.

With more solidly constructed rooms, what others can see when the door is open is important. The door should not open facing a waiting area so that people can see the patient on the ultrasound couch. There are often frequent interruptions to a scan by other staff and the door can open to reveal the patient in an embarrassing position. If this is unavoidable, curtains (fireproof) that cover the opening to the door should be mandatory.

Toilets should be situated nearby, especially for the use of patients requiring a full bladder preparation. The knowledge that toilets are in close proximity helps to give patients confidence in this situation and for those who have to void their bladder in the middle of an examination, the examination time is considerably shortened.

The ultrasound room

The size of the room is an essential element for consideration. With obstetric ultrasound, it is common for relatives to accompany the patient, adding to the need for a larger room. With general medical ultrasound, where relatives do not usually come into the room with the patients, the room itself could be smaller. However, space must account for helpers if the patient is disabled or has special needs, nursing staff, a chaperone if required (a serious consideration owing to the intimate nature of some of the investigations), an interpreter and those in training (radiographers, students, trainee radiologists). Interventional procedures also involve the use of more space (patient's bed or trolley, sterile trolley). The movement of staff around the patient must also be considered, in addition to the movement of equipment within the room and the movement of patients onto or near to equipment.

The size of the door must allow the easy entrance of beds/trolleys/wheelchairs and drip stands and other auxiliary equipment into the room. There must also be sufficient room to turn a bed or trolley into the ultrasound room if the room is situated directly off a corridor.

A drinking water supply must be available for those patients requiring a full bladder for their examination and who may have arrived without or with less than optimal filling. Disposable cups must be available to avoid risk of cross-infection, waste baskets for the empty cups should be made available and the water source should be close to the waiting area to avoid patients trailing backward and forwards with their cups, slopping water onto the floor and posing a danger to others.

Room contents — some considerations

Deciding what to put in the ultrasound room and where it should go requires much thought. The position of couch, scanner, desk, sink, chairs, lights and so on depends on the work practice involved. The idea is to cut down on wasted effort expended by walking round things, going backwards and forwards to reach things; in short to make the room as ergonomic and efficient as possible for staff and patients. This can be done by examining work practices and planning as one would plan a kitchen. Basically, the room requires a scanning area, a reporting/work area and a clean area for interventional procedures.

Scanning area

The ultrasound machine should be chosen specifically for the type of work performed, using dedicated probes for the type of work. It will probably stay in more or less the same place but can be moved if required. It should not require special cooling but if the room becomes uncomfortable owing to the heat dispersed, then the air conditioning, if installed, should be easily regulated to reach the optimum temperature. The monitor should be visible to the patient as well as the sonographer, either by rotating the monitor towards them or by means of a remote monitor. This appertains more to an obstetric ultrasound room, however.

As patients walk into a room that sometimes has quite subdued lighting, electric power cables trailing from the scanner must not pose a safety risk. The use of concealed floor-level sockets (4×13 amp power sockets) placed below the machine can help eliminate this hazard.

The couch should be comfortable, padded, easily cleaned and of the rise/fall type to help elderly patients get on and off, preferably electrically operated to avoid much physical effort pumping the couch up and down. It should have the facility to hold rolls of paper that the patient lies on and to hold a waste bin to take the gel-soaked paper from the previous patient. The couch should also have a raisable backrest to allow patients with breathing difficulties to sit up and should be able to be tilted head up and down as required for flexible technique and for emergencies. Ideally the couch should have the head end towards the door as parts under investigation are then not seen when the door is opened accidently during a scan.

A ceiling-mounted curtain rail and curtain made of fire-retardant material should be suspended between the door and the couch for essential privacy and should be constructed with a curve to the rail so that the curtain can be pulled back out of the way when required. The couch should also be positioned so that patients can enter the room and climb onto the couch from one side and staff have the freedom of movement on the other side.

The machine can be positioned close to the head of the couch on the left-hand side, assuming right-handedness. If the operator is left-handed, the machine and the couch may both be turned round 180°. This will result in the patient's feet being positioned towards the door but the machine will still be on the same side of the room.

A comfortable height-adjustable chair on castors must be available to the operator to give good back support, a comfortable scanning height and freedom of movement. The importance of operator comfort and scanning height must not be underestimated. Time must be taken to find the most comfortable position in order to reduce shoulder and neck strain and the possibility of repetitive strain injury (RSI).

Reporting/work area

A desk is essential with drawers to hide objects that clutter up the workspace. There should be shelving for stationery, videos, floppy disks (unless containing confidential patient information when they should be locked away), thermal paper (away from heat source) and coupling gel.

A computer terminal may be positioned on the desk, if required, for searching old reports or creating new ones. Booking the patient in or making appointments should be carried out outside the room in the reception area. Light boxes for viewing films or scans belonging to the patient should be positioned near the scanning area. A chair is required to work at the desk.

The 'clean' area

This should be at the opposite end of the room to the door, away from the dust of the corridor. There should be as much work surface as possible and wall-mounted cupboards to hold all that is required for any inter-ventional procedures or for any of the patients' needs, e.g. urine bottles, vomit bowels, incontinence pads. Wall-mounted cupboards are advocated for two reasons.

- To reduce strain on the back when retrieving things from floor-mounted cupboards.

- Work surfaces with a clear space below will allow sterile trolleys and couches to be parked under-neath when not required, thus avoiding floor clutter. The couch can be stored away when the patient enters the room on their bed, rather than transferring the patient onto the couch and having to move the bed out of the room into the corridor.

The clean area should also have a sink for scrubbing up before sterile procedures. The sink should have a tiled splashback to avoid early disintegration of the plaster and it should be positioned behind the area where people are walking to avoid slipping on splashed water. Lever action taps and a soap dispenser should be supplied as should a paper towel dispenser and waste paper bin.

Other considerations

- *Lighting.* A dimmer switch is essential to control the amount of lighting in the room. In addition, as much time is spent getting up and sitting down in order to switch lights down, it may be worth considering an infrared light dimming control to reduce this movement.

- A ceiling-mounted spotlight for focused light during interventional procedures.

- A 'do not enter' light on the door to deter visitors mid scan.

- *Fire safety.* In addition to statutory regulations, a CO_2 extinguisher.

- *Power supply.* Sufficient electric sockets around the room for ancillary equipment and for patient-related electrical equipment.

- *Communications.* An intercom between reception desk and ultrasound room. Telephones are intrusive and disrupt a scanning session. The messages sent and received on the intercom should be discreet and confidential.

- *Safety.* A panic button should be discreetly placed for the protection of staff and for emergency situations.

- *Storage.* Lockable wall cupboards for medical requisites.

- *Teaching.* A whiteboard and pens and reference books are important needs when people are being trained in ultrasound and a notice board for copies of protocols, techniques, etc is essential.

- Information for the patients outside regarding the preparation and procedures that they will undergo.

Other items required:

- a chair for the helper, translator, relative

- stainless steel dressing trolley

- sharps bin

- biopsy needles and gun

- all sterile medical equipment as required for inter-ventional work.

Lastly, in a proactive department, a risk analysis should be made of potential hazards in addition to those already mentioned that could occur in the everyday operation of this department. This should include the establishing of written work and reporting protocols that are read, understood and agreed by sonographers, radiologists and the employing authority and a complaints procedure that is flexible and clear to both staff and patients.

A suggested plan of an ultrasound room is shown in Figure 16.1.

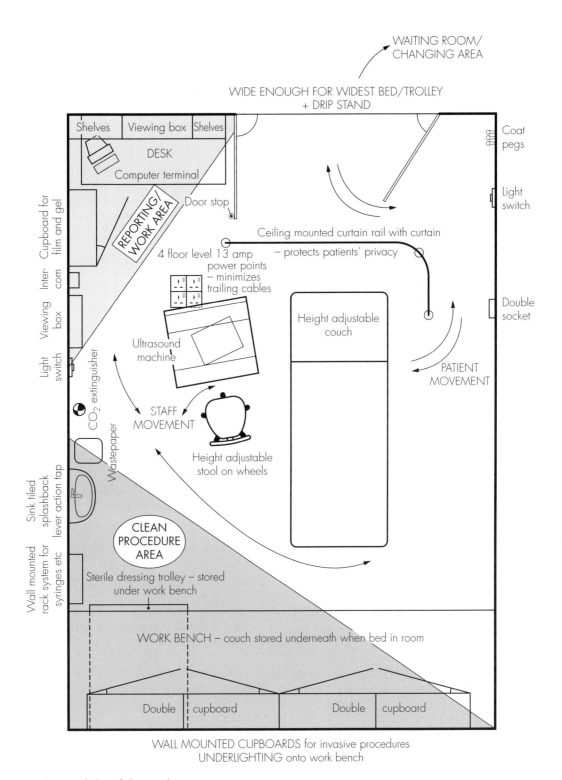

WAITING ROOM/
CHANGING AREA

WIDE ENOUGH FOR WIDEST BED/TROLLEY
+ DRIP STAND

Shelves | Viewing box | Shelves

DESK
Computer terminal

Coat pegs

Light switch

REPORTING/WORK AREA

Cupboard for film and gel

Inter-com

Viewing box

Light switch

Door stop

Ceiling mounted curtain rail with curtain
– protects patients' privacy

4 floor level 13 amp power points
– minimizes trailing cables

Double socket

Height adjustable couch

Ultrasound machine

CO_2 extinguisher

Wastepaper

STAFF MOVEMENT

PATIENT MOVEMENT

Height adjustable stool on wheels

Sink tiled splashback

lever action tap

CLEAN PROCEDURE AREA

Wall mounted rack system for syringes etc

Sterile dressing trolley – stored under work bench

WORK BENCH – couch stored underneath when bed in room

Double | cupboard | Double | cupboard

WALL MOUNTED CUPBOARDS for invasive procedures
UNDERLIGHTING onto work bench

Fig. 16.1 Suggested plan of ultrasound room.

References

1. Bode PJ, Niezen RA, van Vuyt AB, Schipper J 1993 Abdominal ultrasound as a reliable indicator for conclusive laparotomy in blunt abdominal trauma. J Trauma (USA) 34: 27–31

2. Rothlin MA, Naf R, Amgwerd M *et al* 1993 Ultrasound in blunt abdominal and thoracic trauma J Trauma. (USA) 34: 488–495

3. Bennet MK, Jehle D 1997 Ultrasonography in blunt abdominal trauma. Emerg Med Clin North Am 15: 763–787

4. McGahan JP, Rose J, Coates T *et al* 1997 Use of ultrasonography in the patient with acute abdominal trauma. J Ultrasound Med 16: 653–662

5. Lichtenstein D, Axler O 1998 Intensive use of ultrasound in the intensive care unit: prospective study of 150 consecutive patients. Int Care Med (USA) 19: 353–355

6. Stocksley MI 1998 Radiographer participation in abdominal ultrasound. J Diagn Radiog Imag 1: 27–33

7. UKAS 1996 Guidelines for professional working standards – ultrasound practice. UKAS, London

APPENDICES

1 Common abdominal conditions
2 Common blood tests
3 Abdominal aortic aneurysms:
   monitoring intervals
4 Renal failure
5 Reporting
6 General further reading

Common abdominal conditions

Brief non-definitive description of some common conditions and appearances of patients sent for ultrasound scans

Condition	Patients present with	Tests	US appearances	Measurements	Look for	Role of US	Notes
Gallstones	Right upper quadrant pain. Pain severe, colicky, radiating to right shoulder tip, nausea, +ve Murphy's sign, mild jaundice, gallbladder felt below LCM	Raised or slightly raised serum bilirubin, alkaline phosphatase, AST, ALT	Mobile, highly reflective masses in gallbladder, clean posterior acoustic shadow, ?mid-grey sludge	Variable, gallbladder wall can be thickened with cholecystitis >4–5 mm	Impacted stone in neck of gallbladder, thickened gallbladder wall, biliary sludge, obstructed ducts, other stones, other gallbladder pathology – if so, look at liver and enlarged lymph nodes, if present	Confirm presence of stones, condition of gallbladder, confirm if any dilated ducts present, exclude other pathology, assess pancreas	Cystic ducts can produce shadows; ensure this is not a stone. Use a higher frequency and focus carefully for best assessment of stones. Move patient to confirm mobility of stones. Gallstone ileus can make visualizing the pancreas difficult
Acute pancreatitis	Epigastric pain (mild to severe), nausea, vomiting. Movements cause pain and guarding, tender, rigid abdomen, patients double up. Appearances similar to perforated ulcer, abdominal aortic aneurysm leak. Linked with gallstone disease	Raised serum amylase (more specific if 5 times normal levels), raised WBC level	Swollen pancreas with decreased echogenicity, possible fluid exudate in or around pancreas	Generally larger than normal overall (definitive measurements can be misleading)	Gallstones, biliary tree dilatation, pancreatic duct dilatation, fluid (pseudocyst) collection	Exclude pancreatic mass, confirm gallstones, measure ducts, search for pseudocysts, guide for pseudocyst drainage procedure, if required	Use of water load to visualize the pancreas (should not be forced if patient is nauseous)
Obstructed biliary system	Jaundice (possibly intermittent); yellow skin and sclera, itching, pale stools that float, dark foamy urine	Serum bilirubin raised (>30 μm/l for yellowing to be apparent)	Depending on level of obstruction: dilated IHBDs (too many tubes), dilated CD (double-barrelled shotgun sign – portal vein and	Thin wall to gallbladder if dilated, ?IHBDs >3–4 mm, CD >8 mm	Visible IHBDs, rounded gallbladder, shadows from stones in CD, pancreatic head mass (dilated pancreatic duct), ampullary mass	Exclude non-obstructive jaundice, measure size of ducts if dilated, find level of obstruction, attempt to find cause of obstruction,	If ducts are normal size and patient is jaundiced, obstruction may be recent and ducts may not yet be dilated (scan again in 2–3 days' time). Stones and shadowing are

Condition	Patients present with	Tests	US appearances	Measurements	Look for	Role of US	Notes
			CD about the same size), tense spherical gallbladder if obstruction lower than cystic duct level (but normal or smaller if obstruction higher than cystic duct), possible pancreatic duct dilatation			confirm/exclude dilated pancreatic duct	difficult to see in CD when there is little bile around the stone and when duodenal gas lies over the duct. Is the tense gallbladder perhaps a choledochal cyst?
Portal hypertension secondary to liver cirrhosis	Enlarged liver and spleen, weakness, weight loss, fatigue. There may be an enlarged, taut abdomen with enlarged veins visible around the umbilicus	Usually raised AST, ALT and prothrombin time (> 16 s) and lowered serum albumin level	Liver can be enlarged or shrunken, depending on stage of liver disease. Inferior border of liver blunted. Echogenicity increased and intrahepatic portal walls not seen. Coarse echo pattern (micronodular). Nodular appearance if macronodular type. Spleen and extrahepatic vessels enlarged, ascites often present (check for thickened gallbladder wall). Umbilical vein remnant can recanalize	Spleen >14 cm to inferior border, extending below lower pole of kidney. Extrahepatic portal vein >13–14 mm diameter, SMV >12 mm diameter, splenic vein >12 mm diameter	Accompanying mass (?hepatocellular carcinoma), varices around the splenic hilum, porta hepatis and pancreatic bed. Confirm reduced/absent/reversed blood flow into liver with Doppler. As for portal vein, thrombosis can suddenly worsen the patient's condition, exclude portal vein clot and absent PV flow	In this condition, provide as much information as possible about liver, spleen, vessels and blood flow	Caudate and left lobes of liver can be spared the shrinking process. Do not measure portal vessels after eating. Normal portal vessel diameter does not exclude portal hypertension

Condition	Patients present with	Tests	US appearances	Measurements	Look for	Role of US	Notes
Obstructed urinary system	If obstruction by ureteric calculus: colicky flank pain made worse by movement, sweating, pallor, vomiting. If obstruction by enlarged prostate: enlarged bladder, inability to void urine, poor stream, dribbling, pain or urethral blockage	Evidence of blood and/or protein in urine. Raised serum calcium. Enlarged prostate on PR examination	Ureteric obstruction (usually unilateral) either at lower end or at pelviureteric junction causes dilated calyces. Sometimes cortex is thinned. Bladder obstruction from enlarged prostate (echo-poor prostatic mass with or without highly reflective contents indenting bladder) causes enlarged bladder, possible diverticula, thickened bladder wall	Bladder wall often >5 mm thick	Ureteric obstruction: dilated ureter (proximal or distal), echogenic mass in ureter at these points, lack of ureteric jet on affected side, mass at vesicoureteric junction, obstructed upper moiety from ectopic insertion of one ureter in duplex system. Bladder obstruction: stones, diverticula	To confirm obstruction, find level and cause of obstruction, confirm normality or otherwise of calyces and bladder, ascertain unilateral or bilateral obstruction, confirm that bladder is emptying or if there is residual urine, exclude lymphadenopathy or other extrinsic masses as causes of obstruction	Has the patient undergone lithotripsy recently? A full bladder can cause a hydronephrosis so observe the bladder when empty before assessing the kidneys. Ensure that a hydronephrosis is not a collection of cysts. Ensure the patients are not dehydrated as this can mask a hydronephrosis
Abdominal aortic aneurysm	Pulsatile epigastric mass that may not be felt by the patient but found by chance on routine examination, possible persistent aching pain in the epigastrium and central abdomen, backache, pain radiating down one leg (similar to sciatica). If leaking or ruptured aneurysm, severe pain radiated to back.	Clinical examination: BP, pulse, respiration, femoral pulses, etc.	Tapering wedge-shaped enlargement of aorta, atheroma seen as mid-grey echoes, possibly some calcification with posterior shadowing, true lumen seen as echo-free channel in middle of aorta. Aorta may be ectatic	Aneurysm considered when AP diameter >3 cm	Relationship of AAA to renal arteries and other vessels, extension of aneurysm to common iliac arteries? (If there is, look for extension to popliteal arteries.) Atheroma	Measure AAA and relate it to position of renal arteries, possible confirmation or exclusion of leak (difficult). Differentiating between genuine AAA and rebound pulse of normal aorta in thin patient, to exclude other masses mimicking an	Look at aorta when scanning urinary system in the older male. Use of coronal oblique (rosethorn view) to see position of AAA relative to renal vessels (for description, see Chapter 8). There may be paraaortic masses indenting the aorta that make it look like an AAA

Condition	Patients present with	Tests	US appearances	Measurements	Look for	Role of US	Notes
	Blood loss causes tachycardia, hypotension, pallor, sweating and weak femoral pulses					epigastric mass, to follow-up graft postoperatively	

Common blood tests

Common blood tests and their significance, relevant to abdominal pathology. Please note: normal values are not prescriptive as they can vary geographically.

Test	Normal value	Increased	Decreased
Acid phosphatase	1–5 U/l	Prostate cancer, liver disease	
Albumin	36–50 g/l	Diabetes insipidus	Nephrosis, liver failure, metastatic carcinoma
α-fetoprotein (AFP)	<13 μg/l	Hepatoma, hepatitis	
Alkaline phosphatase (ALP)	20–90 U/l	Liver disease, obstructive jaundice, liver metastases, cholelithiasis	
Alanine aminotransferase (ALT)	5–30 U/l	Hepatitis, cirrhosis, liver metastases, obstructive jaundice, liver congestion, pancreatitis, renal disease, alcohol ingestion.	
Amylase	50–300 U/l	Pancreatitis, GI obstruction, renal disease, acute alcohol ingestion, postoperative abdominal surgery	Pancreatic necrosis
Aspartate aminotransferase (AST)	10–40 U/l	Trauma, liver disease, pancreatitis, renal infarct, neoplasia, alcohol ingestion	Terminal liver disease
Bilirubin	2–17 μmol/l	Obstructive jaundice, liver disease, neonatal jaundice	
Calcium	2.1–2.6 mmol/l		Pancreatitis
Cholesterol	<5.2 mmol/(ideal)	Obstructive jaundice, nephrosis, diabetes mellitus, pancreatitis	Malignancy, infection, severe liver damage
Creatinine	62–132 μmol/l	Renal failure, urinary obstruction	
Glucose – fasting	3.6–5.8 mmol/l	Diabetes mellitus, phaeochromocytoma, liver disease, nephrosis, acute or chronic pancreatitis	
Haemoglobin	Male 130–180 g/l Female 115–165 g/l		Anaemia, melaena
Magnesium	0.75–1.0 mmol/l	Renal disease	Renal tubular necrosis, acute tubular necrosis, chronic glomerulonephritis
Potassium (K+)	3.5–5 μmol/l	Acute renal failure	Cirrhosis, nephrosis
Prostate-specific antigen (PSA)	0–4 ng/ml	Prostate cancer, benign prostatic hyperplasia	
Sodium (Na^{2+})	132–144 mmol/l	Chronic renal failure	Acute renal failure
Triglycerides	0.4–2.2 mmol/l	Nephrosis, cholestasis, pancreatitis, cirrhosis, hepatitis	
Urea	2.5–7.0 mmol/l	Renal disease, leukaemia, urinary tract obstruction	
White cell count (WCC)	4–11 × 10^9/l	Infection	

Abdominal aortic aneurysms – monitoring intervals

Table of intervals between scans for monitoring abdominal aortic aneurysm growth (©G. M. Grimshaw 1994)

Diameter	AGE																
	60	61	62	63	64	65	66	67	68	69	70	71	72	73	74	75	>75
27	48	48	48	48	60	60	–	–	–	–	–	–	–	–	–	–	–
28	48	48	48	48	60	60	–	–	–	–	–	–	–	–	–	–	–
29	48	48	48	48	48	60	60	–	–	–	–	–	–	–	–	–	–
30	48	48	48	48	48	48	60	60	–	–	–	–	–	–	–	–	–
31	48	48	48	48	48	48	48	48	60	–	–	–	–	–	–	–	–
32	36	36	36	36	48	48	48	48	48	48	–	–	–	–	–	–	–
33	36	36	36	36	36	36	48	48	48	48	48	–	–	–	–	–	–
34	36	36	36	36	36	36	36	36	48	48	48	48	–	–	–	–	–
35	24	24	24	24	24	36	36	36	36	36	48	48	48	48	–	–	–
36	24	24	24	24	24	24	24	24	36	36	36	36	48	48	48	–	–
37	24	24	24	24	24	24	24	24	24	24	24	36	36	36	48	48	48
38	18	18	18	18	18	18	24	24	24	24	24	24	24	36	36	36	36
39	18	18	18	18	18	18	18	18	18	24	24	24	24	24	24	24	24
40	12	12	12	12	12	12	18	18	18	18	18	18	18	24	24	24	24
41	12	12	12	12	12	12	12	18	18	18	18	18	18	18	18	18	18
42	6	6	6	6	6	12	12	12	12	18	18	18	18	18	18	18	18
43	6	6	6	6	6	6	12	12	12	12	12	18	18	18	18	18	18
44	6	6	6	6	6	6	6	12	12	12	12	12	12	12	12	12	12
45	3	6	6	6	6	6	6	6	6	6	6	6	6	12	12	12	12
46	3	3	6	6	6	6	6	6	6	6	6	6	6	6	6	12	12
47	3	3	6	6	6	6	6	6	6	6	6	6	6	6	6	6	6
48	3	3	3	6	6	6	6	6	6	6	6	6	6	6	6	6	6
49	3	3	3	3	3	6	6	6	6	6	6	6	6	6	6	6	6
50	R	R	R	R	R	3	6	6	6	6	6	6	6	6	6	6	6
51	R	R	R	R	R	R	3	6	6	6	6	6	6	6	6	6	6
52	R	R	R	R	R	R	R	3	6	6	6	6	6	6	6	6	6
53	R	R	R	R	R	R	R	R	3	6	6	6	6	6	6	6	6
54	R	R	R	R	R	R	R	R	R	3	3	3	3	3	3	6	6
55	R	R	R	R	R	R	R	R	R	R	3	3	3	3	3	3	3
56	R	R	R	R	R	R	R	R	R	R	R	3	3	3	3	3	3
57	R	R	R	R	R	R	R	R	R	R	R	R	3	3	3	3	3
58	R	R	R	R	R	R	R	R	R	R	R	R	R	3	3	3	3
59	R	R	R	R	R	R	R	R	R	R	R	R	R	R	3	3	3
60	R	R	R	R	R	R	R	R	R	R	R	R	R	R	R	3	3

☐ Active involvement of vascular specialist

Rescan interval in months
Aortic diameter in mm
R   Consider for elective repair

Renal failure

	Acute renal failure (ARF) (loss of renal function over days or weeks)	Chronic renal failure (CRF) (loss of renal function over months or years)
Causative conditions	Acute glomerulonephritis Acute tubular necrosis Interstitial nephritis Obstruction	Chronic long-term and progressive glomerulonephritis Trauma Tumour Obstruction Pyelonephritis Vascular disease
How serious?	Reversible if damaging stimulus is treated If no damage to basement membranes, regeneration in 2–3 weeks	Irreversible: nephrons permanently destroyed gradually Renal dialysis and transplant necessary to continue life
Biochemical changes	Potassium high Acidosis occurs Possible hypertension Urea increased Creatinine high Creatinine clearance low Haemoglobin low Sodium low Retention of water	Potassium normal or high Acidosis occurs Hypertension High urea Creatinine high Creatinine clearance low Sodium often high Excessive polyuria (10 litres/day) from reduction in reabsorption due to damaged tubules End-stage uraemia
Generalized ultrasound appearances of kidney	Kidney larger and of lower reflectivity	Kidney smaller, thinner cortex, increased reflectivity

Note:

Compensatory hypertrophy can occur (contralateral kidney expands to compensate in function for the damaged kidney). Compensatory mechanisms can fail as glomeruli are subjected to wear and tear from increased filtration pressure and constriction of efferent vessels, leading to progressive renal failure. Damage to endothelial cells leads to platelet thrombosis, hyalinization and fibrosis leading to insufficient renal tissue to maintain life. Complete renal failure, left untreated, can lead to death in 1–2 weeks.

Reporting

United Kingdom Association of Sonographers Guidelines on Reporting in Abdominal Ultrasound
(reproduced with the kind permission of UKAS, 1996)

COMMUNICATION

The sonographer should:

obtain informed consent from the client/patient or their representative

be professional and understanding throughout the examination

be able to explain the scanning procedure appropriately to each client/patient

be aware of the individual client'/patient's special needs including privacy during the examination

be able to obtain sufficient verbal and/or written information to perform the examination correctly

be able to discuss the relative risks and benefits of the examination with the patient/client

be able to explain the findings appropriately to the client/patient and relevant clinical staff in accordance with locally agreed practice.

SCANNING PROCEDURES

The sonographer should:

be able to establish whether the clinical details provided are sufficient and whether the correct examination has been requested

obtain oral informed consent for intracavitary examinations and ensure a chaperon is present where necessary

utilise the information from the case notes/previous investigations and other sources correctly

employ a systematic approach which is modified according to the individual client/patient and the findings relating to that client/patient, in particular:

    respiration
    body habitus
    organ position/acoustic properties
    pathological findings
    client/patient cooperation

proceed to further techniques or examination of additional areas/organs where necessary in accordance with locally agreed practice

be aware that the examination may be incomplete and the implications of this

be able to assist with ultrasound guided invasive procedures

be aware of potential risks involved in the procedure to the client/patient

understand the role of the ultrasound examination in the clinical context of that client/patient

attend to the after care of the client/patient

be aware of the appropriate local Health and Safety regulations.

REPORTING

The ultrasound report should be written by the person performing the ultrasound examination and should be viewed as an integral part of the whole examination.

The report should be written as soon as possible after the examination has been completed.

The name and status of the person issuing the report should be recorded on the report form.

The person issuing the report should take responsibility for the accuracy of the report and ensure that the report is communicated to the appropriate personnel.

Report Style

- The style of the report should be concise, clear and easily understood. Standard reports which are understood and accepted by staff within a hospital may need to be modified for outside referrals.

- Potentially ambiguous phraseology should not be used.

- Acoustic or technical language should be used when it significantly assists in the diagnosis. '*Echogenic*' is, for example, frequently used inappropriately to indicate increased reflectivity. It should be avoided unless qualified by a comparative such as '*increased echogenicity*'.

- Irrelevant information should be avoided.

- The sonographer should be aware of his/her limitations and consequently seek clinical advice when necessary.

- Abbreviations should only be used when the user is confident that they will be clearly interpreted.

Report Worksheets

- The use of worksheets, when used in conjunction with departmental schemes of work, is recommended.

- Where a report proforma is used, it should include a clear definition of what a positive, negative or missing response means. It is essential to ensure that the **precise** meaning of statements made on the proforma is clearly understood. It is recommended that a free-text facility is available on the report form and is used when appropriate.

Clinical Content

- The report should address the clinical question and should generally pertain to the reason for referral.

- The report should be conclusive where possible, indicating when the appearances are consistent with a specific diagnosis. Where no conclusion is possible alternative explanations for the ultrasound appearances may be offered.

- Any limitations should be stated and, if a relevant organ has not been fully examined, the reason(s) should be indicated.

- The exclusion value and significance of the ultrasound appearances should be stated where relevant.

- The sonographer should be aware at all times of the implications for the patient of the contents of the report and act in accordance with local guidelines.

GUIDELINES RELEVANT TO GENERAL ABDOMINAL EXAMINATIONS

Observations

The sonographer should be able to demonstrate:

normal anatomy/variants of abdominal organs and structures including age related appearances of whole organ in at least two planes. This should include assessment of size, outline and ultrasound characteristics

vascular anatomy including position, course and lumen of relevant vessels. Haemodynamic observations including the presence/absence of flow, direction, velocity and variance. Assessment of anastomoses

pathological findings including focal and diffuse processes and associated haemodynamic findings. Pre- and post-operative assessments.

The anatomical structures which the sonographer should normally examine during an abdominal scan are listed below:

liver: size, shape, contour and ultrasound characteristics of all segments. Appearance of intrahepatic vessels and ducts. Porta hepatis and adjacent area. Portal venous, hepatic venous and arterial systems

diaphragm: contour, movement, presence of adjacent fluid, masses, lobulations

ligaments: appearance of falciform, ligamentum teres and venosum

gallbladder: size, shape, contour and surrounding area. Ultrasound characteristics of the wall and the nature of any contents

common duct: maximum diameter and contents. Optimally it should be visualised to the head of pancreas

pancreas: size, shape, contour and ultrasound characteristics of head, body, tail and uncinate process. Diameter of main duct

spleen: size, shape, contour and ultrasound characteristics including the hilum. Assessment of splenic vein blood flow and presence/absence of collaterals

aorta: diameter, course and branches including the bifurcation. Appearance of its walls, lumen and the para-aortic regions

IVC: patency, diameter, appearance of its lumen and the para-caval regions

kidneys: size, shape, position and orientation, outline and ultrasound characteristics of cortex, medulla, collecting system, main and intrarenal arteries and veins

ureters: diameter. Assessment of the presence/absence of dilatation/reflux

bladder: volume and contents, appearance of bladder wall

adrenals: size and ultrasound characteristics. Presence of thickening or nodules

other structures which should also be examined where relevant include: gastrointestinal tract, peritoneum, omentum, muscles, abdominal wall, lymph nodes and sites for potential fluid collection (including upper/lower abdomen and thorax). Proceed to examination of the pelvis where necessary. The emphasis of the examination of the above structures will be altered according to clinical presentation.

GUIDELINES RELEVANT TO GENERAL ABDOMINAL REPORTING

It may be useful to have a standardised reporting format for normal abdominal scans which includes all the organs routinely examined and which is acceptable to the imaging department and referring clinicians.

Where the format contains a tick list an explanation of the possible responses should be included. This is particularly important if this check list forms part of the report issued by the sonographer.

Several 'normal' formats may be required according to the reason for referral in order to answer the relevant clinical question(s) including:

Routine abdominal examination
Oncology
Urology – with/without bladder volume
Liver Transplant – pre- and post-operative
Renal Transplant
Neonatal/Paediatric

NORMAL ULTRASOUND APPEARANCES – SUGGESTED REPORT FORMATS

Referral for suspected biliary disease:

Normal appearances of liver, gallbladder, common bile duct, pancreas, spleen and both kidneys.
No evidence of biliary disease.

Referral for urological symptoms:

- *Normal appearances of both kidneys and bladder. No ureteric dilatation.*

- *Normal appearances of both kidneys and bladder. Pre-micturition volume . . . mls.*
  Post micturition volume . . . mls.

Referral for known primary carcinoma:

Normal appearances of liver, gallbladder, CBD, pancreas, spleen, both kidneys and adrenal glands.
No evidence of lymphadenopathy.

Referral for palpable RUQ mass:

Normal appearances of liver, gallbladder, CBD, pancreas, spleen and both kidneys. Prominent Reidel's lobe noted/no masses identified.

Referral for post-operative pyrexia:

No upper abdominal or pelvic collections seen.

| ABNORMAL ULTRASOUND APPEARANCES – SUGGESTED REPORT FORMAT |

These may be due to either significant or incidental pathology or artefact. Acoustic descriptions should be omitted unless they add to the report. Some cases **may** require an acoustic description e.g. *'attenuates the sound'* and in such cases the significance of these appearances should be indicated.

Referral for fatty intolerance:

Normal appearances of the liver, pancreas, spleen and both kidneys. The gallbladder contains several stones. Normal common duct with no intra-hepatic duct dilatation.

Referral for RUQ pain:

The liver has increased echogenicity with reduced prominence of portal tracts consistent with fatty change.
There is a 30 mm highly reflective focal lesion in the right lobe of the liver. Appearances are most likely to represent an haemangioma.
Normal appearances of the gallbladder, pancreas, spleen and both kidneys.

Where the significance is unclear, the fact that the finding is non-specific should be stated. Possible causes should be suggested.

The report should endeavour to anticipate further clinical questions:

- if gallstones are present in a case of fatty intolerance the size and appearance of the biliary ducts and pancreas should be indicated

- it is usually necessary to comment on spleen size, presence/absence of varices and haemodynamics where possible in cases of chronic liver disease

- the presence/absence of ascites, lymphadenopathy or distant metastases in cases of known primary carcinomas.

Referral for bleeding varices:

Shrunken nodular liver. Enlarged spleen (160 mm) with varices around the hilum.
Reverse flow is present in the portal vein and there is increased intra hepatic arterial flow. Patent right and middle hepatic veins – left technically difficult to demonstrate.
Patent paraumbilical vein is noted.
Gross ascites is present.
Conclusion: Appearances are compatible with advanced liver disease with portal hypertension.

If a relevant organ has not been examined the reason should be indicated:

- *pancreas obscured by bowel gas.*

- *gallbladder is contracted, patient not fasted.*

Clinical features should be included if helpful, for example:

- *non-tender gallbladder.*

- *palpable mass.*

The report should be conclusive where possible, indicating when the appearances are consistent with a specific diagnosis. Where no conclusion is possible alternative explanations for the ultrasound appearances may be offered:

- *Enlarged liver containing multiple focal lesions of increased echogenicity. These probably represent metastases but multiple haemangiomata are also a possibility.*

- *There is a poorly defined 70 mm, mainly solid mass adjacent to, and separate from, the left kidney. This may be bowel or a lymph node mass. Suggest repeat scan tomorrow after bowel preparation.*

It may be appropriate, depending on local practice, to suggest further investigations which may clarify the diagnosis. These include other imaging investigations such as a plain X-ray for renal calculi, CT for staging ovarian carcinoma or invasive procedures.

Irrelevant information should be avoided.

Where serial examinations are being performed it is not usually necessary to comment serially on the normal appearances within the whole upper abdomen:

- *The right subphrenic collection has reduced in size. Maximum diameter now 60 mm.*

ROUTINE ABDOMINAL EXAMINATION WORKSHEET

Name	**Unit No:**
Address:	**DOB:**
Consultant:	*Ward:*
Date of examination:	

Clinical details: **? Abdominal tenderness:**

✔ = *normal U/S appearance & position*   x = *abnormal U/S appearance & position*   *ns = not seen*

Abdomen:

Liver:

Portal venous system	*Hepatic veins*	*Hepatic artery*

Bile Ducts: *Common Bile Duct:*

Gallbladder: *Pancreas:*

IVC: *Aorta:*

Spleen:

Kidneys: *R:*   *L:*

Renal perfusion: *R:*   *L:*

Adrenals: *R:*   *L:*

Pelvis: *Other:*

Sonographer's Report:

Date:

Final Report:

Date:

Equipment: *Scanned by:*   *Reported by:*

Status:

GUIDELINES RELEVANT TO PAEDIATRICS AND NEONATAL EXAMINATIONS

Observations

The sonographer should be aware of the content and implications of The Children's Act (1991).

The sonographer should be able to:

- *consider* the special needs and care of the patient, including the presence of the parent/guardian/accompanying person during the examination where appropriate

- *use* appropriate communication skills

- *make use of* immobilisation, sedation and other techniques where relevant in accordance with local guidelines

- *demonstrate* normal anatomy/variants, including age related appearances of the whole organs and structures examined in at least two planes including size, shape, outline and ultrasound characteristics

- *make the relevant measurements*

- *understand* the differences between the anatomy and pathology of children and adults

- *understand* the role of ultrasound in prenatally diagnosed conditions and its role in the management of the neonate.

The anatomical structures which the sonographer should be able to examine correctly and the observations which he/she should be able to carry out are listed below:

abdomen and pelvis: as for the adult abdomen and pelvis but with particular attention to the different size and ultrasound characteristics of organs in the neonate and child

gastro-intestinal tract: with particular attention to the pylorus and appendix.

Further reading

Allen PL, Dubbins P, Pozniak MA, McDicken WN. 2000 Clinical Doppler Ultrasound. Churchill Livingstone, London

Carty H, Crawford S, Higham J. 2001 Paediatric Ultrasonography. Greenwich Medical Media, London

College of Radiographers. 1998 Occupational Standards for Diagnostic Ultrasound. London: BSC Print Ltd

Kawamura, DM. 1997 Diagnostic Medical Sonography: Abdomen and Superficial Structures Lippincott-Raven, New York

Meire HB, Cosgrove D, Dewbury K. 2000 Abdominal and General Ultrasound Vols 1 and 2. Churchill Livingstone, London

INDEX

A

abdominal aorta, 33, 127–140
  anatomy, 127–128
  dissection, 138–139
  graft monitoring, 139
  measurement
    aneurysms, 136, 138, 259
    normal values, 133
    techniques, 134
  normal appearances, 130–132
  palpation, 128
    aneurysm, 136
  relations, 128
  scanning techniques, 129–132,
    277
  surface markings, 128
  variations in anatomy, 128
  see also aneurysms, abdominal aorta
abdominal wall, 229–230
abscesses
  Crohn's disease, 220
  kidney, 164
  liver, 48–49
    vs necrotic metastases, 47
  postoperative, 240, 241
  prostate, 202
  psoas muscles, 232
  rectus sheath, 230
  renal transplantation, 179
  spleen, 113–114
  subphrenic, 49, 234
  see also fluid collections
acalcular cholecystitis, 77, 78
accelerated rejection, renal transplants,
  177
accessory pancreatic duct, 93, 95
accessory renal arteries, 144

accessory spleens, 110
  lymph node enlargement *vs*, 123
acid phosphatase, 263
  normal levels, 197
acoustic enhancement
  bile duct dilatation, 83
  cysts, 42
acoustic impedance, coupling gels, 7
acoustic shadowing
  cystic duct, 67, 78, 257
  gallstones, 72, 73–74, 78
acoustic windows, 13–14
  bladder as, 12, 198
  liver as, 13, 95
acquired immunodeficiency syndrome
  (AIDS), kidneys, 167
acute alcoholic hepatitis, 53
acute appendicitis, 222, 223
acute bacterial nephritis, 163
acute cholecystitis, 77–79
acute diffuse proliferative
    glomerulonephritis, 165–166
acute fatty liver of pregnancy, 53, 54
acute pancreatitis, 104–105, 257
acute pyelonephritis, 162–163
  diabetes mellitus, 167
acute rejection, renal transplants, 177
acute renal failure, 271
acute tubular necrosis, 165
  renal transplants, 176–177
acute viral hepatitis, 52–53
Addison's disease, 209
adenomas
  adrenal cortex, 210
  eosinophilic (oncocytomas), 157
  gallbladder, 75
  granular cell (oncocytomas), 157
  kidneys, 157

  liver, 44
adenomatous polyps, bladder, 189
adenomyomatosis, gallbladder, 76
adenosquamous carcinoma, pancreas,
  100
adrenal cortex, 205
  adenomas, 210
  normal appearance, 207–208
adrenal glands, 205–212
  anatomy, 205–206
  normal appearances, 208–209
  scanning techniques, 207, 277
adrenal medulla, 205
  normal appearance, 207–208
adrenaline (epinephrine), 205
adult polycystic disease, 155
age
  normal measurements
    common duct, 68
    gallbladder, 69
    spleen, 112
    pancreas, 97, 98
agenesis, renal, 146
AIDS, kidneys, 167
alanine aminotransferase (ALT)
  chronic hepatitis, 53
  cirrhosis, 54
  normal levels, 34
ALARA (As Low As Reasonably
  Achievable) principle, 6
albumin, 263
  normal levels, 34, 95
alcoholic hepatitis, 53
aldosterone, 205
aliasing, 22, 24
alkaline phosphatase (ALP), 263
  normal levels, 34, 65, 197
aloe vera, 7

α-fetoprotein (AFP), 263
    hepatocellular carcinoma, 45
    normal levels, 34
amoebic abscesses, 49
ampulla of Vater *see* hepatopancreatic
        ampulla
amylase, 263
    normal levels, 95
    pancreatitis, 104, 257
anaemia, iron deficiency, 220
analgesic nephropathy, 165
anastomoses, renal transplantation, 175
    stenosis, 178
anatomy *see under specific organs*
androgens, excess, 209
aneurysms
    abdominal aorta, 135–138, 187,
        259–260
        lymph nodes *vs*, 123
        monitoring intervals, 267
    dissecting, 138–139
    renal arteries, *vs* cysts, 154
    splenic artery, pancreatic
        pseudocysts, 103
angiography, portal vein, pancreatic
        carcinoma, 101
angiomyolipomas, kidneys, 157
angioplasty, renal artery stenosis, 178
angle correction, pulsed wave
        Doppler, 23
annular pancreas, 94, 98
antimicrobial ingredients, coupling
        gels, 7
Antimicrobial Preservation
        Effectiveness Test
        (USPXX11), 7
anxiety, intestinal gas, 11
aorta *see* abdominal aorta
aperients, 10
appendicitis, 221–223
arcuate arteries, kidneys, 150
artefacts
    renal cysts, 154
    see also comet-tail artefacts
arteries
    endurance athletes, 133
    see also named arteries
ascariasis, biliary, 80

ascites, 55, 56, 240, 241–242
    as acoustic window, 14, 217
    diagnostic pitfalls, 190
    pancreatic, 105–106
aspartate aminotransferase (AST), 263
    chronic hepatitis, 53
    cirrhosis, 54
    normal levels, 34, 65
asplenia, 110
asthenic type, 13
atheroma, 135
athletes, arteries, 133
ATN *see* acute tubular necrosis

B

bacteria, coupling gels, 7
bacterial nephritis, acute, 163
ball-valve effect, common duct
        obstruction, 82
balloon catheters (Foley), 192–193
baseline
    pulsed wave Doppler, 22–23
    shift, colour Doppler, 25
beam steering, pulsed wave Doppler,
        23
benign prostatic hyperplasia, 201
bezoars, 226
bilateral renal agenesis, 146
bile, 31
    echogenic (biliary sludge), 74–75
    stasis, 71
bile ducts, 33
    anatomy, 63
    normal appearance, 67–69
    obstruction, 81–85, 86, 257–258
    pancreatic carcinoma, 100
    pathology, 80–89
    scanning techniques, 67
biliary atresia, 87–88
biliary sludge, 74–75
biliary stasis, 71
biliary system, 63–89
    patient preparation, 65–66
    reporting normal appearances, 278
    see also bile ducts; gallbladder
bilirubin, 263
    acute viral hepatitis, 52

biliary obstruction, 257
    normal levels, 34, 65
bilirubin stones, 71
biopsy
    haemangiomas, 44
    kidney, 179–180
    liver, 58–59
    pancreatic carcinoma, 100
    see also fine needle aspiration
bladder, 183–193
    as acoustic window, 12, 198
    anatomy, 183, 184
    artificial, 189
    benign prostatic hyperplasia, 201
    carcinomas, 188–189
        vs calculi, 190
        diagnostic pitfalls, 200
    Doppler ultrasound, 27
    diverticula, 190
    fistulas, Crohn's disease, 220
    fluid collections *vs*, renal
        transplantation, 179
    normal appearances, 185
    obstruction, 170, 259
    palpation, 183
    patient preparation, 12, 147,
        184–187
    relations, 183
    scanning techniques, 184–187, 277
        cystitis, 192
blood flow, 21
    hepatofugal, 57
    renal arteries, renal transplantation,
        176
    resistance, Doppler ultrasound, 21,
        22
blood pressure
    kidneys and, 143
    normal, 128
blunt trauma, kidneys, 174–175
Bochdalek hernia, 234
body types, 12–13
bowel, 215–226
    anatomy, 215–216
    fluid collections *vs*, 240
    normal appearances, 217–219
    palpation, 217
    resections, 216

surface markings, 216
bowel gas *see* intestinal gas
box size, colour Doppler, 25
breakfast, 10
breathing, 16–17
'bright' liver, 52
broadband digital beamforming
    technology, 3
Budd–Chiari syndrome, 57–58
    Doppler ultrasound, 27
bull's eye lesions *see* target lesions

C

calcification
    abdominal aortic aneurysms, 136
    chronic pancreatitis, 105–106
    gallbladder, 77
    liver lesions, 41
        metastases, 47
    nephrocalcinosis, 173–174
    renal cell carcinoma, 158
    renal cysts, 154
    splenic cysts, 115
calcium
    levels, 263
        normal, 95
    urinary calculi, 172
calculi
    appendix, 222
    prostate, 202
    urinary, 171–173, 259
        bladder, 189–190
        xanthogranulomatous
            pyelonephritis, 164
    see also gallstones
calyces *see* collecting systems (kidneys)
Candida albicans, 165
caput medusae, 55
carcinoembryonic antigen, normal
    levels, 34
carcinoid tumours, 221
carcinomas
    adrenal glands, 210
    bile duct obstruction, 85, 86
    bladder *see* bladder, carcinomas
    gallbladder, 75–76
        porcelain gallbladder, 77

intestinal, 220–221
kidneys *see* renal cell carcinoma
liver
    Klatskin tumours, 85, 88
    see also cholangiocarcinomas;
        hepatocellular carcinoma
pancreas, 98–102
prostate, 200–201
    prostatitis *vs*, 202
reporting, 278
see also metastases
cardiac failure *see* congestive cardiac
    failure
Caroli's syndrome, 88
    choledochal cysts *vs*, 86
cartwheel cysts, hydatid disease, 50
catheters, urinary, 192–193
caudate lobe, 31
    cirrhosis, 55
    normal size, 39, 40
    variations, 34
cavernous haemangiomas, 43–44
CD (colour Doppler), 24–25
central venous pressure, inferior vena
    cava, 139
Charcot's triad, 84
chenodeoxycholic acid, dissolution
    therapy, 72
chewing gum, 11
children, 282
    acute bacterial nephritis, 163
    biliary system, 67
        patient preparation, 65, 66
    cooperation, 17–18
    kidneys
        normal appearances, 150–152
        normal measurements, 151
        patient preparation, 147
        scanning techniques, 149–150
        transplantation, 175
        tumours, 153
    liver scanning, 35
    pancreas, 95, 98
    patient preparation, 10–11
        biliary system, 65, 66
        bladder scanning, 184
        kidneys, 147
        pancreas, 95

renal artery stenosis, 166
    urinary tract infections, 161–162,
        192
    vesicoureteric reflux, 171, 192
cholangiocarcinomas, 85, 86
    Klatskin tumours, 85, 88
cholecystectomy, 72
    common duct diameter, 68
cholecystitis
    acute, 77–79
    gallstone ileus, 72
    see also chronic cholecystitis
cholecystokinin, 63
choledochal cysts, 42, 65, 86, 87 (Fig.)
choledocholithiasis, 84, 85 (Fig.)
cholelithiasis *see* gallstones
cholesterol, levels, 263
cholesterol gallstones, 70–71
chronic active hepatitis, 53
chronic cholecystitis, 79, 80 (Fig.)
    jaundice, 82
chronic hepatitis, 53
chronic lobular hepatitis, 53
chronic pancreatitis, 105–106
chronic persistent hepatitis, 53
chronic pyelonephritis, 163–164
chronic rejection, renal transplants,
    177–178
chronic renal failure, 271
cine-loop facility, kidneys in children,
    147
cirrhosis, 51, 54–55
    hepatocellular carcinoma, 45, 54
cisterna chyli, 121
cleaning probes, 7–8
clear cell carcinoma *see* renal cell
    carcinoma
clotting of blood
    acute viral hepatitis, 52
    liver and, 31
    liver biopsy and, 58
    see also prothrombin time
coarse needle biopsy, liver, 59
cobra-head deformities, 191
coeliac axis, 127, 130, 132
    liver haemangiomas, 44
coeliac lymph nodes, 121
    enlargement, 122

collateral circulation (portosystemic), 55, 56
collecting systems (kidneys), 150–151
 duplitized, 146
 pelvicalyceal dilatation, 167–168, 169 (Fig.), 170
 transplants, 176
colon
 intussusception, 223
 see also large intestine
colour averaging, 25
colour Doppler, 24–25
colour sensitivity *see* packet size
columns of Bertin, 143, 145, 146, 152
comet-tail artefacts
 adenomyomatosis, 76
 intestinal gas, 219
common bile duct, 63
common duct, 33
 age, normal measurements, 68
 anatomy, 63, 64
 vs gastroduodenal artery, 83
 hepatic artery *vs*, 68–69
 liver transplantation, 60
 measurement
  endoscopic retrograde cholangiopancreatography, 70
  normal values, 37, 67–68, 81
 normal appearance, 37
 obstruction, 81–85, 86
 pancreatitis, 104
 relations, 64
 scanning techniques, 67, 85, 277
common hepatic duct, 63
common iliac arteries, 127
 aneurysms, 137
common iliac veins, 127
communication, 275
compatibility *see* DICOM compatibility
compensatory hypertrophy, kidney, 146, 271
compliance, abdominal aortic aneurysms, 136
compound imaging, real-time, 3
compression, appendicitis, 222
compression (set-up program), 8–9

computed tomography
 hepatopancreatic ampulla carcinoma, 102
 portal vein, pancreatic carcinoma, 101
concretions, intraluminal, 226
congenital muscular dystrophy, 232
congenital Wilms' tumour, 158
congestive cardiac failure
 ascites, 241
 liver, 57
congestive disorders, spleen, 117–118
Conn's syndrome, 209
 tumours causing, 210
contraceptives *see* oral contraceptive pill
controls, setting, 8–9
 abdominal aortic aneurysms, 137
 biliary system, 66
 colour Doppler, 24–25
 pulsed wave Doppler, 22–23
conventions, orientation, 9
cooking smells, patient preparation, 10
coronal oblique position, 130, 132, 133
cortical adenomas, adrenal glands, 210
corticomedullary differentiation, 161, 163
cortisol, normal levels, 207
Couinaud segments, liver, 32
coupling gels, 7–8
Courvoisier's law, 82
creatinine, 263
 normal levels, 146
  urine, 146
creatinine clearance, normal values, 146
Crohn's disease, 219–220
cross-infection, 243
 coupling gels, 7
crura, diaphragm, 233
crystal drop-out test, 6
cubicles, 250
'cuddle' position, kidney scanning, 149
Cushing's syndrome, 208–209
 tumours causing, 210

cyclosporin A
 nephrotoxicity, 177, 178
 renal transplantation, 176
cystadenomas, bile duct obstruction, 85
cystic artery, 64
cystic duct, 63
 acoustic shadowing, 67, 78, 257
 obstruction, 77, 78, 81–82
cystic fibrosis, 106
 gallbladder, 80
 gallstones, 71
cystitis, 192
cysts
 adrenal glands, 209
 choledochal, 42, 65, 86, 87
 hydatid, 50, 115
 kidneys, 153–154
  dialysis, 157
  non-Hodgkin lymphoma *vs*, 161
  pelvicalyceal dilatation *vs*, 170
 liver, 41, 42–43
  metastases, 47
 medullary pyramids *vs*, 152
 ovarian, diagnostic pitfalls, 185, 190, 240
 pancreas, 102
 prostate, 202
 spleen, 114–115

D

'dark' liver, 52
daughter cysts, hydatid disease, 50
diabetes mellitus
 fasting, 11
 kidneys, 167
dialysis, cysts of kidneys, 157
diamond ring appearance, 76
diaphragm, 232–235
 anatomy, 232–233
 hernias, 234–235
 identification pitfalls, 211
 liver metastases *vs*, 48
 normal appearance, 233
 scanning techniques, 233, 277
DICOM compatibility, 5

diffuse liver diseases, 41, 51–58
  hepatocellular carcinoma, 41
  metastases *vs*, 48
  scanning sections, 58
diffuse proliferative
    glomerulonephritis, acute,
    165–166
dimercaptosuccinic acid (DMSA),
    kidney scintigraphy, 161, 162,
    163
dimethyl siloxane, 11
direction of blood flow, 21
display *see* output display standard
dissecting aneurysms, 138–139
dissolution therapy, gallstones, 72
distensibility, abdominal aortic
    aneurysms, 136
diverticula, bladder, 190
  diagnostic pitfalls, 185
DMSA scanning, kidneys, 161, 162,
    163
Doppler ultrasound, 21–28
  cirrhotic nodules, 55
  hepatocellular carcinoma, 45–46
  inferior vena cava filters, 140
  urinary tract infections, 161
  see also pulsed wave Doppler
double barrel shotgun sign, 82–83,
    257–258
double gallbladder, 65
drainage *see* percutaneous drainage
drinking, water, 10, 11, 96, 251
dromedary hump, 145, 146, 152
drop-out *see* crystal drop-out test
drug-induced interstitial nephritis, 165
Duchenne muscular dystrophy, 232
ductal carcinoma, pancreas, 100
duodenum, 215–216, 218
  as acoustic window, 13
  atresia, 98
  vs pancreas, 98
duplex kidney, obstructed moiety,
    171
duplex scanning, 21
duplitized collecting system and
    ureter, 146
dysplastic kidneys, multicystic, 156
dysplastic polyps, bladder, 189

E

echinococcal cysts (hydatid cysts), 50,
    115
echogenic bile (biliary sludge), 74–75
echogenicity, reporting, 276
ectatic aorta, 139
ectopia vesicae, 192
ectopic kidney, 146
ectopic spleen, 110
effusions pleural, 234
ellipsoid method, gallbladder volume,
    70
emergencies, 247
emphysematous cholecystitis, 78
empyema, gallbladder, 78–79
endoscopic retrograde
    cholangiopancreatography,
    common duct diameter, 70
endoscopic ultrasound
  adrenal glands, 212
  hepatopancreatic ampulla
    carcinoma, 102
  pancreas, 96
  portal venous system, pancreatic
    carcinoma, 101
endothelial cysts, adrenal glands,
    209
endurance athletes, arteries, 133
eosinophilic adenomas, kidneys, 157
epidermoid cysts, spleen, 114
epinephrine (adrenaline), 205
equipment, 3–9
  biliary system, 66
  planning for, 251
    image recording, 250
  psoas muscles, 231
  rectus abdominis, 229
  renal transplants, 176
ERCP (endoscopic retrograde
    cholangiopancreatography),
    common duct diameter, 70
erect position, 16, 248
  gallbladder scanning, 67
ergonomics, 3, 251–253
Escherichia coli, acute pyelonephritis,
    162
eventration, 235

external iliac vessels, identification
    pitfalls, 223
extracapsular haematomas, spleen, 116
extracorporeal shock-wave lithotripsy,
    173
extrarenal pelvis, 146, 152, 170
exudates
  abdominal, 242
  pleural, 234

F

faecal masses, 217, 280
falciform ligament, 32, 38
false aneurysms, 136–137
fasting, 10
  biliary system, 65–66
  diabetes mellitus, 11
  glucose levels, 263
  liver, 35
  pancreas, 95
  Phrygian cap, 64
fatty infiltration
  liver, 53–54
    focal tumours, 44, 45
  pancreas, 106
fatty intolerance *see* malabsorption
    syndrome
femoral nerve, psoas haematoma, 232
fetus *see* foetus
fever, renal transplantation, 177
filter (wall filter)
  colour Doppler, 25
  pulsed wave Doppler, 23
filters, inferior vena cava, 140
fine needle aspiration
  abscesses, 48, 243
  hydatid cysts, 50
  liver, 59
    abscesses, 48
fistulas, Crohn's disease, 220
fizzy drinks, stomach contents *vs*
    masses, 10
flatulence *see* intestinal gas
flow rate measurement, urodynamics,
    186, 187
fluid collections, 239–243
  aortic grafts, 139

fluid collections – *continued*
  false aneurysms, 137
  ovulation, pouch of Douglas, 240
  renal transplantation, 176, 178–179
  see also abscesses; cysts; urinomas
fluids (oral), 10, 11, 12
  bladder scanning, 184
  intestinal gas removal, 96
  ultrasound departments, 251
  urinary tract, 147
focal lesions
  liver, 41–51
    scanning sections, 58
  spleen, lymphoma, 113
focal nodular hyperplasia (liver), 44
foetus, lobulation of kidneys, 145,
    146, 164
Foley balloon catheters, 192–193
footprint, transducers, 4
foreign bodies, bladder, 190
fossae, liver, 32
frame averaging, colour Doppler, 25
frame rate *vs* sensitivity
  colour Doppler, 25
  pulsed wave Doppler, 23–24
free fluid (peritoneum), 14
  see also ascites; fluid collections
frequencies, 3
  biliary system, 66
  vs blood flow detection, Doppler
    ultrasound, 21
frequency scale control
  colour Doppler, 25
  pulsed wave Doppler, 23
frusemide, nephrocalcinosis, 173
fungal infection, kidneys, 165
fusiform aneurysms, 135

G

gain *see* receiver gain control; time
    gain compensation
gallbladder
  acute viral hepatitis, 52
  age, normal measurements, 69
  anatomy, 63, 64
    variations, 64–65
  ascites, 56

biliary atresia and, 87, 88
Doppler ultrasound, 26, 27
fasting, 10
functions, 63
intrahepatic, 42, 64
measurement, normal values, 69, 70
Murphy's sign, 77
neonates, 67
  normal measurements, 69
non-visualized, 80
normal appearance, 67, 68
palpation, 65
  Murphy's sign, 77
pancreatic carcinoma, 100
pathology, 70–80
relations, 64
scanning techniques, 66–67, 70,
    277
surface markings, 64
variations in anatomy, 64–65
gallstone ileus, 72
gallstones, 70–74, 257
  acoustic shadowing, 72, 73–74,
    78
  acute cholecystitis, 77
  common duct, 84, 85
  identification pitfalls, 226
  pancreatitis, 103
γ-glutamyl transpeptidase, normal
    levels, 34
gangrenous appendix, 222, 223
gangrenous cholecystitis, 78, 79
gas
  biliary system, 88–89
  common duct, 84
  emphysematous cholecystitis, 78
  kidneys, 173, 178
  pancreatitis, 104
  portal venous system, 57
  urine, 220
  see also air; intestinal gas
gastroduodenal artery, 127
  vs common duct, 83
gastrosplenic ligament, 109
gate cursor, Doppler, 22
gel blocks, 8
giant cell carcinoma, pancreas, 100
glomerulonephritis, 165–166

glucagon, 11
glucocorticoids, 205
glucose
  metabolism, liver, 31
  normal values
    blood, 263
    urine, 146
glycogen, 31
grading, reflectivity of kidneys, 163
grafts, abdominal aorta, monitoring,
    139
granular cell adenomas, kidneys, 157
*Guidelines for professional working
    standards – ultrasound practice*
    (UKAS), 249
*Guidelines on reporting in abdominal
    ultrasound* (UKAS), 275–282

H

habitus (body types), 12–13
haemangiomas
  liver, 43–44
    Doppler ultrasound, 27
  spleen, 115
haematomas
  kidneys, 174–175
  liver, 50–51
  postoperative, 241
  psoas muscles, 232
  rectus sheath, 230
  renal transplantation, 179
  spleen, 116
haemoglobin, 263
  iron deficiency anaemia, 220
  normal levels, 111, 146, 217
haemoperitoneum, 247
haemophilia, psoas haematoma, 232
haemopoiesis, spleen, 109
haemorrhage, 242
  adrenal glands, 209–210
  varices, ultrasound reporting, 279
halo sign, 77
hamartomas, kidneys, 158
hamartomatous polyps, bladder, 189
Hartmann's pouch, 65
heart failure *see* congestive cardiac
    failure

heparin, 31
hepatic adenomas, 44
hepatic artery, 32, 33, 93, 127
    common duct vs, 68–69
    haemangiomas, 44
    normal appearance, 37
    pulsed wave Doppler, normal
        appearance, 40
hepatic ducts, 33
hepatic plexus, 64
hepatic veins, 32–33, 128, 133
    Doppler ultrasound, 26, 27
    haemangiomas, 43–44
    normal appearance, 37, 39
    obstruction, 57–58
    pulsed wave Doppler
        normal appearance, 40
        portal hypertension, 57
hepatitis, 51, 52–53
    viral (A, B, C, D, E), 52
hepatoblastomas, 46
hepatocellular carcinoma, 41, 44–46
    cirrhosis, 45, 54
hepatofugal flow, 57
hepatomegaly
    conditions mimicking, 40
    metastases, 48
hepatopancreatic ampulla, 63
    carcinoma, 102
    obstruction, 81
hernias, 230
    diaphragmatic, 234–235
    inguinal, 226
hiatus hernia, 234
hilum (kidney), 143
hilum (liver), 31–32, 33
    bile duct obstruction at, 81
    Klatskin tumours, 85, 88
HIV infection (AIDS), kidneys, 167
Hodgkin's disease, lymph nodes, 122
honeycomb cysts, hydatid disease, 50
horseshoe kidney, 146
    vs pancreas, 98
hourglass gallbladder, 65
HPS see hypertrophic infantile pyloric
        stenosis
human immunodeficiency virus
        (HIV) infection, kidneys, 167

Hybritech test, normal values, 197
hydatid cysts, 50, 115
hydrocortisone, 205
hydronephrosis, 169, 180, 259
    bladder overfilling, 12
    see also pyonephrosis
hydrops, gallbladder, 77
hyperacute rejection, renal transplants,
        177
hypercholesterolaemia, 70
hyperechoic lesions, liver, 41
    metastases, 48
hypernephroma see renal cell
        carcinoma
hypersthenic type, 13
    pancreas scanning, 95
hypertension
    phaeochromocytoma, 211
    polycystic renal disease, 155
    renal trauma, 174
hypertrophic infantile pyloric stenosis,
        224–226
    scanning technique, 224–225
hypertrophy, compensatory, kidney,
        146, 271
hypoechoic lesions, liver, 41
    metastases, 48
hypoglycaemia, 31
hyposthenic type, 13

I

ileocaecal junction, surface markings,
        216
image recording equipment, 4–5
    planning for, 250
immunosuppression, renal
        transplantation, 176
infantile hypertrophic pyloric stenosis,
        224–226
infantile polycystic disease, 155–156
infants
    biliary system, 66, 67
    kidney, 149–150
    liver, 35, 37
    pancreas, 95, 98
    patient preparation, 10–11
        biliary system, 66

pancreas, 95
    urinary tract infections, 161–162
infarction, spleen, 115
infections
    fungal, kidneys, 165
    HIV, kidneys, 167
    spleen, 117
    urinary tract, 153, 161–165, 192
    wounds, postoperative, 240
inferior adrenal artery, 205
inferior mesenteric artery, 127, 215
inferior mesenteric lymph nodes, 121
inferior pancreaticoduodenal artery,
        93
inferior vena cava, 33, 127–135,
        139–140
    anatomy, 127–128
    Budd–Chiari syndrome, 57
    calibre, 133
    displacement, 140
    filters, 140
    liver transplantation, 60
    normal appearances, 133
    relations, 128
    scanning techniques, 129–132, 277
    surface markings, 128
    tumour involvement, 139, 140,
        159, 160
    variations in anatomy, 128
    Wilms' tumour, 160
inferior vesicular artery, 197
inguinal hernia, 226
inspiration, 17
intensive therapy unit patients, 247
intercostal scanning
    adrenal glands, 207
    gallbladder, 66
    kidneys, 149
    liver, 36
    spleen, 111
interlobar arteries, kidneys, 150
interstitial nephritis, 165
intestinal gas, 215–216, 219
    kidney scanning, 147
    pancreas scanning, 96
    patient preparation, 10, 11
    scanning techniques, 14
intestines, see bowel, 215–226

intestines – *continued*
   fluid collections *vs*, 240
   obstruction, 220
intrahepatic ducts, diameters, 70
intrahepatic gallbladder, 42, 64
intraoperative ultrasound, liver
     transplantation, 60
intussusception, 223–224
iron deficiency anaemia, 220
ischaemic tubular necrosis, 165
islets, pancreas, 93
   tumours, 102

J

jaundice, 81, 84, 257
   chronic cholecystitis, 82
   scanning sections, 58
juvenile nephronophthosis, 156

K

kidneys, 143–180
   abdominal aortic aneurysms, 137,
     138
   adrenal tumours displacing, 210
   anatomy, 143–146
   ascites, 56
   carcinoma *see* renal cell carcinoma
   compensatory hypertrophy, 146,
     271
   Doppler ultrasound, 26, 28, 152,
     176
   failure, 271
   horseshoe, 146
     vs pancreas, 98
   intussusception *vs*, 224
   liver reflectivity *vs*, 51, 52
   normal appearances, 150–152, 163
   palpation, 146
   patient preparation, 147
   power Doppler, 26
   pulsed wave Doppler
     normal appearances, 152
     transplants, 176
   relations, 144–145
   scanning techniques, 147–150, 277
   surface markings, 145

transplantation, 175–179
variations in anatomy, 145–146
volumes, 151
see also polycystic renal disease;
   renal arteries
Klatskin tumours, 85, 88

L

lacerations, kidneys, 175
large intestine
   functions, 215
   obstruction, 220
   see also bowel
laser printers, 5
lateral aortic lymph nodes (paraaortic
   lymph nodes), 121
   enlargement, 122
lateral decubitus positions, 15, 16, 17
   general surveys, 248
   kidneys, 148
   liver, 36, 37
   pancreatic tail, 96
   spleen, 111
lateral plane, abdomen, 216
laxatives (aperients), 10
left gastric artery, 127
leiomyosarcomas, inferior vena cava
   invasion, 140
leukaemia, 116–117
   spleen, 117
lienorenal ligament, 109
   varices, 118
ligamentum teres, 32
   portal hypertension, 56
ligamentum venosum, 32, 38
lighting, ultrasound rooms, 252
lipids (triglycerides), levels, 263
lipomatous pseudohypertrophy of
   pancreas, 106
liposarcomas, inferior vena cava
   invasion, 140
lithotripsy, 72, 173
liver, 31–60
   as acoustic window, 13, 95
   anatomy, 31–34
   body types, 13
   Doppler ultrasound, 26, 27, 40

echogenicity, *vs* kidney, 163
equipment set-up, 8
failure, 51
function tests, 34
   acute viral hepatitis, 52
   chronic hepatitis, 53
neuroblastoma, 211
normal appearances, 37–40
palpation, 34
polycystic renal disease, 42–43, 155
   Caroli's syndrome *vs*, 88
portal hypertension, 258
relations, 33
scanning techniques, 35–37, 58,
   277
surface markings, 33–34
transplantation, 59–60
variations in anatomy, 34
lobulation of kidneys, fetus, 145, 146,
   164
lymph nodes, 121–123
   anatomy, 121
   normal appearances, 121
lymphadenopathy, 121–123
lymphangiomas, 115
lymphocoeles, 241
   renal transplantation, 178, 179
lymphoid organs, spleen as, 109
lymphomas, 113
   kidneys, 161
   lymph nodes, 122
   metastases *vs*, liver, 47, 48
   pancreas, 102
   spleen, 113, 116

M

macronodular cirrhosis, 54, 55
magnesium levels, 263
Magnetic Resonance Imaging,
     hepatopancreatic ampulla
     carcinoma, 102
malabsorption syndrome, 221
   ultrasound reporting, 278
malignant melanomas, gallbladder
     metastases, 76
masses
   faecal, 217, 280

right upper quadrant, reporting, 278
vs stomach contents, 10
MCUG (micturating cystourethrograms), 162
mean corpuscular haemoglobin concentration
   iron deficiency anaemia, 220
   normal range, 217
mean corpuscular volume
   iron deficiency anaemia, 220
   normal range, 217
measurement
   abdominal aorta, aneurysms, 136, 138, 259
   flow rate, urodynamics, 186, 187
   head of pancreas, 101
   hypertrophic infantile pyloric stenosis, 225
   normal values
      aorta, 133
      bowel wall thickness, 219
      common duct, 37, 67–68, 81
      gallbladder, 69, 70
      kidneys, 150, 151
      liver, 38–39
      pancreas, 98
      portal vein, 37, 56
      prostate, 200
      spleen, 112
      splenic vein, 56
      superior mesenteric vein, 56
   portal vein, 56
   setting equipment for, 9
   superior mesenteric vein, portal hypertension, 258
   techniques
      aorta, 134
      bladder, 185–186
      common duct, 67
      kidneys, 151, 152
      prostate, 199–200
mechanical effects, ultrasound, 5
mechanical index, 5
medullary calcinosis, 173–174
medullary cystic disease of kidneys, 156
medullary pyramids (kidneys), 143–144

cysts *vs*, 152
   neonates, 150
   renal transplants, 176
medullary sponge kidney, 156–157
membranoproliferative glomerulonephritis, 166
membranous nephropathy, 166
mesoblastic nephroma, 158
metabolism, liver, 31
metastases
   to adrenal glands, 210–211
   of adrenal tumours, 210
   kidneys, 160
   liver, 46–48, 49
      fatty infiltration *vs*, 54
      necrosis, 45, 47, 48
      malignant melanomas, gallbladder, 76
   prostate carcinoma, 200
   spleen, 114
metronidazole therapy, amoebic abscesses, 49
micro gallbladder, 80
micronodular cirrhosis, 54, 55
micturating cystourethrograms, 162
micturition, urodynamics, 186, 187
middle adrenal artery, 205
mineral oils, as coupling media, 7
mineralocorticoids, 205
mixed echo lesions, liver, 41
monkey puzzle tree appearance, 83
Morgagni hernia, 234
mosaic pattern lesions, liver, 41
mucinous cystic carcinoma, pancreas, 102
mucocoele, gallbladder, 77
multicystic dysplastic kidneys, 156
multiformat imagers, 5
Murphy's sign, 77
muscles
   abdominal, 229–235
   wasting diseases, 232
myolipoma, adrenal gland, 211

N

near-field reverberation, prevention, 8
necrosis, liver lesions, 41

metastases, 45, 47, 48
necrotizing pancreatitis, 104
neonates
   adrenal glands, 208
   gallbladder, 67
      normal measurements, 69
   haemangiomas, 43
   jaundice, 81
   kidneys
      normal appearances, 150
      normal measurements, 151
      scanning techniques, 147, 149
   liver scanning, 37
   nephrocalcinosis, 173
   neuroblastoma, 211
   pancreas, 98
   urinary tract obstruction, 170
nephritic syndrome, 165–166
nephritis, 165
   acute bacterial, 163
nephroblastoma *see* Wilms' tumour
nephrocalcinosis, 173–174
nephronophthosis, juvenile, 156
nephrostomy, percutaneous, 173
nephrotic syndrome, 165, 166
neuroblastoma
   adrenal gland, 211
   Wilms' tumour *vs*, 160, 211
neutrophils, normal counts, 111
nicotine, 11
non-Hodgkin lymphoma
   kidneys, 161
   lymph nodes, 122
non-visualized gallbladder, 80
noradrenaline (norepinephrine), 205
normal appearances
   reporting, 278–279
   see also measurement, normal values; *specific organs*
Nyquist limit, 22, 24

O

obesity, gallbladder scanning, 67, 70
oblique positions, 14–15
   aorta, 130
   biliary system, 67
   gallbladder, 66

oblique positions – *continued*
  general surveys, 248
  kidneys, 148
  liver, 36
  right coronal, 130, 132, 133
  spleen, 111
obstruction
  bile ducts, 81–85, 86, 257–258
    see also jaundice
  cystic duct, 77, 78, 81–82
  hepatic veins, 57–58
  intestinal, 220
  urinary tract *see* urinary tract, obstruction
obstructive chronic pyelonephritis, 164
oesophagitis, hiatus hernia, 234
oils, as coupling media, 7
oncocytomas, kidneys, 157
operators, ergonomics, 3, 251
oral contraceptive pill, hepatic adenomas, 44
organ transplantation *see* transplantation
orientation, 9
  transperineal scanning, 198–199
output display standard, thermal and mechanical indices, 5–6
ovarian cysts, diagnostic pitfalls, 185, 190, 240
ovarian veins, 128
ovulation, pouch of Douglas, fluid, 240
oxalate stones, 172
oxygen, patient preparation, 11

P

packet size, colour Doppler, 25
PACS (picture archiving and communication systems), 5
paediatrics *see* children; infants; neonates
pain, 247
  abdominal aortic aneurysm, 136, 259
  acute cholecystitis, 77
  benign prostatic hyperplasia, 201

chronic cholecystitis, 79
  gallstones, 71, 257
  pancreatic carcinoma, 98
  pancreatitis, 104
  referred, biliary system, 64
  right upper quadrant, ultrasound reporting, 279
testes
  renal disease, 144
  ureteric colic, 172
  urinary calculi, 172
palpation *see under specific organs*
pancreas, 93–106
  anatomy, 93–95
  normal appearances, 97–98
  patient preparation, 95
  polycystic renal disease, 102, 155
  pseudocysts, 103
    choledochal cysts *vs*, 86
  relations, 93–94
  scanning techniques, 95–97, 277
  surface markings, 94
  variations in anatomy, 94–95
pancreas divisum, 94
pancreatectomy, survival rate, 99
pancreatic duct, 93, 97
  carcinoma, 100
  dilatation, 82
  measurement, 98
pancreatitis, 103–106, 257
  choledochal cysts, 86
papilla of Vater *see* hepatopancreatic ampulla
papillary necrosis, diabetes mellitus, 167
papillomas, bile duct obstruction, 85
paraaortic lymph nodes (lateral aortic lymph nodes), 121
  enlargement, 122
paracolic gutters, scanning, 242
parapelvic cysts, 154, 170
parasites
  biliary ascariasis, 80
  hydatid cysts, 50, 115
paraumbilical vein, 56
parents, 17
patient cooperation, 16–18
patient positions, 14–16

biliary system, 66–67
  gallstones, 74
  liver, 35–37
  pancreas, 96
  spleen, 111–112
patient preparation, 10–13
  see also under specific organs
peak flow, urodynamics, 186
pelvicalyceal dilatation, 167–168, 169, 170
pelvis
  patient preparation for scan, 12
  ruptured spleen, 116
pelviureteric junctions, obstruction, 168
penetration depth, 3
percussion, ascites, 55, 240
percutaneous angioplasty, renal artery stenosis, 178
percutaneous drainage
  abscesses, 243
  urinary tract obstruction, 179
percutaneous nephrostomy, 173
perforated appendix, 222, 223
perineum *see* transperineal scanning
perirenal haematomas, 174, 175
peristalsis, 215, 217, 218
peritoneal cake, 226
peritoneum
  free fluid, 14
  haemoperitoneum, 247
  see also ascites; fluid collections
persistence, colour Doppler, 25
pH, urinary calculi, 172
phaeochromocytoma, 211
phosphates, urinary calculi, 172
phrenic nerve paralysis, 233
Phrygian cap, 64, 65
phytobezoars, 226
PI *see* pulsatility index
picture archiving and communication systems (PACS), 5
pigment stones, gallbladder, 71
pixel size, colour Doppler, 25
planning, ultrasound rooms, 249–253
plasma proteins, 31
platelets, normal counts, 111
pleural effusions, 234

pneumaturia, 220
polycystic renal disease
    infantile, 155–156
    liver, 42–43, 155
        Caroli's syndrome *vs*, 88
    pancreas, 102, 155
    pelvicalyceal dilatation *vs*, 170
    spleen, 114, 115, 155
polycythaemia rubra vera, spleen, 117
polyps
    bladder, 189
    gallbladder, 75
popliteal arteries, aneurysms, 137
porcelain gallbladder, 77
porta hepatis *see* hilum (liver)
portal hypertension, 55–57, 258
    spleen, 55, 117–118
portal venous system, 32, 33
    Doppler ultrasound, 26–27, 40, 57
    gas, 57
    hepatocellular carcinoma, 45
    vs liver texture, 51
    measurement, 56
        portal hypertension, 56
    normal appearance, 37
        pulsed wave Doppler, 40
    pancreatic carcinoma, 100–101
    portal hypertension, 258
        measurement, 56
        pulsed wave Doppler, 57
    pulsed wave Doppler, 40, 57
portosystemic anastomoses, 55, 56
    spleen, 111
posterior urethral valves, 171, 191
postoperative scanning
    fluid collections, 240–241
    renal transplantation, 176
potassium, 263
    normal levels, 207
Potter type I (infantile polycystic
        disease), 155–156
Potter type II (multicystic dysplastic
        kidneys), 156
Potter type III (adult polycystic
        disease), 155
Potter's syndrome (bilateral renal
        agenesis), 146
pouch of Douglas, fluid, ovulation, 240

power Doppler, 25
    hepatocellular carcinoma, 46
    kidney, 26
power output, pulsed wave Doppler,
        22
pre-planning, ultrasound departments,
        249–250
preaortic lymph nodes, 121
pregnancy
    acute fatty liver of, 53, 54
    urinary tract
        infections, 161
        obstruction, 170
premature babies, nephrocalcinosis,
        173
prenatal diagnosis, infantile polycystic
        renal disease, 156
PRF (pulse repetition frequency), 23
primary sclerosing cholangitis, 88
printers, 4–5
privacy, 250
probes, 3–4
    biliary system, 66
    cleaning, 7–8
    kidney scanning, 147
    quality assurance tests, 6
    renal transplants, 176
    silicone faces, 7
problem solving, 247
professionalism, 275
proformas, reporting, 276
proliferative glomerulonephritis, acute
        diffuse, 165–166
prone position, 11, 16
    kidneys, 148
propylene glycol, 7
prostate, 197–202
    anatomy, 197
    bladder calculi and, 190
    normal appearances, 199
    palpation, 197
    patient preparation, 197–198
    scanning techniques, 197–200
    urinary tract obstruction, 259
        benign hyperplasia, 201
    urodynamics, 186, 187
prostate-specific antigen (PSA), 197,
        263

prostatectomy (transurethral), 201
prostatitis, 202
proteins
    plasma, 31
    urine, normal values, 146
prothrombin time
    normal levels, 34
    portal hypertension, 258
pseudocysts, pancreas, 103
    choledochal cysts *vs*, 86
psoas muscles, 230–231
    abscesses, 232
    haematomas, 232
    scanning technique, 231
pulsatility index, renal transplantation,
        176, 177
pulse rate, normal, 128
pulse repetition frequency, 23
pulsed wave Doppler, 21–24
    aorta, 134, 135
    kidneys
        normal appearances, 152
        transplants, 176
    liver, normal appearance, 40
    portal hypertension, 57
    renal artery stenosis, 167
    thermal effects, 5
purgatives (aperients), 10
PWD *see* pulsed wave Doppler
pyelonephritis
    acute, 162–163
        diabetes mellitus, 167
    chronic, 163–164
pyloric stenosis, hypertrophic
        infantile, 224–226
pyonephrosis, 164

Q

quadrate lobe, 31
    fatty infiltration and, 45
quadriceps, muscle diseases, 232
quality assurance tests, 6–7

R

radiation nephritis, 165
RAS *see* renal arteries, stenosis

real-time compound imaging, 3
rebound tenderness, 221
receiver gain control
  abdominal aortic aneurysms, 137
  colour Doppler, 24
  pulsed wave Doppler, 23
recording *see* image recording
  equipment
rectus abdominis, 229–230
rectus sheath haematoma, 230
red blood cells
  kidneys and, 143
  spleen functions, 109
redcurrant jelly stool, 224
referred pain, biliary system, 64
reflux, urine *see* vesicoureteric reflux
reflux-associated chronic
  pyelonephritis, 163
reflux oesophagitis, hiatus hernia, 234
rejection, renal transplants, 177–178
renal adenocarcinoma *see* renal cell
  carcinoma
renal agenesis, 146
renal arteries, 127, 151
  abdominal aortic aneurysms, 137,
    138
  anatomy, 144
  aneurysms, *vs* cysts, 154
  inferior vena cava and, 133, 134
  occlusion, 166
  pulsed wave Doppler, 152
  renal transplantation
    anastomoses, 175
    blood flow, 176
  right coronal oblique position, 132
  stenosis, 137, 166–167
    Doppler ultrasound, 28
    renal transplantation, 178
renal cell carcinoma, 158–159
renal cysts in dialysis, 157
renal failure, 271
renal pelvic dilation (*see also*
  hydronephrosis)
renal sinuses, 143, 150, 151
  echogenicity, *vs* cortex, 163
renal veins, 128, 134, 151
  anastomoses, renal transplantation,
    175

anatomy, 144
  thrombosis, 166
    renal transplantation, 178
  tumour involvement, 159
renal volume, 151
reporting, 248–249, 276, 278–281
  work areas for, 251–252
request forms
  use of, 247
  viewing before scan, 12
resections
  bowel, 216
  prostate, 201
resistance to blood flow, Doppler
  ultrasound, 21, 22
resistive index
  blood vessels, 21
  renal transplantation, 176
reverberation artefacts
  near-field, prevention, 8
  see also comet-tail artefacts
Riedel's lobes, 34, 41
right coronal oblique position, 130,
  132, 133
right upper quadrant, ultrasound
  reporting
  masses, 278
  pain, 279
risk analysis, ultrasound departments,
  252
Rokitansky–Aschoff sinuses, 76
rosethorn view (right coronal oblique
  position), 130, 132, 133
rupture
  abdominal aortic aneurysm,
    135–136, 138
  appendix, 222, 223
  liver, 50
  spleen, 116
RVT *see* renal veins, thrombosis

S

saccular aneurysms, 135
safety, 5–7
  ergonomics, 251
sampling frequencies, Doppler
  ultrasound, 22

sandwich sign, 122
Santorini's duct (accessory pancreatic
  duct), 93, 95
scanning techniques, 13–18, 275,
  277
  general surveys, 248
  hypertrophic infantile pyloric
    stenosis, 224–225
  intussusception, 224
  see also under specific organs
scarring, kidneys, 161, 162, 163
screening
  abdominal aortic aneurysms, 136
  polycystic renal disease, 155
sector transducers, 4
  biliary system, 66
seeding of tumours, liver biopsy, 59
segments, liver (Couinaud), 32
seminal vesicles, identification pitfalls,
  200, 201
sensitivity, frame rate *vs*
  colour Doppler, 25
  pulsed wave Doppler, 23–24
septa
  ascites, 242
  pleural effusions, 234
  renal cysts, 154
septate gallbladder, 65
serial examinations
  abdominal aorta aneurysms, interval
    table, 267
  reporting, 280
seromas, 241
shifting dullness, 240
shotgun sign *see* double barrel shotgun
  sign
sickle cell crisis, 115
sickle cell disease
  gallstones, 71
  splenic infarction, 115
silicone faces, probes, 7
sinks, 252
sinus lipomatosis, 150
sitting position, 16
situs inversus *see* transposition
small intestine
  anatomy, 215
  functions, 215

obstruction, 220
see also bowel
smoking, before scan, 11, 65, 95
smoothing, colour Doppler, 25
sodium, 263
   normal levels, 207
sonographers
   professionalism, 275
   reporting, 248–249, 276–282
space requirements, ultrasound rooms, 250–251
sphincter of Oddi, 63
spiral valves of Heister, 63
spleen, 109–118
   as acoustic window, 13
   anatomy, 109–111
   ectopic, 110
   liver transplantation, 60
   normal appearances, 112
   palpation, 110–111
   patient preparation, 111
   polycystic renal disease, 114, 115, 155
   portal hypertension, 55, 117–118
   relations, 110
   scanning techniques, 111–112, 277
   surface markings, 110
   variations in anatomy, 110
   see also accessory spleens
splenic artery, 109
   aneurysms, pancreatic pseudocysts, 103
splenic vein, 93, 109
   normal diameter, 56
   portal hypertension, 258
   thrombosis, pancreatic pseudocysts, 103
splenomegaly, 113
splenunculi *see* accessory spleens
staghorn calculus, 172–173
staging, Wilms' tumour, 160
stand-off gel blocks, 8
standing position, 16
starry sky appearance, 52
starving *see* fasting
stasis, biliary, 71
stenting, urinary tract, 173
sterility, 243

coupling gel, 8
sthenic type, 13
stomach
   as acoustic window, 13
   contents, *vs* masses, 10
stones *see* calculi; gallstones
storage functions, liver, 31
storage space, ultrasound departments, 250
strategic plans, ultrasound services, 249–250
subcapsular haematomas
   kidneys, 174, 175
   liver, 51
   spleen, 116
subhepatic abscesses, 49
subphrenic abscesses, 49, 234
superior adrenal artery, 205
superior mesenteric artery, 127, 130, 132, 215
superior mesenteric lymph nodes, 121
   enlargement, 122
superior mesenteric vein, 93
   measurement
      normal values, 56
      portal hypertension, 258
superior pancreaticoduodenal artery, 93
supine position, 14, 15
   aorta, 129–130
   gallbladder, 66
   general surveys, 248
   kidneys, 148
   liver, 35–36
   pancreas, 96
suprapubic catheter insertion, 193
suprarenal veins, 128
surface markings *see under specific organs*
sweep speed, pulsed wave Doppler, 23

T

target appearances
   acute appendicitis, 222
   bowel, 217

target lesions
   bowel carcinomas, 220
   liver, 41
      metastases, 47, 48
terminal ileum, 219
testes
   lymphatic drainage, 121
   pain
      renal disease, 144
      ureteric colic, 172
testicular veins, 128
thermal effects, ultrasound, 5
thermal index, 5
thermal printers, 4
thoracic duct, 121
thrombosis
   abdominal aortic aneurysms, 136, 137
   inferior vena cava, 139
   renal veins, 166
      renal transplantation, 178
   splenic vein, pancreatic pseudocysts, 103
   varicocoele, renal vein, 166
time gain compensation, 8
tissue harmonic imaging, 3
toilets, 250
tomato juice, 11
toxic tubular necrosis, 165
transducers *see* probes
transitional cell carcinoma, 159–160
   bladder, 188–189
transperineal scanning, prostate, 198–199
transplantation
   kidney, 175–179
      scanning techniques, 176
   liver, 59–60
transposition
   great vessels, 128
   spleen, 110
transpyloric plane, 128
transtubercular plane, 216
transudate, pleural effusions, 234
transurethral resection of prostate, 201
transverse fascia, 229
trauma, 247
   bladder, 191

trauma – *continued*
 diaphragmatic hernia, 234
 kidneys, 174–175
 liver, 50–51
 spleen, 116
Trendelenburg position, gallbladder
  scanning, 66
trichobezoars, 226
triglycerides, levels, 263
trigone, bladder, 183
tuberculosis
 lymph nodes, 122
 spleen, 117
tuberose sclerosis, 157
tubules *see* acute tubular necrosis
tumours
 adrenal glands, 210–212
 bile duct obstruction, 82
 biliary sludge *vs*, 75
 inferior vena cava, 139, 140, 159,
  160
 kidneys, 153
 liver transplantation, 59
 renal veins, 159
 seeding, liver biopsy, 59
 thrombus, inferior vena cava, 139
 see also specific tumours
turbulence, Doppler ultrasound, 21

U

ultrasound rooms, planning, 249–253
uncinate process, 93, 94–95, 97–98
unilateral renal agenesis, 146
United Kingdom Association of
  Sonographers (UKAS)
 *Guidelines for professional working
  standards – ultrasound practice,*
  249
 *Guidelines on reporting in abdominal
  ultrasound,* 275–282
urate stones, 172
urea, 263
 normal levels, 95, 146
 pancreatitis, 104
ureteric colic, 172

ureteric orifices, 185
ureterocoeles, 171, 191
ureters
 anatomy, 144, 183
 assessment, 277
 calculi, 172
 Doppler ultrasound, 28
 duplitized, 146
 normal appearances, 185
 obstruction, 168, 259
 renal transplantation, 175
urethra
 anatomy, 183
 obstruction, 168
  posterior urethral valves, 171,
   191
urinary catheters, 192–193
urinary tract
 infections, 153, 161–165, 192
 obstruction, 167–171, 259
  benign prostatic hyperplasia, 201
  cysts *vs*, 154
  percutaneous drainage, 179
  posterior urethral valves, 171,
   191
  renal transplant complications,
   179
 reporting normal appearances, 278
 stenting, 173
urine
 daily volume, 143
 gas, 220
 normal values, 146
urine jets, 185
urinomas, 158, 241
 renal transplantation, 178
urodynamics, 186, 187
ursodeoxycholic acid, dissolution
  therapy, 72
USPXX11 Antimicrobial Preservation
  Effectiveness Test, 7

V

Valsalva manoeuvre
 inferior vena cava, 130

portal vein measurement, 56
variations in anatomy *see under specific
  organs*
varices
 gallbladder, Doppler ultrasound, 27
 haemorrhage, ultrasound reporting,
  279
 lienorenal ligament, 118
varicocoele, renal vein thrombosis,
  166
velocity of blood flow, 21
velocity scale, colour Doppler, 25
vesicoureteric reflux, 161–162
 children, 171, 192
videoprinters, 4–5
viral hepatitis, acute, 52–53
viscid bile (biliary sludge), 74–75
viscosity, coupling gels, 7

W

wall filter
 colour Doppler, 25
 pulsed wave Doppler, 23
wall thump, pulsed wave Doppler, 23
wandering spleen, 110
warming, coupling gels, 7
wasting diseases, muscles, 232
water, drinking, 10, 11, 96, 251
waterlily sign, 50
Whipple's operation, 99
white cell counts (WCC), 263
 normal, 111, 217
Wilms' tumour, 160
 neuroblastoma *vs*, 211
Wilms' tumour (congenital), 158
Wirsung's duct *see* pancreatic duct
worksheets, reporting, 276, 280–281
worms, bile ducts, 80
wound infections, postoperative, 240

X

xanthogranulomatous pyelonephritis,
 164